Contents

Symposium Organization

ICPFR Board Members

Oded Bar-Or   President
Toshihiro Ishiko   Vice President
Dirk Van Gerven   Secretary-Treasurer
Tetsuo Meshizuka
Han Kemper
Hillel Ruskin
Roy J. Shephard
Henry Montoye
Vassilis Klissouras
C. Chintanaseri

Organizing Committee

Kitsuo Kato   Chairman
Masahiro Kaneko   Secretary General
Kando Kobayashi   Coordinator (The Aged)
Kyonosuke Yabe   Coordinator (The Disabled)
Sadayoshi Taguchi   Coordinator (Ind. Workers)
Toshio Asami
Kihachi Ishii
Toshihiro Ishiko
Toshiyuki Iseki
Yoshio Kuroda
Hideji Matsui
Mitsumasa Miyashita
Tetsuo Meshizuka
Toshio Moritani
Takahisa Yamamoto
Hisao Kotani

Administrative Staff

Masahiro Kaneko
Akira Ito
Hidekazu Fujita
Takafumi Fuchimoto
Munehiko Harada
Jiro Toyooka
Miharu Miyamura
Tetsuo Fukunaga
Kensaku Suei

Symposium Secretariat

Osaka College of Physical Education
1-1 Gakuen-cho, Ibaraki-shi, Osaka 567, Japan

International Series on Sport Sciences
Volume 20

Fitness for the Aged, Disabled, and Industrial Worker

Edited by

Masahiro Kaneko, PhD
Osaka College of Physical Education, Osaka, Japan

Human Kinetics Books
Champaign, Illinois

Library of Congress Cataloging-in-Publication Data

International Council for Physical Fitness Research. Symposium (1988
  : Osaka, Japan)
    Fitness for the aged, disabled, and industrial worker / edited by
Masahiro Kaneko.
        p.   cm. -- (International series on sport sciences, ISSN
0160-0559 ; v. 20)
    "Proceedings of the Symposium of the International Council for
Physical Fitness Research, held on September 5-7, 1988, in Osaka,
Japan"--t.p. verso.
    Includes bibliographical references.
    ISBN 0-87322-262-8
    1. Physical fitness--Congresses.   2. Physical fitness for the
aged--Congresses.   3. Working class--Physical training--Congresses.
4. Physical fitness for the physically handicapped--Congresses.
I. Kaneko, Masahiro, 1938-   . II. Title. III. Series.
    [DNLM: 1. Aged--congresses.   2. Exercise--congresses.
3. Handicapped--congresses.   4. Occupational Diseases--prevention &
control--congresses.   5. Physical Fitness--congresses.   QT 255
I611f 1988]
GV481.I58   1990
613.7'0446--dc20
DNLM/DLC
for Library of Congress   89-24655
                                                                      CIP

ISBN: 0-87322-262-8
ISSN: 0160-0559

Copyright © 1990 by Human Kinetics Publishers, Inc.

Proceedings of the symposium of the International Council for Physical Fitness Research,
held on September 5-7, 1988, in Osaka, Japan.

Developmental Editor: Kathy Kane   Typesetter: Brad Colson
Production Director: Ernie Noa   Text Design: Keith Blomberg
Copyeditor: Julie Anderson   Text Layout: Tara Welsch and
Assistant Editor: Rob King   Denise Peters
Proofreader: Phaedra Hargis   Printer: Braun-Brumfield, Inc.

Printed in the United States of America

10 9 8 7 6 5 4 3 2 1

Human Kinetics Books
A Division of Human Kinetics Publishers, Inc.
Box 5076, Champaign, IL 61825-5076
1-800-747-4HKP

Preface

This volume contains the proceedings of the 1988 Symposium of the International Council for Physical Fitness Research (ICPFR), held on September 5-7, 1988, in Osaka, Japan. The principal theme of this symposium was "Current Topics of Physical Fitness Research." Three sub-themes featured here are the health problems of the aged, the disabled, and the industrial worker. These areas demand considerable attention in industrialized nations, so it seems appropriate to provide a forum whereby participants from different nations can share ideas on such problems of mutual interest. The three sub-themes are nuclei around which other topics cluster. Aging, for example, is not totally dissociated from disability.

The problem of aging has become a popular issue in the media. People are now aware that the proportion of elderly in populations of Western countries is on the increase. For example, in Japan projections indicate that one of every four persons will be a "senior citizen" in the year 2025. Industrial workers also merit attention because they are exposed to various risk factors predisposing them to cardiovascular diseases even before they become elderly.

Physical fitness research is playing an ever more important role in today's world. No longer can we ignore difficulties of the elderly, the disabled, and the industrial worker. Constructive approaches to these problems must be given high priority in the future. We hope the information contained in this volume will be of some help in promoting such advancements. The 1988 symposium was a fortunate occasion because six distinguished guest speakers gave excellent lectures: Professors R.J. Shephard, J.O. Holloszy, the late J. Rutenfranz, P.B. Raven, R.M. Glaser, and O. Bar-Or. Forty-two open papers were also presented at the symposium, which was attended by 388 registered participants. This volume includes all of the lectures and many of the open papers presented at the symposium.

Masahiro Kaneko

Acknowledgments

The organizing committee wishes to thank the sponsors who made the 1988 ICPFR Symposium financially possible. The main sponsors were the Commemorative Association for the Japan World Exposition (1970), Tsuyama MFG Company, Ltd., Namisho Gakuen, Mizuno Corporation, Osaka YMCA, Osaka School of Community Sports, Sogo Company, Ltd., and the Institute of Sangyo-Taiiku of Osaka College of Physical Education. In particular, Kenkokanri-Kaihatsu Center contributed much to the financial management of the Symposium.

PART I

HEALTH AND FITNESS OF THE AGED

The Roles of Exercise
in Health Maintenance and Treatment of Disease
in Middle and Old Age

J.O. Holloszy
Section of Applied Physiology, Department of Medicine, Washington
University School of Medicine, St. Louis, Missouri, USA

Now that the majority of epidemic and endemic infectious diseases and nutritional deficiencies have largely been brought under control in the developed nations, a very high
proportion of the people born in these countries can expect to attain old age. With the
population over the age of 60 years rapidly expanding, degenerative diseases of middle
and old age have become our leading public health problem. In this context, a primary
focus of preventive medicine is now on measures to maintain health and functional capacity
in older people.

There have been many major advances in the medical and surgical treatment of chronic
degenerative diseases associated with aging. Unfortunately, there have not been similar
breakthroughs in the area of health maintenance; diet and exercise are still the most powerful
measures available to us for prevention and reversal of a number of the degenerative diseases that plague older people. These include atherosclerotic coronary heart disease (ASHD),
osteoporosis, and non–insulin dependent diabetes mellitus (NIDDM). While this review
will deal only with the effects of exercise, it should be kept in mind that the effects of
appropriate diet and exercise are often synergistic.

Atherosclerotic Heart Disease

Much epidemiological data has accumulated indicating that men who exercise moderately
vigorously on a regular basis have only 30-50% as great a risk of developing clinical ASHD
compared to sedentary men with an otherwise similar risk factor profile (20, 22). In addition, recent studies employing exercise electrocardiography (7), exercise radionuclide ven-
triculography (6), and myocardial perfusion imaging after maximal exercise (25) have
provided evidence that prolonged, vigorous exercise training, in addition to markedly improving exercise capacity (24), can reverse myocardial ischemia (i.e., improve the supply
of blood and oxygen to regions of the heart to which blood supply was inadequate). Thus,
exercise can reverse or improve angina and abnormal cardiac contractile function in some
patients with clinical ASHD.

Elucidation of the mechanisms by which exercise training mediates its beneficial effects
on ASHD has been hampered by the lack of noninvasive methods for evaluating coronary
artery diameter, atherosclerotic plaque size, and development of coronary collateral vessels. However, a study on monkeys on an atherosclerotic diet has provided evidence that
exercise reduces coronary atherosclerosis and increases the caliber of the coronary arteries (17). Other studies on experimental animals have also shown that exercise results in

an increase in the diameter of the coronary arteries (19, 30). In addition, exercise has a beneficial effect on a number of major coronary risk factors in humans. These include (a) an improvement of plasma lipid-lipoprotein profile with an increase in HDL cholesterol, a decrease in total cholesterol/HDL cholesterol ratio, and a lowering of plasma triglycerides (11, 24); (b) a lowering of elevated plasma glucose and insulin levels (14), which are independent ASHD risk factors; (c) a reduction in elevated blood pressure (26); and (d) weight loss with a decrease in body fat content. The amount of exercise required to produce these protective and therapeutic effects in patients with ASHD appears to be in the range of 16-20 mi of jogging per week or an equivalent amount of some other moderately strenuous form of exercise that results in an increase in energy expenditure of 2,000 Kcal per week or more (6, 7, 22).

Osteoporosis

Evidence is beginning to accumulate indicating that exercise can play an important role in the prevention and treatment of osteoporosis if it is coupled with adequate calcium and vitamin D intake. Recent studies suggest that weight-bearing exercise such as jogging that exerts a compressive force on the bones can not only prevent but can even partially reverse bone loss in osteoporotic middle-aged and elderly women (4).

Glucose Metabolism
and Non–Insulin Dependent Diabetes

Exercise training results in lower plasma insulin concentrations both during fasting and following glucose ingestion in healthy people; despite the blunted insulin response to a glucose challenge, glucose tolerance remains normal or is improved in people who exercise regularly (3, 12, 18). Two separate adaptations are responsible. One results in a diminished insulin response to the same glucose concentration. The other, which involves an increase in sensitivity to insulin, makes possible a sufficiently rapid rate of glucose disposal to result in normal or improved glucose tolerance despite low insulin levels (16).

There is usually a progressive decline in glucose tolerance with aging, largely due to a decrease in sensitivity to the action of insulin. In the United States, this deterioration is sufficiently severe in approximately 15% of people between the ages of 55 and 74 to be classified as NIDDM; an additional 8% of people in this age range have impaired glucose tolerance (10). The vascular and neurological complications of diabetes are major causes of disability and mortality in older people. In its early stages, NIDDM is largely due to resistance to the action of insulin, with insulin deficiency playing a secondary role. As a result, plasma insulin levels are frequently high in response to elevated glucose levels (see Figure 1).

Regularly performed vigorous exercise appears to prevent (27) and also reverse (28), the insulin resistance that develops with aging. Highly trained master athletes in their 60s are often similar to young athletes in terms of excellent glucose tolerance and insulin sensitivity (27). Evidence is beginning to accumulate indicating that regularly performed exercise can normalize glucose tolerance by reducing insulin resistance in patients with early NIDDM who are not severely insulin deficient as well as in people with impaired glucose tolerance (14) (see Figure 1).

As with ASHD, the amount of exercise required to produce this beneficial effect is roughly 16-20 mi of jogging per week or an equivalent amount of some other form of exercise (i.e., an increase in caloric expenditure of 2,000 Kcal per week or more. Figure 1 shows

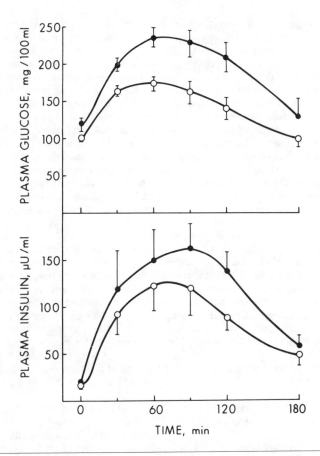

Figure 1. Plasma glucose and insulin responses to a 75-g oral glucose tolerance test in 10 patients, 5 of whom had mild noninsulin dependent diabetes and 5 of whom had impaired glucose tolerance, studied before (closed circles) and after (open circles) 8-12 months of endurance exercise training.

the effect of 8-12 months of endurance exercise training on plasma glucose and insulin levels during an oral glucose tolerance test in 10 patients, 5 with NIDDM and 5 with impaired glucose tolerance. Despite the lower insulin levels after training, glucose tolerance was markedly improved. The beneficial effects of exercise on insulin resistance and glucose tolerance are short-lived, usually being lost within a few days after exercise is stopped (15). It is therefore essential that exercise be performed regularly, at least every other day and preferably 5-6 days per week.

Maintenance of Functional Capacity

Exercise training can induce adaptations that result in increases in functional capacity and run counter to some of the changes that occur with aging. These adaptations include increases in maximal cardiac output, maximal oxygen uptake capacity ($\dot{V}O_2$max), muscle mass, lean body mass, and exercise capacity as well as a decrease in body fat content.

These and other adaptations to exercise that run counter to some of the changes associated with aging could in theory help maintain functional capacity in old age. However, experimental evidence that these adaptations, which have been demonstrated in younger people, can be induced in elderly individuals by means of exercise training is still quite limited. The main reason for this is that most of the studies documenting favorable physiological adaptations to exercise have been done on young and middle-aged people. Of the small number of published studies on older people, most have shown little or no improvement in maximum oxygen uptake capacity ($\dot{V}O_2$max) or cardiac function (2, 5, 21). It now appears that this lack of adaptive response was due to use of too mild an exercise stimulus. A recent study using more vigorous and prolonged endurance training has provided evidence that healthy men and women in their 60s can undergo as large an increase in $\dot{V}O_2$max in relative terms as young individuals if the training is sufficiently frequent, prolonged, and vigorous (29). As this was a preliminary study with a small number of subjects, further research is in progress to determine the extent to which vigorous endurance training can increase aerobic power in the elderly.

Additional evidence that older people can undergo large adaptations to endurance training has come from studies on master athletes, some of whom did not start training until middle age or later (9, 13, 23). One study (13) compared 16 highly trained master endurance athletes aged 59 ± 6 years with 16 young athletes (with whom they were matched on the basis of their training regimens) and with 18 untrained middle-aged men. On echocardiographic evaluation, both groups of athletes had a significantly greater left ventricular volume and mass than the untrained men. $\dot{V}O_2$max averaged 15% less in the masters than in the young athletes (58.7 vs. 69.0 ml $\cdot$ kg^{-1} $\cdot$ min^{-1}). When expressed in terms of lean body mass to correct for differences in body fat content, the $\dot{V}O_2$max of the master athletes was about 60% higher than that of the middle-aged untrained men. Maximum heart rate was 14% lower in the master athletes than in the young athletes (169 vs. 197 beats/min).

The O_2 pulse during maximum exercise (i.e., $\dot{V}O_2$max/heart rate at $\dot{V}O_2$max was identical in the master and young athletes. This finding suggested that the major factor responsible for the lower $\dot{V}O_2$max of the master athletes, compared with the young athletes, is their slower heart rate. Oxygen pulse is the product of stroke volume and arteriovenous O_2 difference (a-$\bar{v}O_2$ diff). The finding that the O_2 pulse during exercise that elicited $\dot{V}O_2$max was the same in the master and young athletes argued against a reduction in maximum stroke volume (SVmax) and maximum arteriovenous O_2 difference (a-$\bar{v}O_2$ diff max) with aging in these highly trained older man. However, one could not be certain that a decrease in SVmax was not compensated for by an increase in a-$\bar{v}O_2$ diff max or vice versa. Therefore, another study was done (9) that compared SVmax and a-$\bar{v}O_2$ diff in master athletes (58 ± 4 years of age), competitive young runners (26 ± 3 years), young runners matched in training and performance to the master athletes (25 ± 3 years), and healthy older sedentary subjects (58 ± 5 years).

The $\dot{V}O_2$max of the master athletes was 9 and 19% lower than that of the matched young and competitive young runners, respectively. When compared at the same relative submaximal work rates, these groups had similar stroke volumes and a-$\bar{v}O_2$ diff, although the master athletes had a lower $\dot{V}O_2$max, cardiac output and heart rate and a higher vascular resistance. Maximal stroke volume and estimated a-$\bar{v}O_2$ diff were the same in the three groups of athletes. These findings support the interpretation that the lower maximal heart rate of the master athletes accounted for their lower $\dot{V}O_2$max. The $\dot{V}O_2$max of the older sedentary subjects was 47% lower than that of the master athletes; this difference was almost equally the result of a lower stroke volume and a lower a-$\bar{v}O_2$ diff. Thus, these older athletes do not appear to exhibit the decline in maximum stroke volume and a-$\bar{v}O_2$ diff that occurs with aging in sedentary individuals; they also appear to have retained a greater peripheral vasodilatory response than healthy sedentary men of the same age.

Muscle mass and strength decline with aging (8). Endurance exercise does not appear to affect this decline. A question of considerable interest is whether heavy resistance exercise such as weight training can counteract the decrease in muscle mass and strength with aging. From the small amount of information available, it appears that heavy resistance exercise training can result in maintenance of a high level of strength in elderly master weight lifters and induce increases in strength and muscle size in previously untrained men in their 70s (1).

In conclusion, evidence is accumulating that regularly performed vigorous exercise can slow the decline in functional capacity and help protect against the development of some of the major chronic diseases that increase with aging. In the case of ASHD, NIDDM, and osteoporosis, it appears that exercise can also play an important therapeutic role.

Acknowledgments

The author's research on the health benefits of exercise in the elderly is supported by Program Project Grant AG05562 and Institutional National Research Service Award AG00078 from the National Institute on Aging.

References

1. Aniansson, A., Gustafsson, E. Physical training in elderly men with special reference to quadriceps muscle strength and morphology. Clin. Physiol. 1:87-98, 1981.

2. Benestad, A.M. Trainability of old men. Acta Med. Scand. 178:321-327, 1965.

3. Bjorntorp, P., Fahlen, M., Grimby, G., Gustafson, A., Holm, J., Renstrom, P., Schersten, T. Carbohydrate and lipid metabolism in middle-aged physically well trained men. Metabolism 21:1037-1044, 1972.

4. Dalsky, G.P. Exercise: its effect on bone mineral content. Clin. Obstet. Gynecol. 30:820-832, 1987.

5. DeVries, H.A. Physiological effects of an exercise training regimen upon men aged 52 to 88. J. Gerontol. 25:325-336, 1970.

6. Ehsani, A.A., Biello, D.R., Schultz, J., Sobel, B.E., Holloszy, J.O. Improvement of left ventricular contractile function by exercise training in patients with coronary artery disease. Circulation 74:350-358, 1986.

7. Ehsani, A.A., Heath, G.W., Hagberg, J.M., Sobel, B.E., Holloszy, J.O. Effects of 12 months of intense exercise training on ischemic ST-segment depression in patients with coronary artery disease. Circulation 64:1116-1124, 1981.

8. Grimby, G., Saltin, B. The aging muscle. Clin. Physiol. 3:209-218, 1983.

9. Hagberg, J.M., Allen, W.K., Seals, D.R., Hurley, B.F., Ehsani, A.A., Holloszy, J.O. A hemodynamic comparison of young and older endurance athletes during exercise. J. Appl. Physiol. 58:2041-2046, 1985.

10. Harris, M.I., Hadden, W.C., Knowler, W.C., Bennett, P.H. Prevalence of diabetes and impaired glucose tolerance and plasma glucose levels in U.S. population aged 20-74 yr. Diabetes 36:528-534, 1987.

11. Haskell, W.L. The influence of exercise on the concentrations of triglyceride and cholesterol in human plasma. Exer. Sports Sci. Rev. 12:205-244, 1984.

12. Heath, G.W., Gavin, III, J.R., Hinderliter, J.M., Hagberg, J.M., Bloomfield, S.A., Holloszy, J.O. Effects of exercise and lack of exercise on glucose tolerance and insulin sensitivity. J. Appl. Physiol. 55:512-517, 1983.

13. Heath, G.W., Hagberg, J.M., Ehsani, A.A., Holloszy, J.O. A physiological comparison of young and older endurance athletes. J. Appl. Physiol. 51:634-640, 1981.

14. Holloszy, J.O., Schultz, J., Kusnierkiewicz, J., Hagberg, J.M., Ehsani, A.A. Effects of exercise on glucose tolerance and insulin resistance. Acta Med. Scand. 711(Suppl.):55-65, 1986.

15. King, D.S., Dalsky, G.P., Clutter, W.E., Young, D.A., Staten, M.A., Cryer, P.E., Holloszy, J.O. Effects of lack of exercise on insulin secretion and action in trained subjects. Am. J. Physiol. 254:E537-E542, 1988.

16. King, D.S., Dalsky, G.P., Staten, M.A., Clutter, W.E., Van Houten, D.R., Holloszy, J.O. Insulin action and secretion in endurance-trained and untrained humans. J. Appl. Physiol. 63:2247-2252, 1987.

17. Kramsch, D.M., Aspen, A.J., Abramowitz, B.M., Kreimendahl, T., Hood, Jr., W.B. Reduction of coronary atherosclerosis by moderate conditioning exercise in monkeys on an atherogenic diet. New Eng. J. Med. 305:1483-1489, 1981.

18. LeBlanc, J., Nadeau, A., Boulay, M., Rousseau-Migneron, S. Effects of physical training and adiposity on glucose metabolism and ^{125}I-insulin binding. J. Appl. Physiol. 46:235-239, 1979.

19. Leon, A.S., Bloor, C.M. Effects of exercise and its cessation on the heart and its blood supply. J. Appl. Physiol. 24:485-490, 1968.

20. Morris, J.N., Pollard, R., Everitt, M.G., Chave, S.P.W. Vigorous exercise in leisure-time: protection against coronary heart disease. Lancet 38:1207-1210, 1980.

21. Niinimaa, V., Shephard, R.J. Training and O_2 conductance in the elderly: II. The cardiovascular system. J. Gerontol. 33:362-367, 1978.

22. Paffenbarger, R.S., Hyde, R.T., Wing, A.L., Steinmetz, C.H. A natural history of athleticism and cardiovascular health. J. Am. Med. Assoc. 252:491-495, 1984.

23. Pollock, M.L., Miller, H.S., Wilmore, J. Physiological characteristics of champion American track athletes 40 to 75 years of age. J. Gerontol. 29:645-649, 1974.

24. Rogers, M.A., Yamamoto, C., Hagberg, J.M., Holloszy, J.O., Ehsani, A.A. The effect of 7 years of intense exercise training on patients with coronary artery disease. J. Am. Coll. Cardiol. 10:321-326, 1987.

25. Schuler, G., Schlerf, G., Wirth, A., Mautner, H.-P., Scheurlen, H., Thumm, M., Roth, H., Schwarz, F., Kohlmeier, M., Mermel, H.C., Kübler, W. Low-fat diet and regular, supervised physical exercise in patients with symptomatic coronary artery disease: reduction of stress-induced myocardial ischemia. Circulation 77:172-181, 1988.

26. Seals, D.R., Hagberg, J.M. The effect of exercise training on human hypertension: a review. Med. Sci. Sports and Exer. 16:207-215, 1984.

27. Seals, D.R., Hagberg, J.M., Allen, W.K., Hurley, B.F., Dalsky, G.P., Ehsani, A.A., Holloszy, J.O. Glucose tolerance in young and older athletes and sedentary men. J. Appl. Physiol. 56:1521-1525, 1984.

28. Seals, D.R., Hagberg, J.M., Hurley, B.F., Ehsani, A.A., Holloszy, J.O. Effects of endurance training on glucose tolerance and plasma lipid levels in older men and women. J. Am. Med. Assoc. 252:645-649, 1984.

29. Seals, D.R., Hagberg, J.M., Hurley, B.F., Ehsani, A.A., Holloszy, J.O. Endurance training in older men and women: I. Cardiovascular responses to exercise. J. Appl. Physiol. 57:1024-1029, 1984.

30. Wyatt, H.L., Mitchell, J. Influences of physical conditioning and deconditioning on coronary vasculature in dogs. J. Appl. Physiol. 45:619-625, 1978.

A Statistical Approach for Physical Senility and Its Control

K. Kikkawa

Institute of Health Science, Kyushu University 11, Kasuga City, Japan

A number of researchers have attempted to measure physiological age in adulthood. Most researchers in biological gerontology have focused on the description of normal aging. Although many scientists agree that there is considerable variation between individuals in the rate of the aging process, only a few studies have explored this area (3). Revealing the characteristics of individuals who retain their functional capacities the longest (i.e., who age most slowly) is one of the primary aims for the gerontologist. Of particular interest are the effects of lifestyle (daily activity, diet, smoking, and economic status), as these can be modified during an individual's lifetime (3).

This study has two purposes. The first purpose is to establish a predictive equation for male chronological age (AGE) through a series of measurements of physical fitness, medical indexes, and physique. The second purpose is to clarify lifestyle factors associated with physical senility, which can be obtained from the developed predictive equation.

Methods

The investigation was based on the data obtained from a study by the Institute of Health Science of Kyushu University, which investigated degrees of health and related factors.

We examined 148 males (mean age 44.6 years [SD 8.85]; range 28-68 years) who performed 10 variables that consisted of six physical fitness tests—grip strength (GRIP), back strength (BACK), single foot blinded balance (BALANCE), standing trunk flexion (FLEX), vital capacity (VITAL) and oxygen intake per body weight (MAP)—of three medical indexes such as systolic blood pressure (SBP), diastolic blood pressure (DBP) and heart rate (HR) at rest and of the percent body fat (FAT) estimated from skinfolds thickness. Six physical fitness tests were taken by general procedures presented by the Japanese Ministry of Education and Tokyo Metropolitan University (17). The blood pressure and heart rate at rest were measured by an automatic blood pressure system (BP103N, Colin, Ltd.). Maximum oxygen intake per body weight was estimated from two heart rate series after stepping tests by Margaria's method (9). Body fat was measured by the body density estimated from skinfold thickness by Nagamine and Suzuki's method (9). Thirty-one members answered a questionnaire that elicited information about past and present physical activity, activity preferences, nutritional intake, satisfaction with life status (economics and environment), and habits promoting wellness.

Statistical Analysis

Since we consider a large number of age-related parameters in multiple regression analysis when predicting chronological age, with the predicted age as the physical age of individual (3), the forward stepwise regression analysis (5) was adopted to establish the predictive equation for chronological age. To obtain an optimal equation with less independent variables, but with a higher multiple correlation coefficient, several statistical information criteria were applied in regression analysis.

In this study, the ratio of predictive age to chronological age × 100 was conceived as physical senility; that is, z=predictive age/chronological age × 100 was used as the degree of senility of each subject, and means of z obtained from subgroups of each item were compared by means of a one-way analysis of variance.

Results and Discussion

As the initial step in the regression analysis, we took into account the following variables in the following order: BACK, MAP, VITAL, SBP, FAT, HR, BALANCE, DBP, FLEX, and GRIP. In the cases where all the variables were used for the analysis, the multiple correlation coefficient showed the highest value but each regression coefficient had many errors. Therefore, the equation is not always appropriate for the multiple regression model. It is desirable to yield an equation composed of few variables but with the least loss of information (10). Many statisticians argued that the stopping rule to select the independent variables should be based on the F-statistics (4, 6, 11, 13).

Several criteria were proposed for variable selections in the regression model: R (multiple correlation coefficient adjusted for degree of freedom), Mallow's Cp, Schwarz Information Criterion (SIC), and Akaike's Information Criterion (AIC) (1, 2, 4, 6, 7, 9, 11, 13, 15, 16). Akaike's Information Criterion is defined as AIC = −2 × log (maximum likelihood) + (2 × number of parameter) (1, 2, 9, 13, 16). SIC is defined as SIC = log (maximum likelihood) − (1/2(log(n)) × (number of estimatable parameters), where n is the number of observations (15), which is not always identically distributed. Mallow's Cp is defined as RSS/MSr − (n−2 × p), where RSS is the residual sum of squares for the equation, p is the number of variables in each equation, and MSr is the residual mean square based on the regression equation using all independent variables (5, 13).

In particular AIC, which is based upon Kullback-Leibler information and considered the most effective criterion, is known to achieve the trade-off between suitability and reliability for statistical models (1, 2, 13). Some scientists empirically support the availability of AIC for regression analysis, because MAICE (minimum AIC estimate) is equivalent to 2.0 of F-to-enter or F-to-remove (13). Figure 1 shows the variable entered at each step of regression analysis and the values of several criteria. The regression equation, which indicates the MAICE, was selected as the optimum regression model. MAICE was achieved in the equation composed of six variables: BACK, MAP, VITAL, SBP, FAT, and HR. The equation is described as follows:

$$\hat{y} = 87.34 - .1439 \times \text{BACK} - .5322 \times \text{MAP} - .00276 \times \text{VITAL} + .1226 \times \text{SBP} - .354 \times \text{FAT} - .117 \times \text{HR}.$$

This was also selected by SIC and Cp as the optimal choice, although the other equation that entered BALANCE as the seventh variable was selected by R*. The multiple correlation coefficient of this equation was 0.6447, the standard error of estimates was 6.97, and F-value was 15.9, which is highly significant. The selected equation seems to be; ustifiable from our empirical observations on the general aging tendency of each variable; that is, the downward trends in such variables as BACK, VITAL, and MAP and the upward trend in SBP from younger to older patients reflected in the equation.

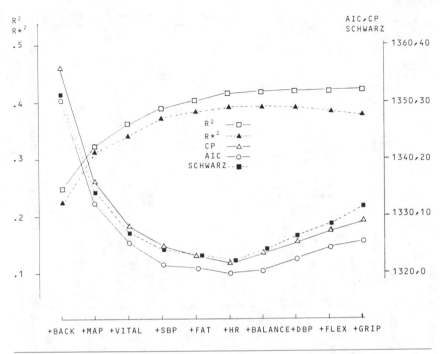

Figure 1. Entered variables at each step by stepwise regression analysis and the changes of criteria.

To check the reliability of this equation, the technique of analysis of residuals was adopted by plotting the predicted age on the horizontal axis and the standardized residuals on the vertical axis (4, 6, 13). Observing the plotted point, they were randomly distributed around zero.

Factors Associated With Degrees of Senility

We conceived a ratio of predictive age obtained from the above equation to chronological age × 100 percent as the degrees of physical senility. And then we tried to find out the factors that affect the degrees of physical senility among lifestyles or life status of individuals who have responded to our questionnaire. Thirty-one members answered the questionnaire: 24 of those were also subjects for regression analysis whereas the other seven males only answered the questionnaire. The analysis of variance was performed by taking the degrees of senility (z) as the dependent variable and the items collected by the questionnaire as independent variables.

The statistically significant ($p < .10$) factors were as follows: sleeping type, commuting mode, physical activity during junior high school, intake of vegetables, smoking, satisfaction with income, conception of life quality, care in keeping regular daily patterns, and satisfaction with home life and personal life (see Table 1). Of those, linear relationships between physical senility and appropriate habitual life and life status, satisfaction with environment and life were observed. The means of degrees of physical senility with-

Table 1   ANOVA of Ratio of Predicted Age to Actual Age for Lifestyle and Life Status Factors

Factors	Subgroup (Ascending order)				F
Type of sleep	Moderate 91.9±12.0(8)	Wake early 97.5±15.7(8)	Wake late 111.6±21.1(15)		3.7
Commuting mode	Walk, bike 87.2±5.8(4)	Walk, driving 90.9±9.7(5)	Driving 110.6±19.7(20)		4.7
Physical activity (J.H.S)	Very active 96.9±16.6(3)	Active 102.4±18.6(9)	Inactive 119.6±18.8(7)		3.0
Intake of vegetables	Enough 84.0±8.2(3)	A little 103.2±16.6(24)	Little 127.2±27.2(3)		4.8
Smoking	<19 pcs. 86.1±7.0(4)	<10 pcs. 94.7±20.0(3)	Not smoking 102.6±17.9(17)	>20 pcs. 116.7±20.7	2.8
Satisfied with income	A little 88.5±9.7(6)	Enough 90.6±1.9(4)	Little enough 106.3±20.5(15)	Undesirable 116.8±18.6(6)	3.6
Level of life	Upper middle 93.4±10.7(15)	Lower 108.2±31.8(3)	Lower middle 112.6±20.4(13)		4.4
Not nervous about irregular lifestyle	NA 83.0±4.8(4)	Little 93.1±7.1(6)	Applicable 93.7±15.6(4)	A little 113.2±19.2(17)	5.5
Satisfied with way of life	Very 95.7±12.8(17)	Enough 98.3±16.1(6)	Little 121.6±22.5(8)		7.2

Note. These factors are statistically significant by ANOVA ($p < .10$). Figures denote $\pm SD$, and the number of observation of each group is shown in the parenthesis.

in groups of subjects who walk to work, consume enough vegetables, are satisfied with their income, conceive of their life levels as better than average, or take care to keep regular life patterns were found lower than in the other group and lower than 100. This reveals that the group of subjects living in these ways are younger in physical functions than their chronological age.

Webster and Logie (18) reported that subjective health perception within nonsmoker groups was associated with differences in functional age. Furukawa (8) reported that the predicted ages from physiological parameters in the patients with hypertension or other diseases were clearly older than their chronological age. Sasaki et al. (12) reported similar results. Shimokata et al. (14) mentioned that an appropriate daily life was associated with the younger physiological age.

The results of the present study concur with previous papers, agreeing that conducting daily life with regularity, being satisfied with daily life and environment, and being careful with diet and physical activity are necessary in order to retain younger physical functions or physiological age.

Conclusion

To assess degrees of physical senility, we established the regression equation for chronological age and conceived the ratio of predicted age to chronological age as the degrees of physical senility. The validity and reliability of the equation were confirmed; however, its coefficient of determination was not enough.

We conceived that individual physical senility depends on the way and consciousness of daily living. In order to confirm the associate factors in delaying senility, a more definitive predictive equation should be established.

References

1. Akaike, H. A new look at the statistical model identification. IEEE Transactions on Automatic Control Ac9(6):716-723, 1974.

2. Akaike, H. What is information criterion AIC? Mathemat. Sci. 153:5-11, 1976. (in Japanese)

3. Borkan, G.A., Norris, A.H. Biological age in adulthood: comparison of active and inactive U.S. males. Human Biol. 52(4):787-802, 1980.

4. Chatterjee, S., Price, B. Regression analysis by example. New York: John Wiley & Sons, 1977. (in Japanese, Sawa and Kano. Kaiki Bunseki no Zissai, Sinyosha, 9-10, 158-239, 1980.)

5. Dixon, W.J., Brown, M.B., eds. BMDP-79, biomedical computer programs P-series. Berkeley: University of California Press, 1979.

6. Draper, N.R., Smith, H. Applied regression analysis. New York: John Wiley & Sons, 1978. (in Japanese, Nakamura. Oyo Kaiki Busenseki, Morikita-Shuppan, 163-216, 1979.)

7. Forsythe, A.B., Englemann, L., Jenrich, R. A stopping rule for variable selection in multiple regression. J. Amer. Statist. Assoc. 68(341):75-77, 1973.

8. Furukawa, T. Model of life span. Mathemat. Sci. 14(1):43-55, 1976. (in Japanese)

9. Kikkawa, K., Ogaki, T., Okabe, H., Matsumoto, J. A statistical approach for physical senility and its control(I). Kyushu J. Phys. Ed. Sports 2:57-66, 1988. (in Japanese)

10. Koizumi, K. The estimation of age from the cranial sutures by means of multivariate methods. J. Anthrop. Soc. Nippon 90(2):109-118, 1982.

11. Okuno, C., Kume, H., Yoshizawa, T. Multivariate analysis. Nikka-Giren 128-158, 1975. (in Japanese)

12. Sasaki, A., Takasaki, Y., Horiuchi, N., Omori, K. 'Expected age' used in evaluation results of multiple health examination. Jpn. J. Geriat. 7(6):323-332, 1970. (in Japanese)

13. Sawa, T. Regression analysis. Asakura Shoten, 1979. (in Japanese, Kaiki Bunseki)

14. Shimokata, H., Shibata, K., Kuzuya, F. Assessment of biological aging status. Jpn. J. Geriat. 24:88-92, 1987. (in Japanese)

15. Stone, M. Comments on model selection criteria of Akaike and Schwarz. J. Roy. Statist. Soc. B. 41(2):276-278, 1979.

16. Sugiyama, K., Ozaki, I., Ushizawa, K., Shimizu, M. Regression analysis of estimating of age in terms of dental defacement. Appl. Stat. 5(3):123-138, 1979. (in Japanese)

17. Tokyo Metropolitan University, ed. Physical fitness standards for Japanese people. 3rd ed. Fumaido, Tokyo: 1980:21-103. (in Japanese)

18. Webster, I.W., Logie, A.R., A relationship between age and health status in female subjects. J. Gerontol. 31:546-550, 1976.

Longitudinal Study on Motor Fitness Tests for the Aged

J. Tahara, S. Sakimoto, K. Uchino, and F. Matsumoto
School of Physical Education, Chukyo Women's University, Yokone-cho, Obu, Aichi-ken, and Yokohama National University, Hodogaya-Ku, Yokohama, Japan

Half of those over 60 years old have diseases such as diabetes and cardiovascular disease. Greater individual differences of physical and motor fitness have also been found among the aged than the young. To exercise without knowing one's fitness status involves some risk, for example, muscular strain, joint sprain, and so on. In order for the aged to avoid such risks, it is necessary to exercise only after a medical checkup. For the medical checkup we also need to prepare more careful applications, especially to base tests on discovering the effect of motor fitness on the aging process.

Methods

Subjects of this study were nine men age 61-81 and 11 women from age 60-79 of the group called the Thursday Exercise Club. All subjects showed no abnormalities in their medical checkups. They exercised regularly, doing rhythm dance, gymnastics, gate ball, and folk dances, meeting every week on Thursday for more than 10 years.

We did not assess their exercise intensity, but they spent 2 hr in the morning and another 2 hr in the afternoon for those activities mentioned. We regarded this group as the "higher-aged regular exercise group."

The importance of the exercise ECG test (treadmill:Bruce) was emphasized in the medical checkup in order to avoid risk in exercises. The study included a motor fitness test for subjects conducted twice a year during the period from December 1983 to December 1987. The items in the motor fitness test were the following: vertical jump, standing trunk flexion, trunk extension, side step, standing long jump, and jumping reaction time.

Results

The ages and sexes of four subjects are shown in Table 1. They conducted the motor fitness test sequentially. Figure 1 shows the measurements of vertical jump. J.A.'s and F.A.'s scores were above those of the physical fitness standards of Japanese (more than 5 cm). We couldn't compare between H.N.'s and T.Y.'s scores and those of the physical fitness standards of Japanese because there were no data for those over 70 years old. Their scores were, however, also above the values for 70-year-olds in the physical fitness standards of Japanese. All of these scores were achieved consistently.

Table 1   The Ages and Sexes of the Subjects Studied Longitudinally

Name	Sex	Age (yr)
J.A.	Male	62-66
H.N.	Male	75-79
F.A.	Female	66-70
T.Y.	Female	70-74

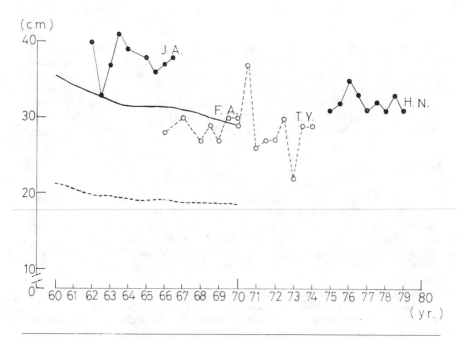

Figure 1. The comparison between the measurements of the subjects (●————● : male, o-----o : female) and the scores of the physical fitness of Japanese (———— : male, --------: female) in the vertical jump.

Also in standing trunk flexion, trunk extension, jumping reaction time, and side step no differences were seen for 4 years. Figure 2 shows the measurements in the standing long jump. All scores in this item significantly declined in average over 4 years. However, they were above those of the physical fitness standards of Japanese (more than 30 cm).

Conclusion

In terms of the elderly subjects who exercised once a week, total average values of the motor fitness tests did not significantly decline over 4 years, to exercise once a week there-

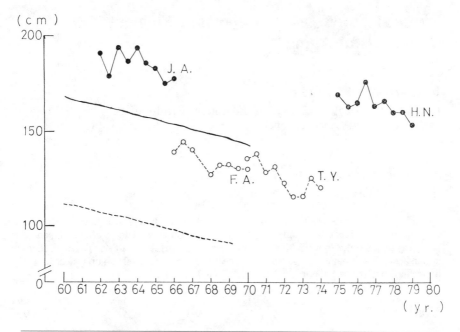

Figure 2. The comparison between the measurements of the subjects (•———• : male, o-----o : female) and the scores of the physical fitness of Japanese (——— : male, --------: female) in the standing long jump.

fore helps maintain motor fitness in spite of the aging process. The reason for the marked decrease in the standing long jump compared to the vertical jump was, perhaps, that the subjects often exercised jumping upward but not forward. More study is needed to discover the reason for the inconsistency in the results of the standing long jump in this study.

Physical Fitness as an Important Element of Successful Aging

K. Moriya and Y. Fukuchi

Department of Health and Physical Education, Faculty of Education, Hokkaido University, Sapporo, Japan

Aging is generally believed to depress physical and mental function. Japanese society is changing as many Japanese people are living longer and the percentage of aged Japanese is increasing. In order to learn how we can age successfully as regards to physical, mental, and social well-being, we surveyed the health and morale levels and physical fitness of septuagenarians in Sapporo in 1984 and from 1987 to 1988.

Methods

In 1984, 221 septuagenarians (110 males, 111 females) who were living at home in "S" area of Sapporo were asked to answer questionnaires on their present health and morale. The health level was evaluated based on 20 questions from Hokudai Health Index (HHI) plus an additional four questions, and the morale level was evaluated based on 20 questions from the modified Philadelphia Geriatric Center Morale Scale (PGM). From the answers to the questionnaires, physical and mental health levels were calculated. Depending on the scores in both categories, the subjects were divided into Groups A (high scores), B (medium scores), and C (low scores), and the health and morale were compared among these groups. Then 30 aged subjects (19 males, 11 females) of Group A and 19 aged subjects (9 males, 10 females) of Group C were asked to have the level of their physical fitness measured. We were able to measure 19 subjects from Group A and 12 subjects from Group C; 2 subjects from Group C declined to participate and the other subjects were absent when we called on them (Group A, 11; Group C, 5). The physical fitness test consisted of measurements of hand grip strength (by hand grip meter, Takei Co.), vital capacity (pulmotester, Fukuda Co.), and squat times for 20 s.

Between 1987 and 1988, we asked the subjects who were examined in 1984 (30 people of Group A and 19 people of Group C) for permission to reexamine their health and morale levels and physical fitness. Of these people, 21 (15 males, 6 females) of Group A and 7 (3 males, 4 females) of Group C agreed to our request. The same methods used in 1984 were used to reexamine the health and morale levels and physical fitness between 1987 and 1988.

Results

In 1984, 28% of the male ($n=31$) and 17% of the female aged ($n=19$) showed higher scores on both health and morale indexes (Group A), while 11% of the males ($n=12$) and 19% of the females ($n=21$) showed lower scores (Group C). The remaining scores were intermediate between both Groups A and C (Group B: male 61%, female 64%). Group A is thought to represent the desirable state of aging. When physical fitness (vital capacity, grip strength, and squat times) was compared between Groups A and C, the male and female aged of Group A demonstrated a higher rating of physical fitness, especially in squat times, than those of Group C (Table 1).

Table 1   Physical Fitness of Septuagenarians Measured in 1984

	Male		Female	
	G.A (n=11)	G.C (n=5)	G.A (n=7)	G.C (n=7)
Vital capacity (cc)	2492±201	2250±364	1445±108	1116±145
Grip strength (kg)	35±1	32±3	21±2	17±2
Squat times (times/20 s)	12±1	7±2*	8±1	1±1**

Note. Mean ±*SE* of the mean. *$p < .05$, **$p < .001$ vs. G.A. (G.A = Group A, G.C = Group C). n = number of aged subjects.

After 3 years, between 1987 and 1988, we followed up on their physical fitness and health and morale levels. Of the subjects in Group A in 1984, 52% remained in that group 3 years later, while the remaining aged people moved to Groups B (38%) and C(10%); those who had been in Group C in 1984 stayed in that group 3 years later. Between 1987 and 1988, Group A had a higher rating of physical fitness, especially in squat times, as compared to those of Group C (Table 2). This is similar to the results in the 1984 experiment shown in Table 1. A significant positive correlation was observed between the successful aging index (the score of health level plus the score of morale level) and squat times in male and female, respectively (see Figure 1).

Table 2   Physical Fitness of the Male Aged Followed Up Between 1987 and 1988

	G.A (n=7)	G.B (n=5)	G.C (n=4)
Vital capacity (cc)	2571±188	2530±232	2163±351
Grip strength (kg)	33±2	31±2	30±2
Squat times (times/20 s)	13±1	12±1	8±2*

Note. Mean ±*SE* of the mean. *$p < .05$ *vs.* G.A (G.B = Group B). Other abbreviations are the same as those used in Table 1.

Conclusion

From the above results, a certain level of physical fitness is inferred to be a basic factor in successful aging. The lifestyles of aged people belonging to Group A were recognized as more active than those of Group C.

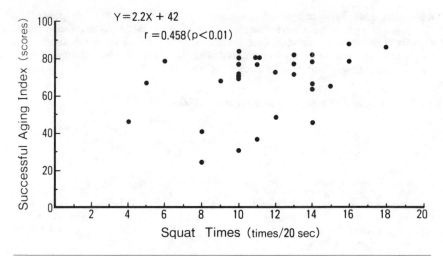

Figure 1. The interrelationship of squat times of the aged males to their index of successful aging (health and morale levels) tested by modified Hokudai Health Index (HHI) and modified Philadelphia Geriatric Center Morale Scale (PGM).

Acknowledgment

We wish to thank Ms. Yukiko Ishida and Ioko Ishizuka for their excellent assistance throughout the research.

Physical Fitness of the People in Taipei Including the Aged

G.-H. Kuo

Taipei Physical Education College, Taipei, Taiwan

In 1987 people over the age of 65 accounted for 5.05% of the Taiwanese population. We estimate that people over the age of 65 will make up 8.3% of Taiwan's population in the year 2000. That is, 1 out of every 12 people in Taiwan will be over the age of 65.

Social costs for the elderly will put an increasing strain on both government and our families. This is a new social problem in Taiwan caused by the advancement of modern science. The purpose of this study was to examine the relationship between exercise and the physical fitness of the aged.

Methods

In 1984 and 1985 during Taipei's sports season (July and August), we held many tests of physical fitness in Taipei. The total number of people participating in this study was 3,562. About 64% of the test participants were male while the remaining 36% were female. The test participants were doing various morning exercise in Taipei at different locations. The contents of the tests included basic tests of physical fitness, a questionnaire survey, and consultation. Figure 1 presents the results of the physical fitness tests.

Physical Fitness Results

1. Static balance test (close one's eyes while standing on one leg): Figure 1A shows that statistical results from 1984 and 1985 are similar. In this test men's ability greatly decreased between the ages of 50-54 while women's ability greatly decreased after the age of 35. This physical fitness test is one example that proves women are aging more quickly than men.

2. Agility test (side step test): Figure 1B shows that in 1984 and 1985 physical fitness measurements were very similar. In the side step test, agility decreased quickly after the age of 40. In this test men scored 68% of the best scores while women's agility was 60% when both groups were above the age of 55. This test also shows that women age faster than men.

3. Power test (standing broad jump): In this test the power of men 55 and over was 66% of their younger counterparts, while older women's abilities were 59% of the best record in the 19-25 age group. So it is clear that women age earlier than men.

4. Flexibility test (trunk flexibility): The flexibility of women was better than men (see Figure 1D). Flexibility of men age 55 and over was 61%, while flexibility in women age 55 and over was 88% of the average in the 25-30 age group. This is one test in which women outperformed men.

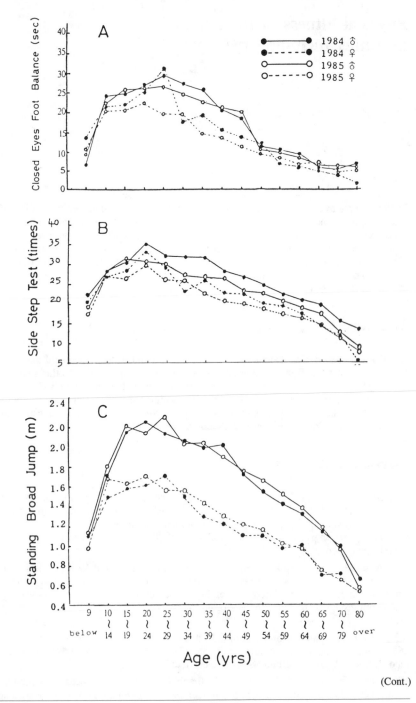

Figure 1.   Physical fitness levels of the people in Taipei in relation to age and sex. A: Balance, B: Agility, C: Power, D: Flexibility, E: Strength, F: Endurance.

(Cont.)

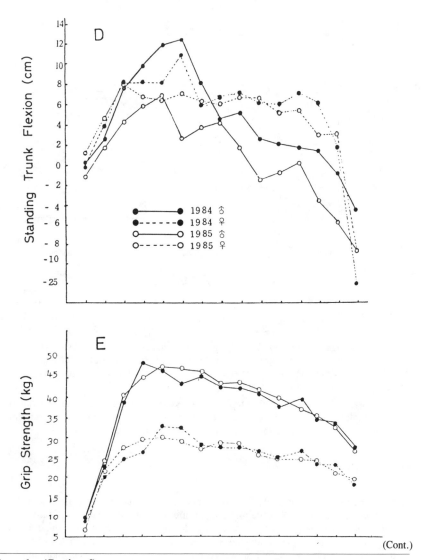

Figure 1.   (Continued)

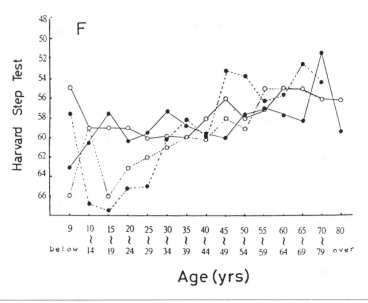

Figure 1.   (Continued))

5. Static strength test (grips): The strength of people age 20-30 was greatest (see Figure 1E). After that time their strength gradually decreased. In this test both men's and women's abilities decreased at about the same rate. In this physical fitness test it appears men and women age at about the same rate.

6. Endurance test (the Harvard step test): As shown in Figure 1F, many of the aged cannot complete the Harvard step test. For this reason, we could not judge endurance. A smaller number of people in Taipei participated in this test.

Discussion

In the physical fitness tests taken by people in Taipei, the majority of people were 45-70 years of age. It was found that the physical abilities of males decrease drastically around the age of 50 and female fitness begins a rapid decline when women are around 40 years old. The aging phenomena of females is about 10 years faster than males. The aging phenomena concerning strength is slower than other areas, and changes in endurance vary greatly from person to person as one grows older. As it was very difficult for older participants to complete the Harvard step test, it is necessary to design a new test. Also, it was found that elderly people prefer leisure types of sports, like jogging, calisthenics, dancing, yoga, "Y Tan Kung," walking, martial arts, hiking, and badminton.

Evaluation of Work Capacity in the Elderly by a Self-Paced Step Test

K. Hirakawa, Y. Oda, T. Okuno, M. Kimura, and T. Morimoto

Department of Physiology Kyoto Prefectural University of Medicine, Kyoto, Japan

Aging is characterized by a loss of functional reserve capacity during exercise (4). To assess physiological responses to exercise, determination of maximal oxygen intake is widely used, but it is not suitable for aged people. The purpose of the present investigation was to explore a test to estimate the reserve capacity of cardiovascular function during exercise in the elderly using submaximal exertion. The test was designed based on the stepping activity in which each subject graded the intensity of his or her performance according to his or her individual fitness level. This test is more relevant to the demands of daily living. The self-paced walking test has been used as an exercise test in the elderly (2, 3), but the step test was chosen because stepping could be readily performed at any place without special tools or training and also because it is convenient for obtaining physiological measurements during the test.

Methods

General Protocol

The present submaximal test developed to evaluate exercise ability of the elderly consists of stepping at three graded paces for 7 min: 3 min at a rather slow pace, 2 min at a normal pace, and another 2 min at rather high pace consecutively, using a platform 20 cm in height. The pace of each step was determined relative to the normal pace, which was defined as the pace used by each subject in everyday life. Heart rate was monitored throughout the step test using an ECG with unipolar chest lead, and blood pressure was measured every 2 min during the stepping. The stepping was terminated when the ST decreased by more than 2 mm, when the blood pressure rose to more than 220 mmHg, or whenever there was a fall of blood pressure with arrhythmia or when a subject claimed muscle fatigue (1).

Calculations

The number of steps at each pace was determined for 30 s at the end of each period, and the work rate at each stage of stepping was determined as kgm/kg of body weight/min from number of steps, body weight, and the height of step (20 cm). From the relationship between work rate (X) and measured heart rate (Y) during stepping, heart rate at a fixed work rate of 4.5 kgm/kg/min was determined and defined as HR 4.5. In addition, heart rate response at this work rate was calculated as follows: percent heart rate increase relative to the predicted maximum heart rate obtained as $220 - \text{age}$ was calculated as (HR 4.5

− resting heart rate) × 100 / (maximum heart rate − resting heart rate) and defined as
% HR 4.5. Similarly, the increase rate of heart rate at normal pace, or HR reserve at
normal pace, was determined as an index of reserve capacity of heart rate response at
normal pace.

Subjects

Subjects were 280 elderly persons ranging in age from 60 to 87 (135 males, 145 females)
living in the Kyoto area, and the mean age was 71.7 ± 5.6 for males and 68.6 ± 5.0
for females. Medical examination including resting ECG was performed before the test
and 94.1% of subjects were able to finish the test.

Results

A typical example of heart rate and blood pressure response during self-paced step test
is shown in Figure 1. Heart rate and systolic blood pressure showed graded response to
the three grades of stepping exercise, although diastolic blood pressure stayed constant.
At each level of step rate, heart rate response was 96.7 ± 13.7, 105.5 ± 15.7, and 120.5
± 17.1 /min, and systolic blood pressure was 150.0 ± 28.1, 162.9 ± 29.8, and 181.0
± 31.2 mmHg, respectively. This indicates that three grades of stepping exercise were
sufficiently different to define the relation between heart rate and exercise and also that
the test is well within the submaximum level.

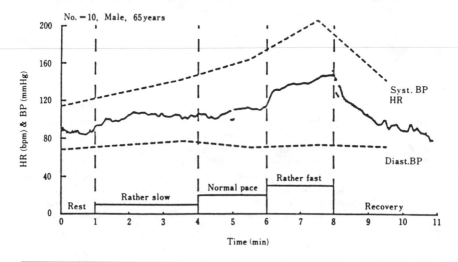

Figure 1. Heart rate and blood pressure during a self-paced step test.

In Figures 2 and 3, the percent increases of heart rate relative to the predicted maximum heart rate are plotted as a function of age for both males and females, respectively.
The results for young adults (male: 23.4 ± 1.4, female: 19.6 ± 1.1 years of age) are
also shown as the open circle in the left end of each figure, which indicate that the increase of heart rate at the exercise level of 4.5 kgm/kg/min was only 23.4 ± 4.2% in

males and 33.0 ± 4.9% in females. The value increased with age, and the increase was significantly correlated with the increase of age, reaching 50% at the age of 75.1 in males and 62.3 in females. In addition, variation of the response increased with age, which indicates that %HR 4.5 can be used to compare the heart rate response to exercise in the elderly.

In Figures 4 and 5, HR reserve at normal pace is shown as the function of age for males and females, respectively. The result for males shows a significant negative correlation with age, while in females significance was not observed due to the large individual variation. Based on these results, it is possible to distinguish elderly persons with high, normal, or low reserve capacity in heart rate response.

Conclusions

Using a graded step test, heart rate response at a fixed exercise load was shown to approach with age to the predicted heart rate maximum, though individual variations were obvious in the change in heart rate response. The reserve capacity of heart rate response observed during stepping at a normal pace was defined as HR reserve, and the value of HR reserve was suggested to be useful for the guidance of the elderly in everyday life and also for prescription of exercise.

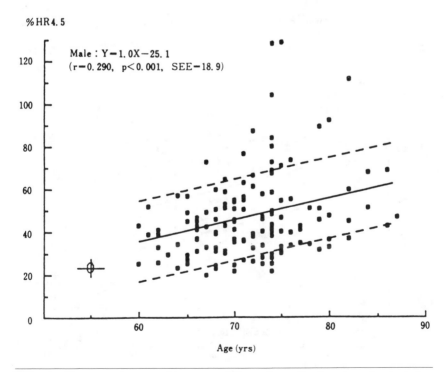

Figure 2.   The percent increases of heart rate relative to the predicted maximum heart rate for males.

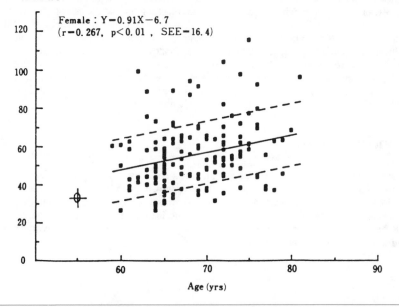

Figure 3.   The percent increases of heart rate relative to the predicted maximum heart rate for females.

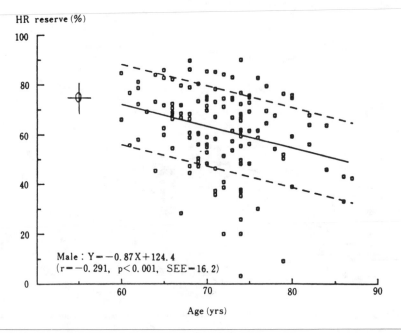

Figure 4.   Heart rate reserve at normal pace for males.

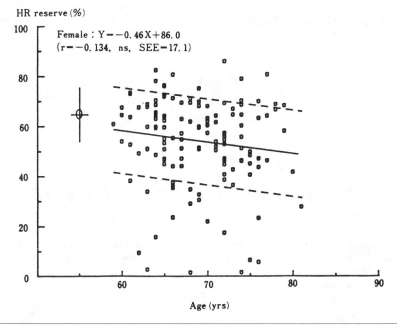

Figure 5.   Heart rate reserve at normal pace for females.

References

1. American College of Medicine. Guidelines for exercise testing and prescription. 3rd ed. Philadelphia: Lea & Febiger, 1986.

2. Bassey, E.J., Fentem, P.H., MacDonald, I.C., Scriven, P.M. Self-paced walking as a method for exercise testing in elderly and young men. Clin. Sci. Molec. Med. 51:609-612, 1976.

3. Bassey, E.J., MacDonald, I.A., Patrick, J.M. Factors affecting the heart rate during self-paced walking. Europ. J. Appl. Physiol. 48:105-115, 1982.

4. Holloszy, J.O. Aging and exercise: physiological interactions. Fed. Proc. 46:1823, 1987.

Application of the Modified Conconi Test in Sports for the Aged

G. Gaisl, P. Hofmann, and V. Bunc
Department of Exercise Physiology, Institute of Sports Sciences, University Graz, Austria

The anaerobic threshold (AT) as well as the maximum oxygen intake capacity are good indicators of the general endurance capacity of a person. In 1982 Conconi (4) introduced a noninvasive field test for the determination of AT at a congress for sports medicine in Vienna. The method developed by Conconi was meant to be used for training top athletes, especially long- and middle-distance runners. The aim of our investigations was to modify this test in such a way that it could be used with untrained persons, children, and the aged in the laboratory on a treadmill or bicycle ergometer (5, 6, 7) and also in the field (8). The modified Conconi tests can now be applied to evaluate general physical fitness and also regulate training (e.g., fitness training and jogging).

Methods and Results

The Conconi test is based on the principle that heart rate curve analysis during a defined load increase (W, km/h) can be used to determine AT, according to Conconi (see Figure 1). It has been shown that the upper deflection from a linear heart rate curve (120-170 beats/min) correlates well with the invasively determined AT (3, 4, 6, 7, 9, 13, 18) and with the ventilatory threshold (1, 2, 16). In order to obtain analyzable heart rate curves, however, it is necessary to adhere to certain loading criteria.

Adjustment of the Initial Load to the Performance Level of the Test Person

The original Conconi test (3) was developed for top athletes. The initial load of the original test procedure (60 s for 200 m = 12 km/hr) is for the aged and for untrained persons already in the range above the AT. Heart rate (HR) has to be the guideline for the initial load. According to Hollmann and Hettinger (11), HR during submaximal loading is independent of the age of a test person. Therefore, the HR for the aged should also be approximately 120-130 beats/min at the end of the first load phase, which would mark the beginning of the range of linear increase of the HR curve (14, 17).

The degree of initial load for the aged and for untrained persons is approximately the following: field test—80-90 s per 200 m, laboratory—bicycle ergometer (40-80 W), and laboratory treadmill (6-10 km/hr at a 5% upgrade).

Coordination of the Rate of Increments of the Various Load Phases With the Performance Capacity of the Test Person

The rates of increment have to be coordinated with each performance level so that the testing time is not too long (exhaustion influence on HR) (2, 10). It has been shown that

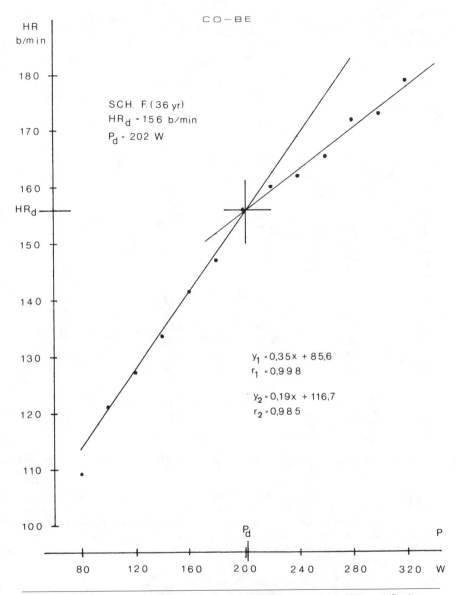

Figure 1. Heart rate curve and anaerobic threshold (bicycle ergometric): HR_d = deflection heart rate, P_d = deflection power, CO-BE = Conconi-bicycle ergometer.

12-16 load phases show the HR curve very well and thus make it easy to analyze. With 12-16 phases, a defined load increment Δ load results from the initial load and the assessable maximum performance (see Table 1):

$$\Delta \text{ load} = \frac{\text{max load} - \text{initial load}}{12 - 16}$$

Table 1   Average Maximum Performance (P_{max}, $P_{max/kg}$) Related to Age and Accompanying Calculated Values for Oxygen Intake ($\dot{V}O_2$max, $\dot{V}O_2$max/kg) for Men and Women

Age (yr)	P_{max} (W)	$P_{max/kg}$ (W/kg)	$\dot{V}O_2$max (L/min)	$\dot{V}O_2$max/kg (ml/kg/min)
M				
29	276	3.7	3.16	41.6
33	268	3.5	3.06	40.0
37	260	3.4	2.96	38.6
41	251	3.2	2.86	37.2
45	242	3.1	2.75	35.8
49	233	2.9	2.65	34.5
53	224	2.8	2.54	33.2
57	215	2.7	2.44	32.0
61	202	2.6	2.29	30.7
65	193	2.4	2.18	29.4
W				
29	181	2.9	2.12	33.5
33	176	2.8	2.08	32.2
37	172	2.7	2.03	31.0
41	168	2.5	1.98	29.7
45	165	2.4	1.93	28.4
49	160	2.3	1.88	27.1
53	156	2.2	1.83	25.9
57	152	2.1	1.78	24.6
61	148	2.1	1.73	23.3
65	144	2.0	1.68	22.0

Example: If a 45-year-old man with an average maximum performance of approximately 240 W is to be tested with an initial load of 80 W and 12 load phases, a load increment of 15 W can be calculated. Guidelines for load phases for the aged and for untrained persons are the following: field—3-5 s per 200 m, laboratory—bicycle ergometer (10-20 W), and laboratory—treadmill (0.5 km/hr at a 5% upgrade).

Proper Choice of Length of Load Phases

It has been shown that at least 60 s are necessary for the first load phase in order for the HR to reach a level adequate to the degree of loading (12). If the first phase is shorter than 1 min, test results are distorted and measured performance levels at the AT are too high (15). After the initial phase, HR adapts more quickly to the following smaller load increments (e.g., 3 s per 200 m). A time of approximately 30 s is a lower limit of load duration per phase. Therefore, we used 1 min per phase on the bicycle ergometer and also on the treadmill in the laboratory, and we reduced the running distance for children, the aged, and untrained persons to 150 or 100 m (reduction of the total testing time).

Testing Time

Considering the criteria given above, a standardized duration of testing of 12-15 min was used for test persons with different physical fitness levels (standardized number of load phases). By adhering to the loading criteria mentioned, we were able to obtain clearly analyzable HR curves in 1,263 cases. Thus, we could prove that the modified Conconi tests are applicable in both the laboratory and the field.

Conclusion

Application of the Modified Conconi Tests
for the Determination of General Physical Fitness

Maximum oxygen intake (see Table 1) and oxygen intake at AT (see Table 2) can be determined by means of the loading data from tests on the bicycle ergometer from the maximum performance (P_{max}) and performance at AT (P_{AT}). These criteria permit a good evaluation of the general physical fitness of the aged and of untrained persons.

Table 2   Average Performance Related to Age (P, P/kg) at the Anaerobic Threshold (AT) and Accompanying Calculated Values for Oxygen Intake ($\dot{V}O_2$, $\dot{V}O_{2/kg}$) for Men and Women

Age (yr)	P_{max} (W)	$P_{max/kg}$ (W/kg)	$\dot{V}O_2$max (L/min)	$\dot{V}O_2$max/kg (ml/kg/min)
M				
29	180	2.4	2.05	27.0
33	174	2.3	1.99	26.0
37	169	2.2	1.93	25.1
41	163	2.1	1.86	24.2
45	158	2.0	1.79	23.3
49	152	1.9	1.72	22.5
53	146	1.8	1.65	21.6
57	140	1.8	1.59	20.8
61	131	1.7	1.49	20.0
65	126	1.6	1.42	19.2
W				
29	118	1.9	1.38	21.8
33	115	1.8	1.36	21.0
37	112	1.8	1.32	20.2
41	109	1.6	1.29	19.3
45	107	1.6	1.26	18.5
49	104	1.5	1.23	17.6
53	102	1.4	1.19	16.9
57	99	1.4	1.16	16.0
61	96	1.3	1.13	15.2
65	94	1.3	1.09	14.3

Application in Fitness Training for the Aged

The modified Conconi tests can also be used for training regulation—for objectively documenting the influence of training—and for performance prognosis. In fitness sports of the aged, the determination of AT and thus the demarcation of an optimal training range (upper and lower limits of intensity) can be carried out with the guidelines for noninvasive Conconi tests. Being given the exact intensity of training, people will largely use aerobic energy, avoid going beyond the maximum intensity, and consequently have a reliable stimulus threshold for improving or stabilizing their endurance level.

References

1. Bunc, V., Hofmann, P., Gaisl, G. Vergleich zweier nichtinvasiven Methoden zur Bestimmung der anaeroben Schwelle. Med. u. Sport. 29:75-77, 1989.

2. Bunc, V., Sprynarova, S., Heller, J., Zdanowicz, R. Possibilities of application of anaerobic threshold in work physiology: II. Methods of determining of anaerobic threshold. Pracovni Lekarstvi 36:127-133, 1984.

3. Conconi, F., Ferrari, M., Ziglio, P.G., Droghetti, P., Codeca, L. Determination of the anaerobic threshold by a noninvasive field test in runners. J. Appl. Physiol. 52:869-873, 1982.

4. Conconi, F., Ferrari, M., Ziglio, P.G., Droghetti, P., Borsetto, C., Casoni, I., Cellini, M., Paolini, A.R. Determination of the anaerobic thereshold by a noninvasive field test in running and other activities. In: Bachl, N., ed. Current topics in sports medicine. Proceedings World Congress, 1982. Vienna. Wien: Urban und Schwarzenberg, 1984:271-281.

5. Gaisl, G., Hofmann, P. Modifications of the CONCONI-test for children and untrained persons in the laboratory and in the field. Proceedings of the International Society of Comparative Physical Education and Sports Conference, 1988, Hong Kong. (in press)

6. Gaisl, G., Wiesspeiner, G. Eine unblutige Methode zur Bestimmung der anaeroben Schwelle bei Kindern. Leistungssport 17(3):27-29, 1987.

7. Gaisl, G., Wiesspeiner, G. A noninvasive method of determining the anaerobic threshold in children. Int. J. Sports Med. 9:41-44, 1988.

8. Gaisl, G., Wiesspeiner, G., Neuhold, C., Hofmann, P. Zur praktischen Durchführung des Conconi-Tests im Feld bei Kindern. Leistungssport 17(6):47, 1987.

9. Herren, D., Charriere, I., Howald, H. Conconi-Test und anaerobe Schwelle. Schweizerische Zeitschrift für Sportmed. 35(3):107-111, 1987.

10. Hofmann, P., Gaisl, G. Der Conconi-Test und seine praktische Anwendung. Condition. 19:18-19, 1988.

11. Hollmann, W., Hettinger, T. Sportmedizin- Arbeits- und Trainingsgrundlagen. Stuttgart-New York: Schattauer, 1980.

12. Israel, S. Sport und Herzschlagfrequenz. Leipzig: J.A. Barth, 1982.

13. Jakob, E., Arratibel, J., Stockhausen, W., Huber, G., Keul, J. Die Herzfrequenz als Kenngröße der Leistungsdiagnostik und Trainingssteuerung. Leistungssport. 18(5):23-25, 1988.

14. Jakob, E., Berlis, M., Huber, G., Glittenberg, K., Keul, J. Die Bestimmung der anaeroben Schwelle mittels des Conconi-Tests in Labor- und Feldversuchen. In: Rieckert, H., ed. Sportmedizin—Kursbestimmung. Heidelberg: Springer, 1987.

15. Sprynarova, S., Bunc, V., Petrzilkova, Z. Influence of a continuously increasing work rate on maximal aerobic power. Physiologia Bohemoslovaca 34:280-281, 1985.

16. Stathus, G., Sucec, A. The reliability of the heart rate deflection point (HRDP) and running speed at the HRDP for male distance runners. Int. J. Sports Med. 8:239, 1987.

17. Tiedt, N., Wohlgemuth, B., Wohlgemuth, P. Die statische Kennlinie der Belastungsfrequenz. Medizin und Sport 13:87-94, 1973.

18. Tokmakidis, S., Leger, L. External validity of the CONCONI's heart rate anaerobic threshold as compared to the lactate threshold. In: Dotson, C.O., Humphrey, J.H., eds. Exercise physiology: current selected research. 3:43-57, 1988.

Acknowledgments

This study was supported by Grant No. 6011 from the Austrian Research Fund.

Computerized Determination Technique of Ventilatory Threshold

Y. Fukuba, S. Usui, M. Munaka, K. Iwanaga, T. Koba, and S. Koga

Research Institute for Nuclear Medicine and Biology, Hiroshima University, Minami-ku, Hiroshima; Faculty of Integrated Arts and Sciences, Hiroshima University, Naka-ku, Hiroshima; Saga Research Institute, Otsuka Pharmaceutical Co., Ltd., Kanzaki-gun, Saga; and Faculty of Education, Akita University, Tegata, Akita, Japan

$\dot{V}O_2$max has traditionally been accepted as a criterion measure of cardiovascular fitness. The direct measurement of $\dot{V}O_2$max in middle-aged and aged men, however, is difficult from a viewpoint of safety. Anaerobic threshold (AT) has also been recognized as a useful measure of submaximal aerobic working capacity. AT is detected by gas exchange parameters (ventilatory threshold; VT) or by blood lactic acid (LA) (lactate threshold; LT). VT is available for application of AT to the practical usage because it is detected by noninvasive measurement. However, the detection of VT has methodological problems: (a) compared with the LA-kinetics, the changes of gas exchange parameters at VT are not clear so that VT detected by visual criteria is less reliable, and (b) when the test is stopped before the work rate becomes the nearly maximal level for some reason, it is difficult to detect VT because the data points above VT become fewer.

In regard to the first problem, we previously examined the relation between VT determined by some objective methods and LT (3). It was found that the best method was to apply nth-order polynomial regression to the kinetics of $\dot{V}_E/\dot{V}O_2$ to $\dot{V}O_2$ and to determine VT as the $\dot{V}O_2$, which showed the minimum value of estimated $\dot{V}_E/\dot{V}O_2$-curve. However, this method was not effective in solving the second problem, because an unstable estimate of VT could be seen sometimes in cases when data points above VT became fewer. Therefore, we applied the smoothing technique to solve this problem in this paper. As a result, we developed a technique to determine VT on real time automatically during an incremental exercise test.

Method

Twenty-one young male students (age 19-27 years) performed an exercise test on a Monark cycle ergometer. Each subject was instructed to begin pedaling at 50 rpm. After a 4-min period of unloaded pedaling, the subject carried out a progressive incremental work rate exercise, in which the work rate was increased by 150 kg every 2 min up to his limit of volitional fatigue. During the exercise test, the expired gas was collected every 1 min (every 30 s at nearly maximal exercise level) by the Douglas bag method. A venous blood sample was taken from a warmed ear lobe during the last 30 s of each work rate and analyzed for LA using the enzymatic method. The Box plot (6) was used for expressing the result of univariate.

The smoothing procedure used in this paper is called Lowess, which stands for locally weighted scatter plot smoothing (2). Lowess is a kind of moving average and has robustness to the outlier. The brief procedure is given as follows.

We define the range within qth nearest neighbor as the local neighborhood at the point (x_i, y_i), with which we intend to compute the smoothed value. We next define neighborhood weight along the x axis. To compute y_i at x_i in the first stage of Lowess, we fit a line to the points within the local neighborhood using weighted least squares. We next define robustness weight along the y axis. Then, it is necessary to define the scale parameter of variation of pure error. In the original procedure of Lowess, the parameter is given by the median of the absolute values of the residuals ($r_i = y_i - \hat{y}_i$, $\hat{y}_i$; smoothed value in first stage). We use the scale parameter (Sr), which was calculated from the nonparametric estimates of residual variation by Ohtaki (4) (see Figure 1), as the alternate value. In the second stage of Lowess, we compute the smoothed value by refitting to the points within the local neighborhood using new weight (neighborhood weight × robustness weight). Here, the question arises, what number of nearest neighbors q should be chosen to use? Increasing the number of q one by one, we computed the scale parameter (Ps) of pure error using mean square error, which results from the smoothing by Lowess at each q. When Ps is smaller than Sr, the smoothing by Lowess at a given q produces overfitting, and when Ps is bigger than Sr, it produces underfitting. The number of q that shows $Sr \fallingdotseq Ps$ is determined as optional nearest neighbors q (q[opt]). Figure 2 shows a typical example of the relation of Ps and Sr to q(opt) is determined as 10. The medians of Ps and Sr to q (opt) in all 21 subjects are 2.0 and 10, respectively (see Figure 1). This modified Lowess is applied to the data set of $\dot{V}_E/\dot{V}O_2$ vs. $\dot{V}O_2$ in each subject as q(opt) = 10, and VT is determined as $\dot{V}O_2$, which shows the minimum value of the smoothed value, and is called VT(q10).

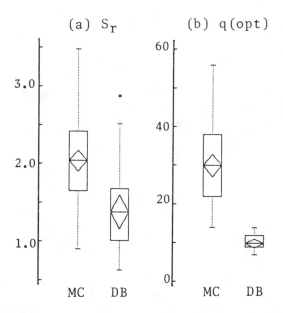

Figure 1. Sr(a) and q(opt)(b) represented by Box plot. MC—measured by mixing chamber in 66 Japanese females, DB—measured by Douglas bag in 21 Japanese young males.

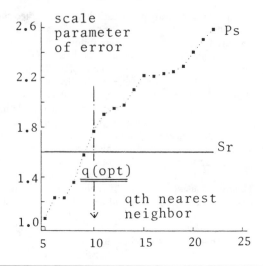

Figure 2. An example of the determination of q(opt).

Determination of VT

Next, we consider the method for solving the second problem, that is, the technique to stop the exercise test in cases when the work rate reaches the level of VT. Every time the gas exchange parameters (GEPs) are supplied to the computer, the computation and decision making based on the rules are applied as follows.

When the number of the supplied GEPs exceeds q(opt), the following procedure is executed.

1. Smoothing the data of $\dot{V}_E/\dot{V}O_2$, which is supplied to the computer up to date, using the modified Lowess: (a) The point for determining the smoothed value is set as the point which divides the range from the maximum value to the minimum value of $\dot{V}O_2$ at intervals of 0.025(L/min), and (b) search for the point that shows the minimum value $(\dot{V}_E/\dot{V}O_2(\text{min}))$ of the smoothed value is executed.

The determination of VT and the rules for stopping the exercise test: (a) The smoothed value within $\dot{V}_E/\dot{V}O_2(\text{min}) \pm Sr$ is considered to be random fluctuation of $\dot{V}_E/\dot{V}O_2(\text{min})$ (b) the smoothed value of $\dot{V}_E/\dot{V}O_2$ is compared to the value of $\dot{V}_E/\dot{V}O_2(\text{min}) + Sr$ successively, and (c) in case there is no point where the smoothed value is higher than the value of $\dot{V}_E/\dot{V}O_2(\text{min}) + Sr$ in the range of the points, which is higher than the point of $\dot{V}_E/\dot{V}O_2$ (min), we do not decide that the work rate during the exercise test has passed the level of VT. Then, the procedure returns to Step 1. On the other hand, in the case that the point that has the higher smoothed value than $\dot{V}_E/\dot{V}O_2(\text{min}) + Sr$ is found, the procedure goes on to Step 2.

2. We stop the exercise test based on the decision that the work rate has passed the level of VT. $\dot{V}_E/\dot{V}O_2(\text{min})$ here is determined as VT. The lower and upper boundaries, which show nearly equal smoothed value to $\dot{V}_E/\dot{V}O_2(\text{min}) + Sr$, are defined as VT(1b) and VT(ub), respectively.

Results

In the relation between VT(q10) and LT, inconsistency was found in some cases. One of the causes was considered to be the following. The data points measured by the Douglas bag method were somewhat few to describe the trend of $\dot{V}_E/\dot{V}O_2$ sufficiently in the location where the trend had a high curvature. One of the ways to solve this problem is to substitute the line fitting in the procedure of the modified Lowess into a quadratic fitting. The other is to increase the points of the data by a measurement system such as the breath-by-breath or mixing-chamber method. By the application of the computation and decision making based on the rules applying to the data set of each subject in the real-time mode, the determination of VT and the decision to stop the test during the exercise test was simulated. Figure 3 shows an example of the time-serial features in the simulation. Figure 4 shows VT, VT(1b), and VT(ub) determined by the simulation for all subjects. The VT had a good consistency with VT(q10). Our computerized technique was able to stop the exercise test below about 70% level of $\dot{V}O_2$max (see Figure 5).

Application

We applied our technique to GEPs measured by the mixing chamber system during the exercise test. The subjects were 66 Japanese females ages 22-57 who were instructors

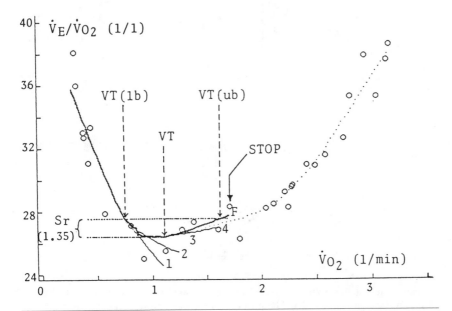

Figure 3. An example of the real-time simulation by our computerized determination technique of VT. The numbers of solid lines show the time-serial smoothing curves computed successively every time one data point is supplied. The bold solid line (F) shows the smoothing curve by final computation at the time the exercise test was stopped. VT, VT(1b), and VT(ub) can be determined from the curve F.

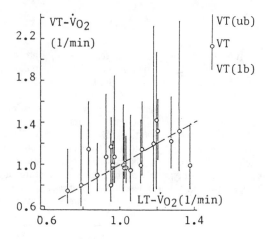

Figure 4.   VT, VT(lb), and VT(ub) computed by our technique from 21 young Japanese males, in relation to LT.

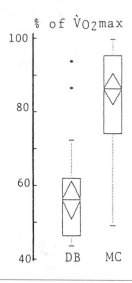

Figure 5.   Percent of $\dot{V}O_2$max at the time the exercise test was stopped.

and participants at an aerobics club. GEPs were measured at 10-s intervals by the Magna 88 system (Morgan Co., Ltd.). The protocol of the exercise test was the same one described in the Experimental Method. The exercise test was stopped by the volition or some symptom of the subject. The maximum value of $\dot{V}O_2$ during the exercise test was defined as peak $\dot{V}O_2$. The medians of Sr and $q(opt)$ in all 66 subjects were 2.0 and 30, respectively (see Figure 1). We executed the simulation by our technique, and the exercise test stopped before the determination of VT was made by the rules for 7 cases out of 66. All peak $\dot{V}O_2$ were below 1.2 (L/min) for these 7 subjects. Figure 6 shows VT, VT(lb), and VT(ub) determined for 59 subjects. The exercise test could be stopped below the level of 90%

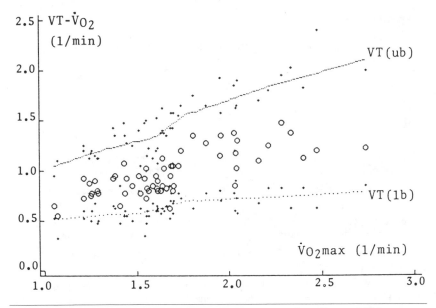

Figure 6. VT, VT(lb), and VT(ub) computed by our technique from 59 out of 66 Japanese females, in relation to $\dot{V}O_2$max.

of peak $\dot{V}O_2$ (Figure 5). Compared with the level of young males, the level when the exercise test halted was relatively higher for females. One cause of this was thought to be the lower peak $\dot{V}O_2$.

Comments

To clear up the subjective uncertainty on VT detection, some objective methods are suggested (1, 3, 5, 7). However, in any case, it is very difficult to estimate VT when the data above VT become less (this occurs often in middle-aged and aged patients). Almost all methods are based on the computerized technique and determine VT by fitting particular parametric models to the data. We developed the computerized technique to describe the trend of $\dot{V}_E/\dot{V}O_2$ during the exercise test by the nonparametric smoothing procedure and to stop the exercise test as soon as VT is determined according to the specific rules. The similar procedure using a spline smoothing was reported by Wade et al. (7). We used the modified Lowess, as its procedure of computation is quite easier than that of the spline smoothing. The defect of the current version is that computing takes a long time. Especially when the data is measured by a system such as breath-by-breath or the mixing-chamber method, q(opt) becomes a large value, and the interval from current data to the next data (= computing time) becomes short. It will be necessary to reexamine the technique and check the algorithm for shortening of the computing time. In conclusion, by the use of our technique, VT could be determined on real time automatically during the exercise test. This technique has two main advantages: (a) avoiding the subjective variation of VT due to visual inspection and (b) making it possible to stop the exercise test at the time of VT determination during the test. The latter advantage makes the exercise test safer and is valuable especially for the purposes of the prediction of aerobic working capacity in middle-aged and aged men and the evaluation of exercise tolerance capacity in patients during cardiac rehabilitation.

Acknowledgments

A part of this study was supported by Grant for Life Science Research from Uehara Memorial Foundation in 1985. The authors greatly acknowledge the assistance of Dr. M. Ohtaki and Ms. K. Komori, Dept. Biometrics, Res. Inst. Nuclear Med. Biol., Hiroshima University.

References

1. Beaver, W.L., Wasserman, K., Whipp, B.J. A new method for detecting anaerobic threshold by gas exchange. J. Appl. Physiol. 60:2020-2027, 1986.
2. Cleaveland, W.S. Robust locally weighted regression and smoothing scatterplots. JASA 74:829-836, 1979.
3. Fukuba, Y., Munaka, M., Usui, S., Sasahara, H. Comparison of objective methods for determining ventilatory threshold. Jpn. J. Physiol. 38:133-144, 1988.
4. Ohtaki, M. A nonparametric estimate of residual variance in one-dimensional regression. Bull. Biometric Soc. Jpn. 8:39-51, 1987.
5. Orr, G.W., Green, H.J., Hughson, R.L., Bennett, G.W. A computer linear regression model to determine ventilatory anaerobic threshold. J. Appl. Physiol. 52:1349-1352, 1982.
6. Tukey, J.W. Exploratory data analysis. London: Addison-Wesley, 1977.
7. Wade, T.D., Anderson, S.J., Bondy, J., Ramadevi, V.A., Jones, R.H., Swanson, G.D. Using smoothing splines to make inferences about the shape of gas-exchange curves. Comp. Biomed. Res. 21:16-26, 1988.

Study on Whole-Body Endurance Test Using Submaximum Exercise Loading

M. Nakanishi, M. Kuwamori, Y. Iwasaki, M. Isokawa, and I. Kita

Tokyo Metropolitan University, Yakumo, Meguro-ku, Tokyo, and Meiji University, Sugirami-ku, Tokyo, Japan

The adequate whole-body endurance test using submaximum exercise loading is indispensable especially for middle-aged and aged persons to measure their endurance safely. Varied step tests have been made and applied for this purpose in the field of physical fitness measurements. However, most of these step tests use the responses of pulse rate as the index to evaluate the level of whole-body endurance, and many researchers have come to realize that these step tests show inferior validity in testing children and aged persons (1, 3, 4).

The test of PWC_{170}, which is well known as a submaximum test using a bicycle ergometer, has also been believed to have problems in validity in the case of testing children and aged persons (5, 7). Generally, these tests are made on the assumption that well-trained subjects show smaller acceleration of heart rate (HR) during a certain intensity of submaximum exercise and their HR decreases more quickly after the exercise. However, this assumption seems inadequate for the middle-aged and aged persons, because among aged groups, there are some subjects who show high acceleration of HR during the exercise though the level of their whole-body endurance is superior (2, 6). Taking these facts into consideration, this study was designed to examine the possibility of assessing the whole-body endurance of middle-aged and aged persons by observing the responses of ventilatory volume ($\dot{V}_E$) during exercise, rather than observing HR.

Methods

Experiments were made in the physical fitness laboratory at Tokyo Metropolitan University in 1987 and 1988, employing 30 healthy male adults (22 subjects submitted to the first experiment) age 19-57 years. The age and physical characteristics of each subject are shown in Table 1. For the loading exercise, a Monark-type bicycle ergometer was used. After the measurements of resting state, exercise for warming up was performed for 2 min at load lkp and pedaling speed 60 rpm. Then, after 2 min rest the exercise test was started, beginning at 0 kp, increasing 0.5 kp every minute, and continuing until exhaustion (see Figure 1). In the meantime, gas metabolism was measured continuously with the Respiro-monitor RM-300 system made by Minato Medical Science Co. Also, a chest lead ECG telemeter system (made by NEC • SANEI Co.) and a blood pressure monitoring system (made by Colin Co.) were used to avoid unexpected accidents during the exercise test.

As shown in Figure 2, in this exercise test $\dot{V}_E$ increases exponentially along with the time axis and finally reaches the maximum point ($\dot{V}_E$max) at the time of exhaustion. If

Table 1   Age and Physical Characteristics of Each Subject

Subject No.	Age (years)	Height (cm)	Weight (kg)	VC (L)	MVV (L/min)	$\dot{V}_E$max (L/min)	$\dot{V}O_2$ (ml/min)
1	32	173	105	4.10	245.0	117.0	3937
2	55	161	61	3.50	176.5	106.7	2172
3	57	167	59	4.55	180.0	100.3	2208
4	42	165	52	4.60	219.5	101.5	2389
5	26	174	66	5.85	214.0	116.6	3129
6	44	165	70	3.30	130.0	97.9	2680
7	19	178	60	4.00	215.0	94.2	2718
8	49	164	62	4.45	192.5	114.0	2409
9	37	168	52	4.00	200.0	113.8	2313
10	49	156	60	2.65	107.5	83.8	2197
11	33	172	68	5.10	240.0	156.8	3879
12	39	163	68	3.90	145.0	91.2	2475
13	38	177	71	4.70	205.0	91.4	2595
14	22	167	75	5.40	185.0	150.2	3567

15	20	168	56	5.00	170.0	99.3	3221
16	21	178	70	5.30	190.0	97.9	2806
17	19	172	55	4.60	205.0	99.4	2520
18	29	165	58	4.40	130.0	93.9	2342
19	24	173	60	4.65	185.0	101.6	2802
20	45	163	60	4.15	191.0	93.2	2162
21	41	167	80	4.20	185.0	128.7	2786
22	40	163	72	3.40	185.0	107.8	2278
23	34	170	66	4.25	160.0	101.8	2271
24	22	178	73	5.35	210.0	131.9	3137
25	25	171	58	4.15	200.0	112.0	2323
26	46	172	72	3.90	187.5	108.1	2306
27	39	167	59	4.05	180.0	98.3	2345
28	49	161	61	4.20	185.0	97.9	2172
29	20	178	74	4.60	175.0	136.1	3508
30	23	167	62	4.65	160.0	101.7	2840
N	30	30	30	30	30	30	30
Mean	34.6	168.8	65.5	4.365	185.12	108.17	2682.9
SD	11.4	5.7	10.2	0.667	29.95	17.04	506.4

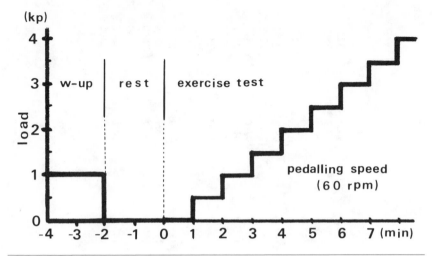

Figure 1. Protocol of bicycle ergometer loading test.

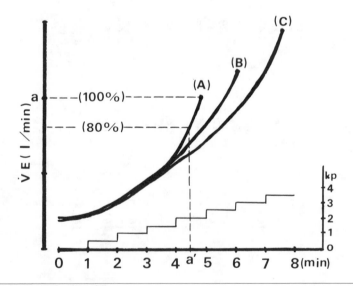

Figure 2. Changes of ventilation volume ($\dot{V}_E$): When $\dot{V}_E$maxpred. of subject (A) is a, a' is obtained as the subject's 80% value.

the $\dot{V}_E$ reaches the maximum point while testing, the test cannot be submaximum. Therefore, the $\dot{V}_E$max is predicted in advance, then the time $\dot{V}_E$ requires to reach $X\%$ of the predicted $\dot{V}_E$max is measured. For example, when the predicted $\dot{V}_E$max ($\dot{V}_E$maxpred.) of subject (A) is a, the time required to reach 80% of the prediction becomes a', which is used as an index (called 80% value) in this test.

Results

At first, in order to predict the $\dot{V}_E$max of each subject, correlations between measured $\dot{V}_E$max and many items were examined. As the body weight and the age were considered to show comparatively high correlations with $\dot{V}_E$max, the multiple regression equation between measured $\dot{V}_E$max and these two items was induced.

$$\dot{V}_E\text{max} = 0.50427 \times \text{Wt.} - 0.39879 \times \text{Age} + 86.986$$

Using the above equation, $\dot{V}_E$max of each subject was predicted. And significantly high correlation between $\dot{V}_E$maxpred. and measured $\dot{V}_E$max was recognized ($r=0.45$). Then, the time $\dot{V}_E$ of each subject required to reach 60, 70, 80, and 90% of $\dot{V}_E$maxpred. was measured, and the correlations between each value (required time) and measured $\dot{V}O_2$max were investigated. Table 2 is the list of correlation coefficients obtained.

Table 2   Correlation Coefficients Between Each Value and Maximum Oxygen Intake ($\dot{V}O_2$max)

	60%	70%	80%	90%
r	0.453*	0.661**	0.728**	0.809**
n	(22)	(21)	(20)	(16)

$*p < .05$, $**p < .001$.

As in the table, the lowest correlation was shown at 60% value and the highest at 90% value. That is, if the submaximum test is developed using the 90% value the test will be able to predict the $\dot{V}O_2$max most accurately. However, in practice, it was also found that 6 out of 22 subjects would reach exhaustion during the test for 90% value, 2 out of 22 subjects would reach exhaustion during the test for 80% value, and 1 out of 22 subjects would reach exhaustion in the test for 70% value. Therefore, it was concluded that 60% value must be used for a complete submaximum exercise test, although the accuracy of the $\dot{V}O_2$max prediction would be inferior.

As a result of the first experiment, it was thought that increasing the accuracy of the $\dot{V}_E$maxpred. is necessary in order to obtain an index that closely correlates with $\dot{V}O_2$max. So, the second experiment was designed to find out another equation for a more accurate $\dot{V}_E$max prediction.

At first, varied items that might correlate with the measured $\dot{V}_E$max were examined, and a correlation matrix was made. As shown in Table 3, it was clear that (a) $\dot{V}_E$max does not closely correlate with the age but with the body weight, (b) the correlation coefficient to the vital capacity is almost as high as the coefficient to the MVV, and (c) the correlation coeffiecients between body weight and ventilatory items are not so high. Finally, it was concluded that predicting $\dot{V}_E$max from body weight and vital capacity is the most reasonable, and the following equation was induced.

$$\dot{V}_E\text{max} = 0.64810 \times \text{Wt} + 11.51084 \times \text{VC} + 15.47318$$

Using the above equation, it was confirmed that to increase the accuracy of predicting $\dot{V}_E$max the correlation coefficient (r) between $\dot{V}_E$max pred. and measured $V_E$max was increased ($r=0.450$ to 0.607). As in the first experiment, 60, 70, 80, and 90% values were obtained for each subject, and the correlations between each value and the measured $\dot{V}O_2$max were investigated. Table 4 shows the result of the investigation.

Table 3 Correlation Matrix Among Six Items

	$\dot{V}_E$max	Age	Height	Weight	VC	MVV
$\dot{V}_E$max	—	−0.265	0.313	0.408*	0.468**	0.465**
Age	—	—	−0.677***	−0.082	−0.574***	−0.232
Height	—	—	—	0.294	0.597***	0.556**
Weight	—	—	—	—	0.047	0.259
VC	—	—	—	—	—	0.493**
MVV	—	—	—	—	—	—

$*p < .05$, $**p < .01$, $***p < .001$.

Table 4 Correlation Coefficients Between Each Value and Maximum Oxygen Intake ($\dot{V}O_2$max)

	60%	70%	80%	90%
r	0.656*	0.703*	0.752*	0.755*
n	(30)	(30)	(29)	(26)

$*p < .001$.

After all, the correlation coefficients between the indexes and the $\dot{V}O_2$max did not increase so much beyond expectation. However, the numbers of subjects who reached exhaustion during the test decreased: 4 out of 30 subjects would exhaust to obtain 90% value, and 1 out of 30 would exhaust to obtain 80% value, but none would exhaust to obtain 70 and 60% values. So, we came to the conclusion that the 70% value would be the most appropriate to use as an index to make the submaximum test. Figure 3 shows the result of the correlation analysis between the 70% value and the $\dot{V}O_2$max.

Conclusion

In order to develop a whole-body endurance test using submaximum exercise that can be applied to middle-aged and old aged persons, responses of ventilatory volume ($\dot{V}_E$) during stepwise exercise loading with bicycle ergometer were investigated. A tentative test using the response of $\dot{V}_E$ was designed, and its validity was examined. As a result,

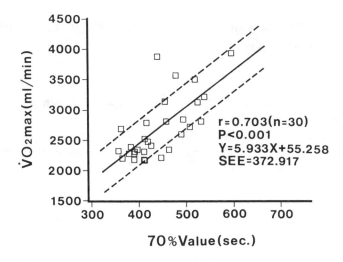

Figure 3. Correlation between the index (70% value) and the maximum oxygen intake ($\dot{V}O_2$max).

the possibility of developing such a test with which the level of $\dot{V}O_2$max can be estimated to some extent, was confirmed, although much testing and modification seem to be needed for the improvement of the test.

References

1. Ishiko, T., Katamoto, S., Yoshida, T. Validity of evaluating endurance capacity in young boys and girls from cardiac response to the step test. Report of the Research Center in Physical Education (Japan) 2:42-51, 1974.

2. Katsuki, S. A review of studies on the step tests for evaluating respiro-circulatory endurance. Bulletin of the Physical Fitness Research Institute (Meiji Life Foundation) 29:23-57, 1974.

3. Matsui, H., Miura, M., Kobayashi, K. The relation between maximum oxygen intake and modified Harvard Step Test index for elementary school boys and girls. Report of Research Center of Physical Education (Japan) 2:33-41, 1974.

4. Meshizuka, T., Nakanishi, M., Iwasaki, Y. Study on the general endurance test for the middle aged. Re-examination of the step test. Research Bulletin of Physical Education (at TMU) 2:43-58, 1968.

5. Nakagawa, A., Ishiko, T. Assessment of aerobic capacity with special reference to sex and age of junior and senior high school students in Japan. Jpn. J. Physiol. 20:118-129, 1970.

6. Nakanishi, M., Iwasaki, Y., Nagata, A., Isokawa, M., Sakai, N. Heart rate responses of middle aged persons during the submaximum and maximum exercise. Research Bulletin of Physical Education (at TMU) 9:7-14, 1983.

7. Nakanishi, M., Meshizuka, T., Iwasaki, Y., Isokawa, M. Study on the general endurance test for the middle aged (3). Research Bulletin of Physical Education (at TMU) 5:21-28, 1974.

Plasma Lipoprotein and Apolipoprotein Metabolism in Elderly Runners

T. Tamai, H. Takai, T. Nakai, S. Miyabo, M. Higuchi,
K. Iwaoka, and S. Kobayashi

The Third Department of Internal Medicine, Fukui Medical School,
Matsuoka-Cho, Fukui and The Division of Health Promotion, National
Institute of Nutrition, Tokyo, Japan

It has been reported that physical exercise decreases plasma cholesterol (Ch), plasma triglyceride (TG), very low density lipoprotein (VLDL)-TG, and low density lipoprotein (LDL)-Ch, and increases high density lipoprotein (HDL)-Ch in young and middle-aged men (1, 2). Although there are several reports about the effects of exercise on plasma lipoprotein concentrations in older athletes (5), the metabolism of plasma apolipoprotein (apo) has not been extensively investigated in elderly subjects. In the present study, we examined plasma apolipoprotein and lipoprotein metabolism in not only well-trained elderly male runners but also in female runners.

Subjects and Methods

Runners and sedentary controls of both sexes from 30 to 70 years old volunteered for this study. Each person was informed of the design and risks of this project prior to obtaining a written consent. No subject had suffered any disorders that would influence the lipoprotein metabolism. No subject took a specific diet or drug.

Blood was obtained from the subjects, who had fasted for more than 14 hr. Plasma lipoproteins were fractionated by ultracentrifugation at a density of 1.006 g/ml for 22 hr at $105,000 \times g$. The infranatant solution was applied to heparin-Mn^{++} precipitation method according to Lipid Research Clinics Program (3) for separation of HDL (Result 1). In Result 2, plasma lipoproteins were fractionated by ultracentrifugation at densities of 1.006, 1.019, 1.063, and 1.125 g/ml. The 1.006 g/ml top fraction, the 1.125 g/ml bottom fraction, and the fractions of 1.006-1.019 g/ml, 1.019-1.063 g/ml, and 1.063-1.125 g/ml were designated VLDL, HDL$_3$, intermediate density lipoprotein (IDL), LDL, and HDL$_2$, respectively. Ch and TG were meadured by enzymatic methods. Plasma concentrations of apo A-I, A-II, B, C-II, C-III, and E were measured by a single-radial immunodiffusion method using 1% agarose plate that contained specific goat antisera. Apo B subspecies in VLDL (d < 1.006 g/ml) were analyzed by SDS-3.5% or 3-15% gradient polyacrylamide gel electrophoresis. After staining, the protein bands were evaluated by densitometer and the peak area was measured. Apo B-48 ratio (percent of apo B-48 in total apo B) was calculated.

All subjects completed a progressive test on a motor-driven treadmill to determine their $\dot{V}O_2$max. Total body fat composition was estimated by the method using skinfold thickness according to Nagamine and Suzuki (4).

Results and Discussion

Effects of physical exercise on plasma lipoprotein and apolipoprotein metabolism in male subjects: Table 1 represents profiles of the subjects studied and concentrations of lipoproteins and apolipoproteins. Although there were no significant differences in plasma concentrations of Ch and TG between two old groups and between two young groups, old runners (OR) and young runners (YR) had decreased levels of VLDL-Ch and LDL-Ch and increased levels of HDL-Ch, apo A-I, and apo A-II.

In old runners, both HDL-Ch as a part of HDL-lipids and apo A-I and apo A-II as HDL-proteins were higher than in the old controls (OC). But the relative increment of lipid and protein in HDL was greater than that of protein, as estimated from the ratio of apo A-I/HDL-Ch and/or apo A-I +apo A-II/HDL-Ch. On the other hand, the composition of LDL was not different between OR and OC. Similar results were obtained between YR and the young controls (YC). Therefore, physical activity appears to affect both HDL-lipids and proteins.

Effects of physical exercise on metabolism of apo B subspecies in female subjects: Plasma lipids, lipoproteins, apolipoproteins, and VLDL-apo B subspecies were studied in 19 fasted female runners (R) and 23 age-matched sedentary control women (S). Plasma concentrations of Ch, apo A-I, and apo E were significantly higher in runners than controls (see Table 2). In lipoprotein fractions, runners had lower VLDL concentrations and higher HDL concentrations mainly due to higher levels of HDL_2 than controls. Apo B-48 ratios in VLDL were significantly ($p < 0.05$) lower in runners ($2.86 \pm 0.39\%$) as compared to controls ($4.6 \pm 0.54\%$) (see Figure 1).

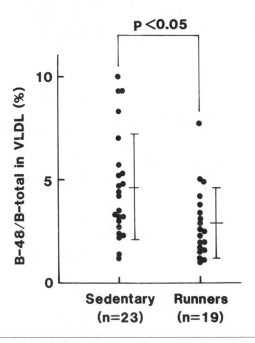

Figure 1. Apolipoprotein B-48 ratio (percentage of apo B in total apo B) in VLDL prepared from sedentary women and female runners.

Table 1 Profile of Male Volunteers

	Old runners (n = 12)	Old controls (n = 12)	Young runners (n = 16)	Young controls (n = 15)
Age	62.5 ± 0.7	64.0 ± 0.9	34.7 ± 0.7	34.0 ± 0.7
Body mass index (kg/m²)	21.1 ± 0.4	22.6 ± 0.7	21.1 ± 0.4	22.1 ± 0.6
$\dot{V}O_2$max (ml/min)	2.71 ± 0.08*	1.78 ± 0.10	3.86 ± 0.09*	3.08 ± 0.13
Plasma-Ch (mg/dl)	207.7 ± 8.3	211.2 ± 9.4	191.3 ± 6.2	194.1 ± 7.2
Plasma-TG (mg/dl)	76.2 ± 6.5	106.2 ± 14.6	61.3 ± 3.1	88.0 ± 8.0
VLDL-Ch (mg/dl)	4.6 ± 1.1*	10.9 ± 2.7	4.1 ± 0.6	6.9 ± 1.2
VLDL-TG (mg/dl)	23.0 ± 4.8	47.8 ± 13.1	16.8 ± 2.0*	33.0 ± 6.0
LDL-Ch (mg/dl)	134.7 ± 8.1	149.0 ± 8.8	122.4 ± 5.3	130.2 ± 6.4
HDL-Ch (mg/dl)	68.4 ± 4.7**	51.3 ± 3.1	61.4 ± 2.2	54.8 ± 2.4
apo A-I (mg/dl)	156.1 ± 4.7*	143.7 ± 3.6	148.5 ± 4.1	146.5 ± 4.1
apo A-II (mg/dl)	34.8 ± 1.2*	31.8 ± 0.7	36.3 ± 0.9	34.7 ± 1.0
apo B (mg/dl)	77.2 ± 4.2	79.6 ± 5.0	73.8 ± 1.8	79.1 ± 2.5
apo C-II (mg/dl)	3.8 ± 0.2	4.4 ± 0.4	4.2 ± 0.2	4.2 ± 0.3
apo C-III (mg/dl)	10.0 ± 0.5	9.5 ± 0.8	9.8 ± 0.5	9.1 ± 0.5
apo E (mg/dl)	3.6 ± 0.2	4.2 ± 0.2	4.3 ± 0.2*	3.8 ± 0.2

Each value represents mean ± SEM. *$p < .05$ vs control, **$p < .01$ vs control.

Table 2   Concentrations of Triglyceride, Cholesterol, and Apolipoprotein in Sedentary Women and Female Runners

	Sedentary women (n = 23)	Runners (n = 19)
Ch: Plasma	164.4 ± 5.9	189.4 ± 5.6**
VLDL	7.7 ± 1.0	4.8 ± 0.9*
IDL	1.4 ± 0.4	0.9 ± 0.1
LDL	86.3 ± 4.6	99.9 ± 4.4*
HDL$_2$	36.6 ± 2.8	46.9 ± 3.0*
HDL$_3$	32.4 ± 1.3	36.9 ± 1.8*
TG: Plasma	78.5 ± 7.1	66.7 ± 4.4
VLDL	29.6 ± 4.2	17.3 ± 3.3*
IDL	2.7 ± 0.6	1.8 ± 0.2
LDL	26.4 ± 3.1	25.1 ± 1.2
HDL$_2$	10.3 ± 0.7	12.7 ± 0.8*
HDL$_3$	9.0 ± 0.6	9.8 ± 0.5
Apolipoproteins		
A-I	160.9 ± 5.0	183.3 ± 5.2**
A-II	35.2 ± 0.9	36.9 ± 0.9
B	94.6 ± 3.2	101.5 ± 2.7
C-II	3.2 ± 0.2	3.3 ± 0.2
C-III	7.8 ± 0.4	8.6 ± 0.4
E	3.5 ± 0.1	4.6 ± 0.3**

Note. (mg/dl, mean ± SEM). *$p < .01$, **$p < .005$, Sedentary women vs. Runners.

In sedentary controls, an age-related rise in apo B-48 ratio was observed. However, such an increment was not found in runners. Runners showed a tendency for a positive correlation between apo B-48 ratios and concentrations of VLDL-TG. These data indicated that endurance-type exercise decreased exogenous lipoprotein especially in older runners, which is most likely mediated by the increase of lipoprotein-lipase activities.

Conclusion

In this cross-sectional study, physical exercise decreased triglyceride-rich lipoprotein and LDL and apo B-48 ratios, increased HDL, and changed HDL composition. Physical exercise may have more favorable effects on plasma concentrations and compositions of lipoproteins and apolipoproteins in older runners than in younger runners.

References

1. Kiens, B., Lithell, H., Vessby, B. Further increases in high density lipoproteins in trained males after enhanced training. Europ. J. Appl. Physiol. 52:426-430, 1984.

2. Leclerc, S., Allard, C., Talbot, J., Gauvin, R., Bouchard, C. High density lipoprotein cholesterol, habitual physical activity and physical fitness. Atherosclerosis 57:43-51, 1985.

3. Lipid Research Clinics Program. Manual of laboratory operations. Lipid and lipo-protein analysis. U.S. Dept. of Health, Education and Welfare, publication No. (NIH) 75-628, 1974.

4. Nagamine, S., Suzuki, S. Anthropometry and body composition of young Japanese men and women. Human Biol. 36:8-15, 1964.

5. Seals, D.R., Allen, W.K., Hurley, B.F., Dalsky, G.P., Ehsani, A.A., Hagberg, J.M. Elevated high density lipoprotein cholesterol levels in older endurance athletes. Am. J. Cardiol. 54:390-393, 1984.

Physical Performance Survey in 900 Aged Individuals

M. Kimura, K. Hirakawa, and T. Morimoto

Osaka College of Physical Education Ibarakishi, Osaka and Kyoto Prefectural University of Medicine, Kyoto, Japan

Appropriate exercise is necessary for aged individuals to maintain health and mobility. We have attempted to assess components of physical fitness in individuals above 60 years of age for the purpose of exploring a method for quantitation of the fitness level of the elderly, thus facilitating prescription of exercise programs and evaluation of training effects for them (2, 5). In this study, the fitness level of the elderly was evaluated by an exercise battery test.

Methods

The subjects of this study consisted of 368 males and 527 females aged 60-89 years, living in or around the cities of Kyoto and Osaka, who voluntarily applied for enrollment in our battery exercise test through senior citizen's clubs and schooling clubs for the elderly. Some subjects had not participated in any sports for 40-50 years or were apparently at a low fitness level.

The fitness tests for adults (60 years old or below) formulated by the Ministry of Education (6) were modified into the present battery test, which consisted of six tests with relatively mild physical exertion: one-leg balancing with the eyes closed, stepping in the sitting position, sit-and-reach trunk flexion, vertical jump, hand grip strength (mean of the bilateral measurements), and breath holding.

Among these items, vertical jump and hand grip strength were evaluated similarly to the tests for middle-aged subjects. Anterior trunk flexion was performed in the sitting position instead of in the standing position and was evaluated, as was one-leg balancing, with the eyes closed, by the method commonly employed in Japan. The number of steps in the sitting position was counted over a 20-s period, and breath-holding time was measured after about 20% exhalation from full inhalation (2). The battery test was performed after confirmation of the health of the subjects by a medical check.

Results

Table 1 shows the mean and standard deviation of the age, body build parameters, and blood pressures in each age group at 5-year intervals together with the results of the analysis of variance for the significance of intergroup differences. No difference was observed in systolic or diastolic blood pressure among the age groups, but both the height and weight decreased with age. Significant intergroup differences were observed in the weight of both sexes and in the height of only females.

Table 2 summarizes the results of the tests. The performance tended to deteriorate with age in both sexes, with the differences in the mean values among age groups being significant except for breath holding of both sexes and one-leg balancing of females.

Table 1   Physical Characteristics of Subjects in 5-Year Age Groups

Age group	60-64	65-69	70-74	75-79	80-84	85-89	Total
Male							
No. of subjects	20	113	130	66	32	7	368
Age (years)	62.4(1.5)	67.1(1.4)	72.1(1.5)	76.5(1.3)	81.5(1.2)	87.1(1.2)	71.9(5.5)***
Height (cm)	161(5)	161(6)	160(5)	160(5)	159(4)	154(4)	160(5)
Weight (kg)	56.3(6.1)	57.4(8.5)	56.0(8.0)	57.4(9.2)	53.2(7.6)	49.1(8.0)	56.3(8.4)*
Systolic blood pressure (mmHg)	131(24)	137(19)	140(21)	140(20)	145(24)	137(30)	139(21)
Diastolic blood pressure (mmHg)	77(11)	79(11)	79(12)	77(12)	78(13)	71(6)	78(12)
Female							
No. of subjects	55	232	172	59	9		527
Age (years)	62.7(1.3)	67.0(1.3)	71.6(1.3)	76.6(1.2)	81.0(1.2)		69.4(4.3)***
Height (cm)	150(4)	149(4)	149(5)	147(6)	147(6)		149(5)**
Weight (kg)	53.0(7.0)	49.1(6.9)	49.0(7.2)	47.7(7.8)	44.7(7.2)		49.3(7.3)***
Systolic blood pressure (mmHg)	138(23)	137(19)	139(19)	146(20)	141(26)		139(20)
Diastolic blood pressure (mmHg)	82(16)	78(11)	78(11)	80(11)	80(9)		79(11)

Note. Mean $\pm$ *SD*. *$p < .05$, **$p < .01$, ***$p < .001$.

Table 2 Results of Fitness Tests

Age group	60-64	65-69	70-74	75-79	80-84	85-89	Total
Male							
One-leg balancing (s)	9.4(6.3)	7.4(7.5)	6.1(4.8)	4.0(2.7)	3.2(2.3)	2.7(1.4)	6.0(5.6)***
Stepping (times/20 s)	32.0(4.8)	29.5(6.5)	28.4(5.4)	27.1(5.9)	23.8(6.3)	26.3(9.3)	28.2(6.2)***
Flexibility (cm)	3.2(7.9)	1.6(8.0)	1.2(8.3)	-1.0(9.5)	-3.7(8.8)	0.6(7.1)	0.6(8.6)*
Vertical jump (cm)	32.9(7.6)	27.3(6.4)	25.4(6.7)	22.2(7.6)	18.3(6.2)	13.4(6.0)	25.0(7.6)***
Grip strength (kg)	34.5(7.8)	32.3(7.0)	31.5(5.8)	29.4(6.7)	24.8(5.2)	22.1(9.6)	30.8(6.9)***
Breath holding (s)	34.6(14.3)	33.3(11.5)	32.6(13.4)	33.7(18.3)	30.3(9.0)	30.1(9.6)	32.9(13.5)
Total score	20.9(3.8)	18.5(4.6)	17.5(3.8)	15.7(4.0)	12.8(2.7)	12.6(3.4)	17.2(4.4)
Female							
One-leg balancing (s)	7.2(5.0)	6.5(6.1)	5.6(7.6)	5.2(8.8)	3.5(2.5)		6.1(6.8)
Stepping (times/20 s)	29.3(5.1)	29.5(4.1)	27.7(4.0)	26.8(5.2)	21.1(5.9)		28.4(4.5)***
Flexibility (cm)	9.5(7.4)	8.1(7.3)	6.8(7.1)	7.9(7.5)	3.5(8.8)		7.7(7.4)*
Vertical jump (cm)	21.2(4.5)	18.7(4.8)	16.5(5.1)	14.6(4.6)	11.5(4.5)		17.7(5.2)***
Grip strength (kg)	21.9(4.1)	19.9(4.1)	19.0(4.5)	18.3(3.6)	15.5(4.2)		19.6(4.3)***
Breath holding (s)	27.7(8.9)	28.2(8.7)	27.4(10.2)	21.2(10.0)	21.4(5.6)		27.6(9.4)
Total score	20.5(3.1)	18.7(3.9)	17.0(3.8)	16.4(3.7)	12.6(3.9)		18.0(4.0)***

Note. Mean ± *SD*. *$p < .05$, **$p < .01$, ***$p < .001$.

Table 3 shows correlation coefficients between the age and the score of each test. The results of all tests showed negative correlations with age. The correlation coefficients were significant in all items except for breath holding of both sexes, and the values were particularly high in the vertical jump and the total score.

Table 4 shows the percentage of the performance level of our subjects compared with the level of the young Japanese in their peak of fitness. The levels of grip strength and stepping of our subjects remained at 50-70% of the respective peak values, but that of vertical jump was reduced to 20-50% and that of one-leg balancing to 5-20%.

Table 3   Pearson's Correlations Between Age and Components of Fitness

	One-leg balancing	Stepping	Flexibility	Vertical jump	Grip strength	Breath holding	Total score
Male	−0.28**	−0.29**	−0.16**	−0.47**	−0.35**	−0.07	−0.435**
Female	−0.13**	−0.29**	−0.10*	−0.41**	−0.27**	−0.06	−0.375**

$*p < .01$, $**p < .001$.

Discussion

The level of physical fitness is known to change with age. The report of Fitness and Exercise Ability Survey by the Ministry of Education (1) and the *Physical Fitness Standards of Japanese People* (6), in which the results of a number of fitness tests are recorded, illustrate age-related changes in fitness from adolescence to about 60 years of age. Among the components of physical fitness evaluated in our study, muscular strength (grip strength) reaches a peak at around 20 years of age, and agility (repetitive side steps) and trunk flexibility (forward bending in the standing position) peak at 18 years. All these abilities decrease thereafter with age, but the pattern of the decrease differs among the items. Some items (e.g., vertical jump) show nearly linear decreases at constant rates, while others (grip strength and repetitive side steps) exhibit steep declines after certain ages. The results of the present study appear to overlap with the extrapolation of the changes observed in those less than 60 years of age.

Kobayashi (4) noted that the performances in grip strength and repetitive side steps of individuals in their 60s were 70-80% of the peak levels, but those in muscular strength of the back, vertical jump, and chin-lifting from the prone position were reduced to less than 50% of the peak levels. He speculated that these differences were due to the relatively early onset of weakening of the muscle strength in the dorsal regions. Our study indicated that the deterioration in the performance of the elderly is more remarkable in the items requiring complex neural control or support or shift of the body weight. The mean performance levels of our subjects in their early 60s were low, particularly in males, as compared with those in other reports, and these differences appeared to persist in higher age groups.

Breath holding was adopted as a test of endurance, but it has been shown to actually reflect the degree of perseverance (6). While the performance of other tests decreased with age in our study, this item alone showed no correlation with age, with the values being very high even in some subjects above 80 years old. However, the results of breath holding show significant negative correlations with resting and exercising blood pressures

Table 4   Performance of Our Subjects as Compared With the Peak of the Japanese

	Male (%)							Female (%)					
	Peak values of Japanese	Age group						Peak values of Japanese	Age group				
		60-64	65-69	70-74	75-79	80-84	85-89		60-64	65-69	70-74	75-79	80+
One-leg balancing	45.6 s (18 years)	20.6	16.2	13.4	8.8	7.0	5.9	37.4 s (18 years)	19.3	17.4	15.0	13.9	9.4
Stepping	41.5 times/20 s (18 years)	77.1	71.1	68.4	65.3	57.3	63.4	39.3 times/20 s (18 years)	74.6	75.1	70.5	68.2	53.7
Vertical jump*	61.5 cm (18 years)	53.5	44.4	41.3	36.1	29.8	21.8	43.5 cm (18 years)	48.7	43.0	37.9	33.6	26.4
Grip strength*	48.6 kg (22 years)	71.0	66.5	64.8	60.5	51.0	45.5	30.3 kg (22 years)	72.3	65.7	62.7	60.4	51.2
Breath holding	70.0 s (18 years)	49.4	46.6	48.1	43.8	43.3	42.9	38.7 s (18 years)	71.6	72.9	70.8	54.8	55.3

*Standard values of the Japanese. Other values are the mean of high school third graders (65 males and 63 females) determined by the same method as in this study.

and heart rate, suggesting that this parameter may be of value as an index of the risk in exercise loading (3).

Long-term retention of the abilities to sufficiently carry out activities of daily life and to enjoy life is an important factor related to the fitness of the elderly. Which aspects of physical fitness are most important for the elderly has yet to be clarified. However, considering that retention of an adequate cardiopulmonary reserve and exercise ability is particularly vital, we have attempted to quantitatively assess these abilities in individuals aged above 60 years by a method that is safe and appropriately reflects the life of the elderly. The present study performed on about 900 aged individuals allowed evaluation of the fitness level of the elderly with relatively mild physical stress and provided reference values for future evaluation by this method. We further intend to redefine fitness required for the elderly and also to clarify the exercises suitable for them by comparing the results of our tests according to exercise habits of the subjects and geographic regions as well as by examining their relationship to other health parameters.

References

1. Health and Welfare Statistics Association. Hygienic Status of the Japanese. Tokyo: Kosaido, 1987:440-443.

2. Kimura, M., Arai, T., Tsutsui, Y., Kojima, T., Kitamura, T., Nagata, H. Physical strength and fitness tests in aged individuals: I. Profile of physical strength in individuals aged above 65 years. Jap. J. Pub. Health 34:33-40, 1987.

3. Kimura, M., Hirakawa, K., Oda, Y., Morimoto, T. Estimation of physical fitness of aged subjects. Jap. J. Phys. Fitness Sports Med. (in press).

4. Kobayashi, H., Kondo, T. The exercise and fitness of the aged people. Tokyo: Asakura, 1985:57-88.

5. Morimoto, T., Ito, T., Kimura, M., Hirakawa, K. A new method to evaluate the capacity of physical activity in the elderly. In: Report of Osaka Gas Group Welfare Foundation survey. Osaka: Osaka Gas Group, 1988, 1:123-128.

6. Physical Fitness Laboratory, Tokyo Metropolitan University. Physical fitness standards of Japanese people. 3rd ed. Tokyo: Fumaido Shuppan, 1980.

7. Research Center in Physical Education. Prescription of exercise for promotion of health with sports: RCPE method. Tokyo: Kodansha, 1983:50-60.

Effects of Aging, Physical Fitness, Gender, Neural Activation, Exercise, and Practice on CNS Speed of Functioning

M. Vercruyssen, M.T. Cann, J.E. Birren, J.M. McDowd, and P.A. Hancock

Human Factors and Safety Science Depts, ISSM; Dept of Psychology
Laboratory of Attention and Motor Performance, University of Southern
California, Los Angeles, U.S.A.

Most central nervous system (CNS) functions slow with age. Variations of simple and choice reaction time (RT) have been used to measure the capacity and functional integrity of the CNS to process stimuli and quickly activate appropriate motor programs (7). Results from 26 studies of subjects 20-60 years of age showed that simple RT slows by 20% (4). Such slowing can account for many of the deficits found in psychometric tests (19). Physical fitness and health can account for a sizeable portion of the variance produced by aging on human speed of behavior, particularly the rate of processing information through the CNS. However, one cannot simply examine the effects of physical fitness on cognitive aging without also considering some of the interacting factors.

The purpose of this paper is to present relevant findings from experiments conducted at the University of Southern California and elsewhere designed to examine the relative contributions of physical fitness, gender, neural activation, exercise, intratask variables, and practice on the aging of cognitive processes, particularly speed of responses.

Results and Discussion

While slowing with age is a robust effect, it may be wise to view it in terms of some of the vast individual differences, which are usually collapsed or confounded into the average responses reported in the literature. Most noteworthy of these are physical fitness, gender, neural activation, exercise, and practice.

Physical fitness, as measured by aerobic capacity, $\dot{V}O_2max$, or lifestyle involving regular physical activity, improves physical and mental performance. While the locus of age-related psychomotor slowing is a hotly disputed issue, as is the nature of the variables presumed to mediate the relationship between age and speed of response, physical fitness is a very important variable in determining the extent of the presumed slowing. Older physically fit individuals have faster RT than their sedentary counterparts and are often as fast as, or faster than, young sedentary or below average fitness individuals (9, 16, 19, 27, 31, 46, 49, 52, 55, 56, 60). These effects have been also shown in animal models (50). Not only do older fit subjects react faster than their unfit peers, but they do so with less within- and between-subject variability (52). Furthermore, simple reaction time (SRT) appears more sensitive to age by fitness effects than choice reaction time (CRT) with the difference between SRT and CRT being greatest in the physically fit (55), especially in the elderly

(60). Several studies have failed to replicate these findings, but each experiment may require special interpretation due to methodological limitations (50).

Simple RT and $\dot{V}O_2$max are correlated (56), and there is even evidence showing that aerobic training of the elderly (55-70 years) for 4 months significantly increases aerobic capacity and quickens reactive capacity (19). Barry et al. (2) found similar effects following a 3-month exercise program. Such RT effects were not present in flexibility or strength training programs, nor were there exercise and age effects on peripheral processes such as visual, auditory, and somatosensory thresholds or visual acuity.

In an assessment of human biological age, SRT and CRT have been directly related to the age of death in the elderly; those individuals who were faster on these tasks tended to live longer than their slower counterparts (6). The relationship between fitness, RT, and biological age supports the use of RT as a viable and sensitive measure of the level and quality of cognitive functioning (5, 10).

At least two general mechanisms have been proposed to explain how physical activity is presumed to mediate reactive capacity: cellular mechanisms and system mechanisms. Cellular mechanisms operate at the level of motor control and initiation, while system mechanisms operate at the level of the system (e.g., circulatory or musculoskeletal). In the examination of one cellular mechanism, electrophysiological techniques have been used to fractionate RT into central and peripheral components, finding that most of the increase in RT with age is due to central rather than peripheral processes (13, 14, 15).

Another cellular mechanism is the nerve cell usage hypothesis (59), which proposes that continuous firing of action potentials, as induced by chronic exercise, postpones the natural decay of the cell while increasing synaptic efficiency. Muscular contractions have a trophic effect on their neurons and neuronal connections (20). Continuous enervation of muscle tissue is likely to modulate the efficiency of synaptic connections and the amount of neurotransmitter that is secreted. It seems that through constant activity, motor program control, motor neurons, and muscle fibers can stay biologically young (50).

The cardiovascular system is principally implicated as the major system mechanism to modulate age effects on the rate and quality of psychomotor performance. Birren et al. (5) have suggested that exercise may have a positive effect upon cognitive processes (e.g., RT) because of its influence on cerebral blood flow and oxygen level. It seems that decreased circulation to the brain, whether due to disease or simply to sedentary lifestyle, induces slowed responses, particularly in older subjects. Control of blood pressure may be viewed as one aspect of fitness and is related to speed of response; uncontrolled hypertension is related to tapping (22), although the relationship between uncontrolled hypertension and elevated SRT is controversial (32, 33, 47, 48). Subjects suffering from cardiovascular disease show a disproportionate slowing relative to their healthy age-matched counterparts (3, 8, 28, 48). Personality may be another confounding factor; Type A personalities without cardiovascular disease are slower than normal on both SRT and CRT tasks, disproportionately so for CRT when the effect of age is covaried (1).

The neurotransmitter system is another system mechanism that helps explain the effect of chronic exercise in postponing the age-related slowing of RT. Of the numerous neurotransmitters in the brain, (e.g., dopamine, norepinephrine, and serotonin) (53), the catecholamine system, particularly the nigrostriatal dopamine system, decreases with age in both neurotransmitter levels and receptor numbers (34). This decline, especially in Parkinson's disease, has become associated with deterioration of the motor system (51).

Gender interacts with age and previous experience in RT tasks. Pubescent girls and elderly women have generally faster RT than their male counterparts, but gender differences in the middle period are controversial. Generally, men are thought faster than women (42), but these differences decrease and may even disappear with practice. Rikli and Busch (43) found physical fitness and age effects on RT similar to other studies using an all female subject pool. In general, for both men and women, older active individuals behave more like young controls than like their sedentary age-matched counterparts.

Neural activation and exercise can improve performance via stimulation of the ascending reticular activating system—the RAS (17, 30). Activation theory places emphasis on the RAS as the principle source of excitation to the cortex and thereby responsible for maintaining activation or arousal (18, 26, 60). Activation refers to the release of energy into various physiological systems in preparation for action with the amount of energy released serving to control the force and speed of response (18). From this point of view, activation must play a crucial role in the determination of speed of response. Woods (60) has shown that older individuals respond faster when their level of arousal is increased through postural stimulation; older subjects have faster SRT when standing than when sitting or lying but posture does not seem to affect young subjects. Using exercise to increase activation, the old unfit have faster RT when cycling at 20% $\dot{V}O_2$max than at rest, whereas the old fit are faster at 40% $\dot{V}O_2$max, but RT does not improve with exercise for young subjects (60). While SRT is more sensitive than CRT at rest, the reverse becomes true during exercise at 40% HR_{max}. This seems to indicate that the older CNS may function at a generally lower level of activation than the younger CNS but that exercisers function at a slightly higher level of activation than their sedentary counterparts. This fitness-related increased activation may actually facilitate higher attention levels and thus yield decreased RT. Furthermore, limb movement, an inherent confounding variable with exercise, has been found to affect interpretation of exercise effects. Exercise and movement effects depend most on which type of reaction time task is employed (e.g., choice, simple, serial, or discrete) and which component is analyzed (e.g., mean correct trials, or percentage errors) (25, 26, 35, 36, 37).

Practice improves and stabilizes psychomotor performance but at different rates depending on age; older subjects generally take longer to adapt to novel tasks and new situations (24, 39, 44, 45, 54). There is evidence that continuous practice of the elderly can minimize (11, 33, 37, 38) and even eliminate (23, 29, 39, 40, 41) age differences in RT. Cerella and Lowe (12) reanalyzed 27 studies showing cognitive deficits with age and concluded that the age deficit came from a practice component (33%) that was reversible and a nonreversible component (66%) that was assumed to be biological.

A major problem with understanding the specific nature of the effects of physical fitness and exercise on reactive capacity is that the subjects are rarely well practiced on the specific performance tasks. Consequently, the performance of the various groups on psychomotor tasks reflects not only the effects of age and exercise history but also the degree to which the subject groups have benefited (learned) on the test trials. Using fit and unfit (from self-report of daily exercise) subjects from four age groups (20-30, 50-60, and 70-80 years) and performing psychomotor tests over 5 days, Spirduso (51) found exercisers to be faster than nonexercisers across age groups on SRT and CRT tasks during Day 1, but by Day 5 only the youngest exercisers were significantly faster than the other groups.

In summary, the effects of aging on CNS functioning, as measured by RT, depend in part on the physical fitness, gender, level of neural activation, and skill level of the performer. High fitness subjects perform better than those with low fitness; females do better than males in childhood and old age with the reverse true during middle age; and older subjects perform better when standing than when sitting or lying, although postural activation does not substantially impact young subjects. Exercise (at 20% $\dot{V}O_2$max) improves performance in the older unfit and older fit (at 40% $\dot{V}O_2$max) but degrades performance for young subjects, and there is less of an influence of all of these factors when the older subjects are brought to a higher level of skill on the criterion task. As data become available the multiple interactions will be further elucidated.

Conclusions

Evidence is mounting that while the rate of biological deterioration may be largely genetically determined, moderate and chronic physical exercise can serve to alter the natural decay of the integrity of the CNS. It seems that even of moderate level of physical fitness can enhance an organism's performance on many psychomotor tasks even when the tasks reflect few characteristics of the type of exercise practiced. However, the authors of this paper warn that while the effects mentioned herein are relatively robust, actual experimental results depend upon the specific methodology employed, particularly the subject and task characteristics.

In short, the effects of aging on CNS functioning, as measured by RT, depend on the interaction of many factors, not the least of which are the physical fitness, gender, level of neural activation, and skill of the performer as well as the nature, characteristics, and criterion measures of the performance task employed. Research on the multiple interactions of experimental variables is absolutely essential, as until we better understand the whole picture it seems naive to consider any one of these factors in isolation. Choice reaction time shows promise of being a valid, reliable, and sensitive measure of CNS integrity, but only when properly administered and interpreted.

References

1. Abrahams, J.P., Birren, J.E. Reaction time as a function of age and behavioral predisposition to coronary heart disease. Los Angeles: University of Southern California, 1973. Dissertation.

2. Barry, A., Steinmetz, J., Pagh, H., Rodahl, K. The effects of physical conditioning on older individuals: II. Motor performance and cognitive function. J. Gerontol. 21:192-199, 1966.

3. Birren, J.E., Spieth, W., Age, response speed, and cardiovascular functions. J. Gerontol. 17:390-391, 1962.

4. Birren, J.E., Woods, A.M., Williams, M.V. Speed of behavior as an indicator of age changes and the integrity of the nervous system. In: Hoffmeister, F., Muller, C., eds. Brain function in old age. New York: Springer-Verlag, 1979.

5. Birren, J.E., Woods, A.M., Williams, M.V. Behaviorial slowing with age: causes, organization, and consequences. In: Poon, L.W., ed. Aging in the 1980s. Washington, DC: American Psychological Association, 1980.

6. Borkan, G., Norris, A. Assessment of biological age using a profile of physical parameters. J. Gerontol. 35:177-184, 1980.

7. Botwinick, J. Theories of antecedent conditions of speed of response. In: Welford, A.T., Birren, J.E., eds. Behavior, aging, and the nervous system. Springfield, IL: Charles C Thomas, 1965.

8. Botwinick, J., Storandt, M. Cardiovascular status, depressive effect, and other factors in reaction time. J. Gerontol. 29:543-548, 1974.

9. Botwinick, J., Thompson, L.W. Components of reaction time in relation to age and sex. J. Genetic Psychol. 108:175-183, 1966.

10. Botwinick, J., West, R., Storandt, M. Predicting death from behavioral test performance. J. Gerontol. 33:755-762, 1978.

11. Carlton, B.L., Vercruyssen, M., McDowd, J.M., Birren, J.E. Effects of age and practice on attention and stages of information processing using choice reaction time with fixed and variable foreperiods. In: Proceedings of the 1988 Human Factors Society annual meeting. Santa Monica, CA: Human Factors Society, 1988.

12. Cerella, J., Lowe, D. Age deficits and practice: 27 studies reconsidered. The Gerontologist 24:76, 1984.

S

13. Clarkson, P.M. The effect of age and physical activity level on simple and choice fractionated response time. Europ. J. Appl. Physiol. 40:17-25, 1978.

14. Clarkson, P.M. The relationship of age and activity level with the fractionated components of patellar reflex time. J. Gerontol. 33:650-656, 1978.

15. Clarkson, P.M., Kroll, W. Practice effects on fractionated response time related to age and activity level. J. Motor Behav. 10:275-286, 1978.

16. Clarkson-Smith, L., Hartley, A.A. Cognitive benefits from life-style activities: physical exercise and bridge playing. Manuscript submitted for publication, 1988.

17. deVries, H.A. Physiological effects of an exercise training regimen upon men aged 52 to 88. J. Gerontol. 25:325-336, 1970.

18. Duffy, E. Activation. In: Greenfield, N.S., Sternbach, R.A., eds. Handbook of psychophysiology. New York: Holt/Rinehart/Winston, 1972.

19. Dustman, R.E., Ruhling, R.O., Russell, E.M., Shjearer, D.E., Bonekat, H.W., Shigeoka, J.W., Wood, J.S., Bradford, D.C. Aerobic exercise training and improved neuropsychological function of older individuals. Neurobiol. Aging 5:35-42, 1984.

20. Eccles, J.C. Tropic influences in the mammalian central nervous system. In: Rockstein, M., ed. Development and aging in the nervous system. New York: Academic Press, 1973:89-104.

22. Enzer, N., Simonson, E., Blankenstein, S.S. Fatigue of patients with circulatory insufficiency, investigated by means of fusion frequency of flicker. Ann. Int. Med. 16:701-707, 1942.

23. Falduto, L., Baron, A. Age related effects of practice and task complexity on card sorting. J. Gerontol. 41(5):659-661, 1986.

24. Grant, E.A., Storandt, M., Botwinick, J. Incentive and practice in the psychomotor performance of the elderly. J. Gerontol. 33:413-415, 1978.

25. Hancock, P.A., Mihaly, T., Vercruyssen, M. Temporal information feedback utility before, during, and after physical activity. In: Proceedings of the 1988 Human Factors Society annual meeting. Santa Monica, CA: Human Factors Society, 1988.

26. Hancock, P.A., Mihaly, T., Vercruyssen, M., Chignell, M.H. Stress and the efficiency of performance: an evaluation and reinterpretation of the inverted-U function. In: Ergonomics International 88. Proceedings of the International Ergonomics Association Congress, 1988 August, Sydney, Australia. London: Taylor & Francis, in press.

27. Hart, B.A. The effect of age and habitual activity on the fractionated component of resisted and unresisted response time. Med. Sci. Sports Exer. 13:78, 1981.

29. Hoyer, W.J., Labouvie, G.V., Baltes, P.B. Modification of response speed deficits and intellectual performance in the elderly. Human Dev. 16:233-242, 1973.

30. Isaac, W. Arousal and reaction time in cats. J. Comp. Physiological Psychol. 53:234-254, 1960.

31. Kroll, W., Clarkson, P.M. Age, isometric knee extension strength and fractional resisted response time. Exp. Aging Res. 4:389-409, 1978.

32. Light, K. Slowing of response time in young and middle-aged hypertensive patients. Exp. Aging Res. 1:209-227, 1975.

33. Light, K. Effects of mild cardiovascular and cerebrovascular disorders on serial reaction time performance. Exp. Aging Res. 4:3-22, 1978.

34. Mcgeer, P.L., Mcgeer, E.G. Enzymes associated with the metabolism of catecholamines, acetylcholine, and gamma-aminobutyric acid in human controls and practice with Parkinson's disease and Huntington's cholera. J. Neurochem. 26:65-76, 1976.

35. Mihaly, T. Effects of exercise—movement and elevated heart rate—on four measures on CNS speed: before, during and following work on a cycle ergometer, 1988. Thesis.

36. Mihaly, T. Arousal effects on cognition: new strategy which isolates movement and heart rate effects inherent in physical work. In: Proceedings of the 1988 Human Factors Society annual meeting. Santa Monica, CA: Human Factors Society, in press.

37. Mihaly, T., Hancock, P.A., Vercruyssen, M., Rahimi, M. Time estimation performance before, during, and after physical activity. In: Proceedings of the 1988 Human Factors Society annual meeting. Santa Monica, CA: Human Factors Society, in press.

38. Mowbray, G.H., Rhoades, M.V. On the reduction of choice reaction time with practice. Q. J. Exp. Psychol. 2:16-23, 1959.

39. Murrell, K.F.H. Effect of extensive practice on age differences in reaction time. J. Gerontol. 25:268-274, 1970.

40. Murrell, K.F.H., Powesland, P.R., Forsaith, B. A study of Pillar-drilling in relation to age. Occ. Psychol. 36:45-52, 1962.

41. Nebes, R.D. Vocal versus manual response as a determinant of age differences in simple reaction time. J. Gerontol. 33:884-889, 1978.

42. Noble, C.E., Baker, B.L., Jones, T.A. Age and sex parameters in psychomotor learning. Percept. Motor Skills 19:935-945, 1964.

43. Rikli, R., Busch, S. Motor performance of women as a function of age and physical activity. J. Gerontol. 41(5):645-659, 1986.

44. Salthouse, T.A Speed of behavior and its implications for cognition. In: Birren, J., Schaie, K.W., eds. Handbook of the psychology of aging, Vol. 2. New York: Van Nostrand Reinhold, 1985:400-416.

45. Salthouse, T.A., Somberg, B.L. Skilled performance: effects of adult age and experience on elementary processes. J. Exp. Psychol.: Gen. 11:176-207, 1982.

46. Sherwood, D.E., Selder, D.J. Cardiovascular health, reaction time, and aging. Med. Sci. Sports Exer. 11:186-189, 1979.

47. Spieth, W. Cardiovascular health status, age, and psychological performance. J. Gerontol. 19:277-284, 1964.

48. Speith, W. Slowness of task performance and cardiovascular disease. In: Welford, A.T., Birren, J.E., eds. Behavior, aging, and the nervous system. Springfield, IL: Charles C Thomas, 1965.

49. Spirduso, W.W. Reaction and movement time as a function of age and physical activity level. J. Gerontol. 30:435-440, 1975.

50. Spirduso, W.W. Physical fitness in relation to motor aging. In: Mortimer, J.A., Pirozzolo, F.J., Maletta, G.J., eds. The aging motor system. New York: Prager, 1982.

51. Spirduso, W.W. Age as a limiting factor in human neuromuscular performance. Manuscript submitted for publication, 1988.

52. Sirpduso, W.W., Clifford, P. Replication of age and physical activity effects on reaction time and movement time. J. Gerontol. 33(1):26-30, 1978.

53. Spirduso, W.W., Farrar, R.P. Effects of aerobic training on reactive capacity: an animal model. J. Gerontol. 36:654-662, 1981.

54. Surburg, P.R. Aging and effect of physical and mental practice upon acquisition and retention of a motor skill. J. Gerontol. 31:64-67, 1976.

56. Tredway, V. Mood effects of exercise programs for older adults. Los Angeles: University of Southern California, 1978. Dissertation.

57. Vercruyssen, M., Cann, M.T., McDowd, J.M., Birren, J.E., Carlton, B.L., Burton, J., Hancock, P.A. Effects of age, gender, activation, stimulus degradation, and practice on attention and visual choice reaction time. In: Proceedings of the 1988 Human Factors Society annual meeting. Santa Monica, CA: Human Factors Society, in press.

58. Vercruyssen, M., McDowd, J.M., Ynclino, V., Hancock, P.A., Birren, J.E. Human attention: implications for health and safety. In: Proceedings of the 1988 American Industrial Hygiene Conference. San Francisco, in press.

59. Vogt, C., Vogt, O. Aging of nerve cells. Nature 58:304, 1946.

60. Woods, A.M. Age differences in the effect of physical activity and postural changes on information processing speed. Los Angeles: University of Southern California, 1981. Dissertation.

Intraarterial Blood Pressure Regulation During Ramp Exercise and Recovery in Aged Individuals

T. Yoshida, M. Udo, J. Eguchi, M. Chida, M. Ichioka, and K. Makiguchi

Faculty of Health and Sport Sciences, Osaka University, Toyonaka, Osaka; Department of Physical Education, Komazawa University, Tokyo; and School of Medicine, Tokyo Medical and Dental University, Tokyo, Japan

Compared to the classic, prolonged steady-state exercise test, the short non–steady–state incremental exercise test is able to more rapidly obtain the simultaneous determinations of the cardiovascular and respiratory systems' abilities (14). Combining an electrically-braked cycle ergometer with a computerized control system, a ramp incremental exercise testing can be applied for exercise prescription or clinical exercise testing. Although there is some documentation of gas-exchange kinetics during ramp exercise, less attention has been paid to blood pressure regulation during ramp exercise and during recovery (3, 11).

The purpose of the present study is to investigate the relationship between blood pressure and heart rate during a ramp exercise and recovery in aged individuals. In addition, we determined whether the cardiac contractile property might be affected by the point at which blood lactate increases during a ramp exercise (lactate threshold).

Methods

Nine middle-aged males (age 42.5 years, 8.4 years SD; height 165.1 cm, 6.4 cm SD; weight 62.6 kg, 8.6 kg SD) and nine middle-aged females (age 46.7 years, 5.2 years SD; height 151.5 cm, 4.7 cm SD; weight 48.6 kg, 6.3 kg SD) voluntarily participated in the study. They were well informed of the purpose of this study and possible risks and signed the consent form. Prior to the experiment, each subject underwent a complete medical examination including ECG, blood pressure (a cuff method), spirometry, and a general medical checkup; none of them showed any abnormalities.

The incremental exercise test was performed on an electrically braked cycle ergometer (Siemens, 380B) at 50 rpm in the upright position. The test consisted of 4 min of pedaling at the intensity of 20 W for a warm-up, and thereafter ramp function work rate was generated at 1-W increments per 3 s (i.e., $20 \text{ W} \cdot \text{min}^{-1}$ ramp) by the ramp slope controller (Fukuda, Japan).

Ventilation and gas exchange were monitored breath by breath. Inspired and expired gas volumes were measured by a hot-wire respiratory flow meter (16). Fractional gas concentrations were monitored by a zirconia solid electrolyte oxygen analyzer and an infrared carbon dioxide analyzer. After compensation for a time delay of gas concentrations and a gas flow, a dedicated microcomputer processed data for each breath (8). Data were stored on a diskette for later analysis.

To obtain the changes in blood lactate concentration (HLa) and intraarterial blood pressure, a teflon catheter was inserted into the right brachial artery. At the end of the catheter a three-way stop cock was attached to connect a continuous flush device and a pressure transducer (intelligent monitor SMW 104, Hellinge). The intraarterial blood pressure was recorded continuously during the exercise and following the exercise (30-min recovery period). The catheter-transducer system was calibrated before and after each experiment. Blood samples were taken each 30 s from the time at the last 1 min of warming up to the time when RER value reached the 1.0 value during the ramp exercise. Assay of blood HLa was performed by an enzymatic method (Boeringer, Mannheim, FRG). ECG was continously monitored throughout the experiment.

Lactate threshold (LT) is defined as the point at which blood lactate begins to increase above the resting level (14). Unpaired t test was used to evaluate the differences between male and female subjects. Paired t test was used to compare intraindividual analyses. Regression analysis and correlation analysis were performed on the appropriate data.

Results

Table 1 shows mean values in intraarterial systolic blood pressure, mean blood pressure, diastolic blood pressure, pressure-rate production and heart rate at rest, during warm-up, at the lactate threshold, at the LT point, at maximal exercise, and at 5th, 10th, and 15th min of recovery. Figure 1 indicates the time course of systolic blood pressure, mean blood pressure, diastolic blood pressure, heart rate, pressure-rate product, and blood lactate during exercise in female and male subjects. In females the systolic blood pressure, heart rate, and pressure-rate product rose gradually. The regression analysis indicates significantly different slope below and above the lactate threshold (see Figure 1). In male subjects, the determined parameters increased in a linear fashion below and above the LT.

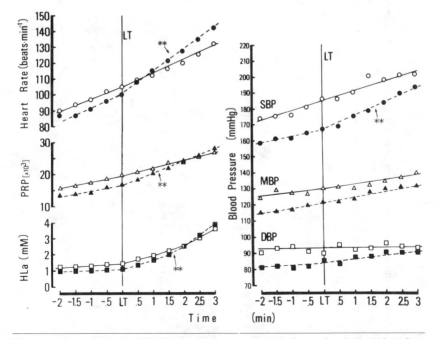

Figure 1. Average values of determinants that are based on the lactate threshold and best-fit regression lines before and after the lactate threshold. Asterisks show the significantly different slope-of-regression line obtained before and after the lactate threshold. Open symbols indicate the mean values in male subjects, and closed symbols indicate those in females.

Table 1   Mean Values with *SD* of Determinants Taken at Rest, During Warming Up, at Lactate Threshold, During Maximal Exercise, and During Recovery

	At rest	During exercise			During recovery		
		W-up	LT	MAX	5 min	10 min	15 min
Male							
Heart rate (beats/min)	70 ± 10	81 ± 13**	105 ± 17**	174 ± 14**	107 ± 21**	99 ± 17**	97 ± 11**
SBP (mmHg)	150 ± 16	169 ± 19***	186 ± 19***	232 ± 32***	153 ± 16	134 ± 10**	132 ± 10**
MBP (mmHg)	112 ± 11	124 ± 13**	130 ± 12**	153 ± 20**	110 ± 9	105 ± 11	106 ± 10
DBP (mmHg)	89 ± 9	91 ± 15	90 ± 12	101 ± 12**	84 ± 6	86 ± 10	85 ± 9
PRP (×10³)	10 ± 2	14 ± 3**	20 ± 5**	40 ± 5**	16 ± 4**	13 ± 3**	13 ± 2
Female							
Heart rate (beats/min)	65 ± 8	84 ± 3**	101 ± 9**	158 ± 16**	80 ± 15**	80 ± 9**	82 ± 5**
SBP (mmHg)	148 ± 13	158 ± 14**	167 ± 11**	196 ± 13**	134 ± 10**	127 ± 12**	120 ± 12**
MBP (mmHg)	108 ± 8	117 ± 7**	121 ± 6**	132 ± 17**	96 ± 13	96 ± 12	98 ± 9
DBP (mmHg)	82 ± 6	84 ± 7	86 ± 8	89 ± 12	71 ± 12**	73 ± 10**	77 ± 7
PRP (×10³)	10 ± 1	13 ± 1**	18 ± 4**	31 ± 4**	11 ± 2*	10 ± 1	10 ± 1

Data are expressed as mean with *SD*. *$p < .05$, **$p < .01$ (compared to the resting value).

Figure 2 indicates the recovery time course of systolic blood pressure, diastolic blood pressure, heart rate, and pressure-rate product and compares these with the resting value. Table 1 and Figure 2 indicate that the systolic blood pressure returned abruptly to the resting value and then decreased below the resting value. Statistical analysis indicates that a significant down drift is observed at the 9th min of recovery in males and the 5th min of recovery in females. On the other hand, heart rate remains still significantly higher than the resting value even in the 30th min of recovery. The pressure-rate product, which is a function as heart rate and systolic blood pressure, returned to the resting value at the 6th min of the recovery period in females but remained significantly higher even in the 15th min of recovery in male subjects (see Table 1 and Figure 2).

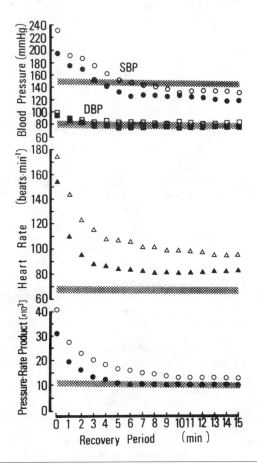

Figure 2. Time course of systolic blood pressure, diastolic blood pressure, heart rate, and pressure-rate product during recovery. Open symbols indicate the mean values in male subjects, and closed symbols indicate those in females. Shadowed area indicates resting values.

Figure 3 illustrates the individual relationship between systolic blood pressure and heart rate during ramp exercise and recovery. Although there is a larger individual difference in the slope of the systolic blood pressure–heart rate relationship during exercise, statistical analysis indicates that this relationship during exercise is significantly different to that during recovery both in males and females.

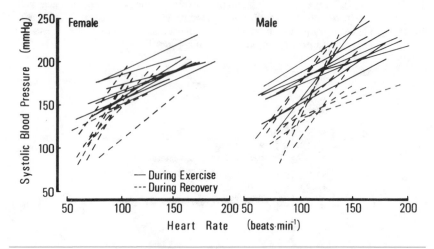

Figure 3. The relationship between heart rate and systolic blood pressure during exercise (solid lines) and during recovery (dashed lines). Each line indicates an individual's regression and its range. Statistical analysis indicates a significantly different slope during exercise and during recovery.

Discussion

The major findings of the present study are that (a) in female subjects, there are disproportionate increases in systolic blood pressure, heart rate, and pressure-rate products between, below, and above the lactate threshold, but in male subjects the cardiovascular parameters increase proportionally to the work rate; (b) there is a specific time course of heart rate, systolic blood pressure, and pressure-rate product during recovery period; and (c) there is a significantly different relationship of heart rate–systolic blood pressure during exercise and during recovery.

The summarized data obtained at rest, during ramp exercise, and during recovery are listed in Table 1. At rest, at the lactate threshold, and at maximal exercise the values of systolic blood pressure, mean blood pressure, and diastolic blood pressure agreed well with the reports by Hansen et al. (3) and Robinson et al. (10), who determined intraarterial blood pressure during a 1-min incremental exercise mode.

Recently, the computerized control system for exercise testing has been well developed. Especially, a ramp exercise mode in which work rate increased by a few watts in a few seconds had been used for clinical exercise testing and/or exercise testing for the prescription on aged individuals. This kind of ramp exercise mode has merit in that exercise testing time may be reduced because the work rate increases more rapidly and in that the incremental rate of exercise intensity is subjectively insensitive. Consequently, it is thought that the blood pressure–heart rate regulation during ramp exercise mode may alter the steady state exercise mode. Åstrand et al. (1), Eklund and Holmgren (2), and Robinson et al. (10) observed that the intraarterial systolic, diastolic, and mean blood pressures increased in a relatively linear fashion with cardiac output and $\dot{V}O_2$. In the present study, the average intraarterial blood pressure in male subjects increased in a relatively linear fashion during a ramp incremental exercise.

On the other hand, in female subjects the time course of systolic blood pressure, heart rate and pressure-rate product during exercise indicated a disproportional increase above the lactate threshold, when data were based upon the lactate threshold (see Figure 1). The findings in female subjects agrees with the recent reports by Spence et al. (11) and Yoshitake et al. (15), who reported that when using middle-aged male or female subjects, the systolic blood pressure and pressure-rate product steeply increased at the exercise levels above the lactate threshold. One of the possible explanations for steeper increases of systolic blood pressure and pressure-rate product above the lactate threshold might be partly contributed by the concentrations of catecholamine. Numerous studies have shown that plasma catecholamine levels increased exponentially during incremental exercise. Subsequently, a close linear relation between concentrations of plasma catecholamine and blood lactate was observed during the incremental exercise (6). The steeply elevated concentration of catecholamine at the exercise intensity above the lactate threshold might increase the sympathetic nervous activity as hypertensive cardiac regulation. In this context, it is of interest that stroke volume during the incremental exercise reached maximally at the exercise intensity corresponding to the lactate threshold (13). Subsequently, the disproportional increase of systolic blood pressure and heart rate increment above the lactate threshold has been ascribed to elevated cardiac sympathetic nervous activity.

Furthermore, not only disproportional increase of cardiac contractile properties but also myocardial oxygen utilization might be increased above the lactate threshold, because pressure-rate product as a predictor of myocardial work increased steeply above the lactate threshold in female subjects (see Figure 1).

There is a discrepancy as to whether intraarterial pressure increased in a linear fashion or in a disproportional fashion during a ramp exericse. Although the reasons for this difference in time course of intraarterial blood pressure during ramp exercise are not precisely known, the fact in the present study that the lactate threshold in females is significantly lower than that in males might be owing to more hypoxic condition in skeletal muscle and cardiac muscle tissue. Then, it might also be considered that hypoxic production of blood lactate and/or catecholamine activities would result in more hypertension in females.

In the present study, during the recovery period from maximal exercise, there is a specific recovery curve in systolic blood pressure, heart rate, and pressure-rate products (see Figure 2). There is a large drop in cardiac output immediately after exercise. Compared to the time course in cardiac output, peripheral resistance during recovery showed interesting characteristics. Tamaki et al. (12) demonstrated the diametrical changes of finger nailfold capillaries during submaximal and maximal cycle exercise and recovery. After submaximal and maximal exercise, vasodilation in finger nailfold capillaries was observed even until the 30th min of recovery. This is the same general trend seen in skin temperature (7) and blood flow (4, 5, 9) during recovery. In other words, peripheral resistance during recovery might remain as low as during exercise. As a result, because blood pressure is a function of cardiac output and peripheral resistance, systolic blood pressure decreased a down drift in spite of significant higher heart rate during recovery (see Figure 2). Figure 3 shows a significant difference in the regression slope of the heart rate–systolic blood pressure relationship during exercise and recovery. As observed in trends of heart rate and systolic blood pressure during recovery, the vasodilation might be due to a reflex release of vasoconstriction tone caused by the increase in body temperature. There may exist a quite different blood pressure regulation system during exercise and recovery.

It is concluded that during ramp exercise the average intraarterial blood pressure elevated in a linear fashion in male subjects but rose gradually in female subjects, that the inflection point of intraarterial blood pressure in females is concurrent with the lactate threshold, and that during recovery the heart rate–systolic blood pressure relationship is apparently different from the rate during exercise, especially in female subjects who tended to exhibit decreased systolic and diastolic blood pressures.

References

1. Åstrand, P.-O., Ekblom, B., Messin, R., Saltin, B. Intra-arterial blood pressure during exercise with different muscle groups. J. Appl. Physiol. 20:253-256, 1965.

2. Eklund, L.G., Holmgren, R.J. Central hemodynamics during exercise. Cir. Res 20(Suppl.1):33-44, 1967.

3. Hansen, J.E., Sue, D.Y., Wasserman, K. Predicted values for clinical exercise testing. Am. Rev. Respir. Dis. 129(Suppl.):S49-S55, 1984.

4. Johnson, J.M., Rowell, L.B., Brengelmann, G.L. Modification of the skin blood flow-body temperature relationship by upright exercise. J. Appl. Physiol. 37:880-886, 1974.

5. Kamon, E., Beldang, H.S. Dermal blood flow in the resting arm during prolonged leg exercise. J. Appl. Physiol. 26:317-320, 1969.

6. Lehmann, M., Keul, J., Huber, G., Da Prada, M. Plasma catecholamines in trained and untrained volunteers during graduated exercise. Int. J. Sports Med. 2:143-147, 1981.

7. Mathews, D.K., Fox, E.L., Tanzi, D. Physiological responses during exercise and recovery in a football uniform. J. Appl. Physiol. 26:611-615, 1969.

8. Noguchi, H., Oguchi, Y., Yoshiya, I., et al. Breath-by-breath VCO_2 and $\dot{V}O_2$ require compensation for transport delay and dynamic response. J. Appl. Physiol. 52:79-84, 1982.

9. Roberts, M.F., Wenger, C.B. Control of skin blood flow during exercise: thermal and nonthermal factors. J. Appl. Physiol. 46:780-786, 1979.

10. Robinson, T.E., Sue, D.Y., Huszczuk, A., Weiler-Ravell, D., Hansen, J.E. Intra-arterial and cuff blood pressure responses during incremental cycle ergometry. Med. Sci. Sports Exer. 20:142-149, 1988.

11. Spence, D.W., Peterson, L.H., Friedewald, Jr., V.E. Relation of blood pressure during exercise to anaerobic metabolism. Am. J. Cardiol. 59:1342-1344, 1987.

12. Tamaki, N., Kuwana, S., Ogawa, Y. The diametrical changes of the hand's nailfold capillaries due to bicycle exercise. J. Yokohama City Univ. Ser. Sport Sci. Med. 8:7-13, 1979. (in Jananese)

13. Tanaka, K., Yoshimura, T., Sumida, S., et al. Transient responses in cardiac function below, at, and above anaerobic threshold. Europ. J. Appl. Physiol. 55:356-361, 1986.

14. Yoshida, T. Current topics and concepts of lactate and gas exchange threshold. J. Human Ergol. 16:103-121, 1987.

15. Yoshitake, Y., Zaiki, N., Shinkai, S., Hino, S., Watanabe, T. Hemodynamic and biochemical responses during exercise at the intensity equivalent to lactate threshold for middle-aged and elderly women. J. Human Ergol. 16:137-143, 1987.

16. Yoshiya, I., Nakajima, T., Nagai, I., Jitsukawa, S. A bidirectional respiratory flow meter using the hot-wire principle. J. Appl. Physiol. 38:360-365, 1975.

Physiological Responses to Snow Shoveling Observed in Aged Men

T. Suda, S. Miyake, T. Sasaki, and M. Kato

Department of Health and Physical Education, Faculty of Education, Hokkaido University, Sapporo; Hokuseigakuen University, Sapporo; Hokuseigakuen Women's Junior College, Sapporo; and Hokkaido Women's Junior College, Hokkaido, Japan

Although snow shoveling is a common task for the inhabitants of snowy regions, little is known about its physiological effects. The strenuous nature of shoveling sand (8) and coal (7) has been reported previously, but little data has been collected regarding snow shoveling. There are many variables that regulate the performance and intensity of the work involved in shoveling snow; for example, snow quality, depth of snow, throwing height and distance, shovel design (4), postures used, body size (3), fitness, and emotional make-up of the workers. For example, shoveling wet or heavy snow has occasionally caused death in people with cardiovascular diseases (5). Of course, this is most likely to happen to aged people of delicate health. Given that this is the case, the present paper concerns itself with the physiological responses of aged men during the act of shoveling snow.

Methods

Fourteen men between the ages of 65 and 81 volunteered to be subjects in this experiment. The physical characteristics of the subjects are presented in Table 1. Clinical examination revealed no signs of cardiovascular disease in any of the subjects. Of the 14 men, 8 had been engaging in physical activities two or three times a week, such as gateball or jogging in snowless times and voluntary snow shoveling for the infirm in times of snow. The other 6 men took no regular exercise. For the experiment, each subject engaged in snow shoveling, designed to closely match his usual snow shoveling behavior, for a period of 10 min. The subjects used a 1.4-kg snow shovel 75 cm in length. Depth of the snow was 0.4-0.7 m, and its density was approximately 0.2. The ambient temperature was between $-3°$ and $+1$ °C. The experiment covered an initial 5 min of sitting rest, 10 min of work, and a final recovery period. Expired air was collected in Douglas bags while subjects were at rest and during the last 2-3 min of work.

The gas was analyzed using a direct reading polarographical high-response oxygen analyzer (AIC, RAS31) and the same type of carbon dioxide analyzer (AIC, RAS41). The weight of snow per shovel was estimated from the strain curves of the gauges attached to the root of the shovel's shaft. Heart rate was calculated from a continuous recording of the ECG. The ECG and strain curves were amplified by a 600 g portable multichannel amplifier designed for this experiment, and they were recorded on a portable multichannel data recorder (TEAC, HR30J). The recorded data were played back and traced by pen recorder. Blood pressure measurements were taken by auscultation during the resting period and the first 2-3 min of the recovery period using a mercury manometer.

Table 1   Physical Characteristics of the Subjects

Number	Sex	Age (yr)	Height (cm)	Weight (kg)
14	Male	74.3 ± 4.6	159.2 ± 5.3	58.8 ± 7.5

Note. Values are mean ± *SD*.

Results

Mean value of the heart rates at rest was 72.4 beats/min, ranging from 53 to 84. During the work, the average value rose to about 125 beats/min at 3 min from the onset of the task and finally reached almost 130 beats/min by the end of the work period (see Figure 1). Heart rate at the highest point of work was estimated to about 80% of average value of maximum heart rate of Japanese in their sex and age (Kobayashi 1982). The highest recorded rates varied widely between individuals ranging from 93 to 155 beats/min.

Systolic blood pressure changed from 161.6 mmHg at rest to 169.6 mmHg during the recovery period. Diastolic blood pressure also increased slightly, from 86.5 to 88.2 mmHg.

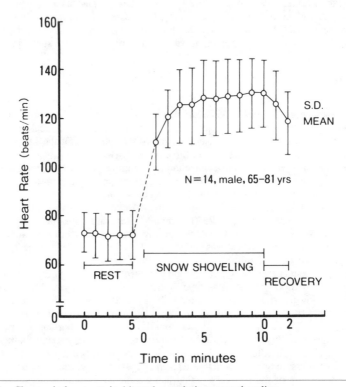

Figure 1. Changes in heart rate in 14 aged men during snow shoveling.

There was a positive significant correlation ($r = .80$, $p < .01$) in the change in diastolic blood pressure between the resting time and recovery period. Judging from the fact that systolic blood pressure in the first 2-3 min of the recovery period was nearly 200 mmHg in some subjects, the value during the work would almost certainly be over 200 mmHg. The resting values for oxygen uptake range from 0.19 to 0.30 L/min, averaging 0.22 L/min. As the expired air of one subject was not collected, due to a technical error, data on oxygen uptake was only available for 13 subjects. During the work period, the data varied widely, from 0.82 to 1.43 L/min. The average $\dot{V}O_2$ at work was 1.14 ± 0.16 L/min in absolute value and 19.3 ± 2.4 ml/min/kg in relative value. These levels correspond to about five times the resting values. Energy expenditure as calculated from oxygen consumption was 5.7 kcal/min. This puts snow shoveling at the same level as the industrial tasks of shoveling coal (7) or sand (8). Although snow shoveling is usually a domestic task and does not continue over as long a time as shoveling in industrial work, the task should be classified as heavy work in terms of oxygen uptake and heart rate response (1, 2) considering the age and physique of the subjects. Oxygen uptake during the work corresponded to approximately 70% of the average Japanese $\dot{V}O_2$max for their sex and age (6). As these levels seem to exceed the anaerobic threshold of the subjects, aged men would be performing the task using anaerobic metabolism, and early fatigue would occur.

There exist large differences in shoveling performance among individuals. Mean value of the rate of shoveling, snow weight per shovel, and performance (amount shoveled per minute) were 9.8 times/min, 5.3 kg, and 58.6 kg/min, respectively. It was noticed that a positive significant correlation ($r = .914$, $p < .001$) was found between the weight of a scoop of snow and the shoveling performance, while there was no significant correlation ($r = -.497$) between the rate of shoveling and the shoveling performance. A positive significant correlation was observed between the shoveling performance and the volume of oxygen uptake during the task, both in absolute value (Figure 2, $r = .768$, $p < .01$)

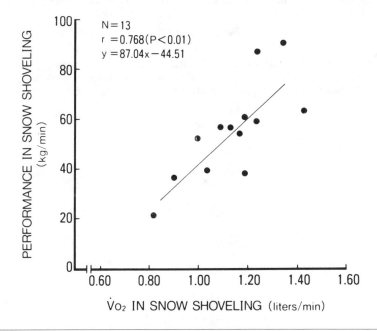

Figure 2. Performance in snow shoveling in relation to oxygen uptake during snow shoveling in 13 aged men.

and in relative value ($r = .727, p < .01$). Energy expenditures corresponding to shoveling performances of 40, 60, and 80 kg were estimated to be about 5, 6, and 7 Kcal, respectively.

Conclusion

Although the subjects were asked to engage in snow shoveling at their usual pace, their responses in terms of heart rate, oxygen uptake, and blood pressure demonstrated that this activity is quite demanding to aged men.

References

1. Andersen, K.L., Masironi, R., Rutenfranz, J., Seliger, V. Habitual physical activity and health. Copenhagen: WHO Regional Publications. 1978:19.
2. Åstrand, P.O., Rodahl, K. Textbook of work physiology. 3rd ed. New York: McGraw-Hill, 1986.
3. Cooper, J.M., Adrian, M., Glassow, R.B. Kinesiology. 5th ed. St. Louis: Mosby. 1982:374-375.
4. Freivalds, A. The ergonomics of shoveling and shovel design—an experimental study. Ergonomics 29(1):19-30, 1986.
5. Karpovich, P.V., Sinning, W.E. Physiology of muscular activity. 7th ed. Philadelphia: W.B. Saunders, 1971:138-140.
6. Kobayashi, K. Aerobic power of the Japanese—growth and development, aging and effect of physical training. Tokyo: Kyorin, 1982:311-313.
7. Lehmann, G., Muller, E.A., Spitzer, H. Der Kalorienbedarf bei gewerblicher Arbeit. Arbeitphysiol. 14:166, 1950.
8. Wyndham, C.H., Morrison, J.F., Williams, C.G., Heyns, A., Margo, E., Brown, A.N., Astrup, J. The relationship between energy expenditure and performance index in the task of shoveling sand. Ergonomics 9(5):371-378, 1966.

Occurrence of Entrainment of Heart Beat Into Endurance Running Pitch and Its Significance in Energy Consumption

M. Udo, T. Yoshida, T. Nakazumi, K. Kinugawa, and A. Watanabe

Laboratory of Exercise Physiology, Department of Sport Science, Faculty of Health & Sport Science, Osaka University; College of General Education, Osaka University of Economics and Law, Osaka, Japan

Endurance running is characterized by alternating movements of four limbs and up-and-down movements of the body trunk. These rhythmic movements, including those of muscle pumps and vertical accelerations acting on the blood flow, may possibly influence the rhythm of the heart beat (1) and possibly influence the energy consumption during endurance running. If this is the case, such results may suggest a certain basic mechanism interacting between running movements and cardiovascular activity and may serve for prescription of efficient, safe running for the purpose of health care. It will be shown that for a period lasting 1-4 min during endurance running, each ECG appears in each step cycle and cumulative interval of ECG follows closely that of step cycles, thus the ECG interval seems to be entrained into the trend in step cycles. It will also be shown that $\dot{V}O_2$ during such a period is less as compared with before and after. Some of the present results have appeared in abstract form (3, 5).

Methods

The running test was made on a treadmill and in free space to determine if the heart beat is entrained into the running pitch and if the $\dot{V}O_2$ during the entrainment differs from that before and after. During both types of running the subject wore a hat, on an occipital part of which an accelerometer (frequency band 0-100 Hz) was affixed. The output of the accelerometer and the ECG was fed into an A/D converter (Canopus ADX98), sampled at a rate of 1 KHz, stored in a hard disc, and displayed on personal computer (NEC PC9801VM2) and XY-plotter (Graphtec FP5301). An interval (T) from the lift-off of one leg to the lift-off of the other leg and an interval (t) from lift-off of one leg to the peak of R wave of an ECG were always measured, and phase (Φ) was calculated according to $\Phi = (t/T) \times 360$.

Treadmill Running

Seven healthy subjects (5 male, 2 female, age 20-33 years) were studied during 20-50 min of treadmill exercise ($\cong$ = 70% $\dot{V}O_2$max; speed, 130-220m/min; slope, 0-4%). The Φ values could be displayed on line using the telemetric ECG and the accelerometer signal.

In the present experiment only the experimenter, not the subject, could see the Φ values during running. The $\dot{V}O_2$ was usually measured by the Douglas bag method ($\dot{V}O_2$ for 60 sec), and in some experiments, the breath-by-breath $\dot{V}O_2$ was measured by the respiro-monitor (Minato, RM-300) at each period of 10-60 s (4).

Free-Space Running

Two healthy subjects (1 male, 1 female, age 25-26 years) were studied during 18-40 min of free-space running ($\cong 60 \sim 70\%$ $\dot{V}O_2$max; distance, 3-9 km; slope 0-5%), the speed being determined arbitrarily by the subjects. The output of the accelerometer and ECG were recorded into a portable data recorder (Teac HR30E, frequency band, DC-1250 Hz) and analyzed off line.

Results

For the purpose of studying the entrainment between the ECG and the running pitch, we analyzed their relation in a period in which the heart rate was close to the running pitch during endurance running. In an example of the treadmill running illustrated in Figure 1A, the heart rate became nearly 160/min, which was close to the running pitch in the period of 7-12 min after the start of the running. In Figure 1B, the phase is shown during 3.9-13.9 min after the start. In the part shown by K (3.9-6.5 min), the heart rate was slower than the running pitch so that the phase (Φ) was increasing with each step. In the part shown by N (12.5-13.9 min), the heart rate became faster than the running pitch so that the phase was decreasing with each step. During a period from 6.7-11 min, the phase persisted at a certain phase somewhat below 180, and during this period each of the R existed in each of the step cycles.

In Figure 1A, we plotted $Xn = T1 + T2 + \text{-----} + Tn$ as the abscissa and Yn, Zn as the ordinate. Taking To as the mean step cycle, $To = (1/n) (T1 + T2 + \text{-----} + Tn)$, Yn was the sum of Ti-To values for the step cycle (Ti), and Zn was the sum of Ri-To values for the R-R interval (Ri) of the ECG ($i = 1, 2, 3, \text{-----}, n$). In other words, Yn and Zn show the trends of rhythm of running and heart beat, respectively, as compared with a rhythm composed of a fixed interval of To. Clearly, in the period from E to F, corresponding to the period from L to M in Figure 1B, Yn and Zn resembled each other in the time course, Yn several seconds preceding Zn. Similar observation was made in the other subjects both on the treadmill and in the free-space running. From Figure 1A it can be assumed that the occurrence of an R wave in each step cycle observed in Figure 1B is not an accidental phenomenon, but that there would be mechanisms in which the running pitch entrains the heart beat.

In view of Figure 1, some mechanisms for entrainment may be considered at work to lengthen the R-R interval in the phase less than 90 ($\Phi < \sim 90$) and shorten the R-R interval in the phase larger than 270 ($\Phi > \sim 270$). To examine such an effect depending on different phases, we made the following study. The R wave of the ECG was used to trigger a pulse generator so as to make a brief sound after a certain delay from the R wave. The subject was directed to step in coincidence with the sound. In Figure 2, when the delay time from the R wave to the actual step was adjusted to induce Φ of about 90 (during 37-39 min and 44-46 min), the heart rate became slightly above 160/min. When the delay time was changed to induce Φ of near 270 (during 39-43 min and after 46 min), the heart rate increased up to near 170/min. The test of this kind was performed repeatedly on the same subject as well as on the other subjects, and the result was reproducible. This result indicates that there is some mechanism that controls the heart rate depending on the phase of the step cycle, and according to the mechanism the phase of the R wave persisted at a certain phase.

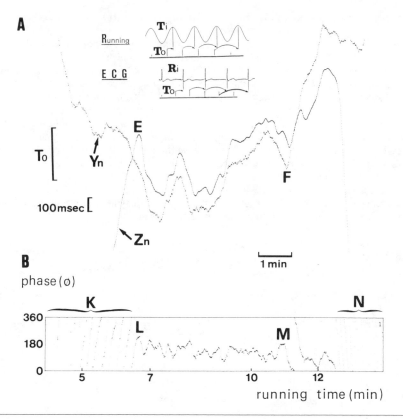

Figure 1.   Entrainment of heart beat into running pitch (see text).

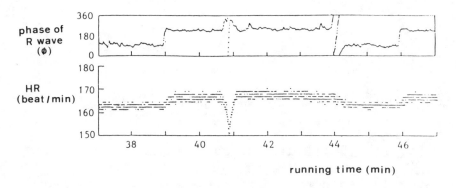

Figure 2. $\dot{V}O_2$ before, during, and after entrainment (see text).

Energy Consumption (V̇O₂) Before, During, and After the Entrainment

To determine if the entrainment has a significant relationship to energy consumption, we measured $\dot{V}O_2$ before, during, and after the entrainment. In the present study, the entrainment was induced using the feedback from ECG as described in Figure 2. Figure 3 shows that during 6-11 min and 18-21 min the subject made his step in coincidence with the sound that was delayed from the R wave to make $\Phi \sim 180$. $\dot{V}O_2$ was measured during each 2 min shown by a, b, and c. During 11-16 min, the sound was given at a fixed interval slightly less than during entrainment (6-11 min and 18-21 min) so as to induce shorter step cycles compared with ECG interval. Figure 3 shows that $\dot{V}O_2$ during entrainment (a and c) was less than either before or after the entrainment (b), while the heart rate was higher during entrainment. The decrease in $\dot{V}O_2$ during entrainment did not seem to be due to decrease in accelerations as far as observed from the accelerometer signal. This type of test was performed repeatedly on the same subject as well as on the other subjects, and the result was reproducible. Thus, certain mechanisms may be working during entrainment to decrease the $\dot{V}O_2$ while increasing the heart rate.

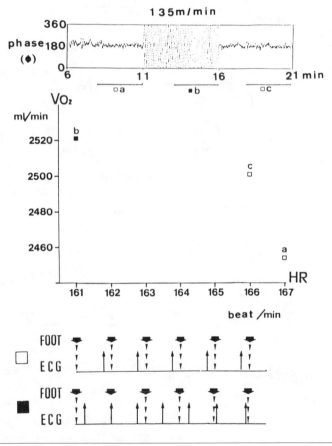

Figure 3. Effect of different phase (Φ) on the heart rate as studied using biofeedback from ECG (see text).

Discussion and Conclusion

We have found an entrainment of heart beat into endurance running pitch and have observed the fact that $\dot{V}O_2$ during the entrainment was less than before and after. Although these examinations were made only on young subjects, the occurrence and the significance of the lower energy consumption may be expected for the aged, thus implying an efficient, safe prescription for the aged.

Some mechanisms for the entrainment may be considered to lengthen R-R interval in the phase less than 90 and shorten R-R interval in the phase larger than 270. One may speculate, for instance, that cardiac output into ascending aorta might be counteracted in the phase shortly after lift-off of one leg producing upward acceleration of the body and might be facilitated in the phase shortly before lift-off of one leg producing downward acceleration. Such phase effect may be a factor that may contribute to changes in R-R interval and $\dot{V}O_2$.

A speculation on the phase effect from venous return is much more complex, because venous return is a time-consuming process. It might rather be possible to infer that the effect on the venous return arising at each step from vertical acceleration of the body and muscle pumps may be accumulated over many steps and that such a cumulative effect may be reflected in the cumulative R-R interval (2). However, to identify the mechanisms responsible for the entrainment and $\dot{V}O_2$ effect presently observed, precise phase effect from each relevant factor should be determined experimentally.

References

1. Bhattacharya, A., Knapp, C.F., McCutcheon, E.P., Evans, J.M. Modification of cardiac function by synchronized oscillating acceleration. J. Appl. Physiol. 47(3):612-620, 1979.

2. Bishop, V.S., Malliani, A., Thoren, P. Cardiac mechanoreceptors. In: Handbook of physiology, Section 2, Vol. 3, Part 2. 1983:497-556.

3. Nakazumi, T., Watanabe, A., Kinugawa, K., Udo, M. Entrainment of the heart beat into the running pitch during endurance running (I). Jpn. J. Phys. Fit. Sports Med. 35(6):340, 1986.

4. Norman, L., Whipp, B.J., Ward, S.A., Wasserman, K. Effect of inter-breath fluctuations on characterizing gas kinetics. J. Appl. Physiol. 62(5):2003-2012, 1987.

5. Udo, M., Watanabe, A., Nakazumi, T., Kinugawa, K. Entrainment of the heart beat into the running pitch during endurance running (II). Jpn. J. Phys. Fit. Sports Med. 35(6):341, 1986.

Biomechanical Analysis of Walking and Fitness Testing in Elderly Women

M. Kaneko, K. Fuchimoto, T. Fuchimoto, Y. Morimoto, M. Kimura, T. Kitamura, Y. Tsutsui, and T. Arai

Osaka College of Physical Education, Ibaraki, Osaka and Central Office of the Geriatric Welfare Center, Kyoto City, Japan

Aging can be characterized as a diminished capacity to regulate the internal environment (5). From a behavioral point of view walking speed might be a good measure of aging, since it declines with aging linearly (1, 2) or curvilinearly (3). However, few studies have dealt simultaneously with biomechanical analysis and fitness testing on the same population of elderly female subjects. The present study aimed to assess (a) how biomechanical parameters affect walking speed and (b) how fitness level relates to walking ability in elderly women.

Method

The subjects were 57 normal elderly females 45-82 years of age who regularly went to a senior citizens' welfare center. The subjects were grouped by age into four age groups: G-50 (48-54 years), G-60 (55-64), G-70 (65-74), and G-80 (75-82). The mean values of age, body height, and weight in each group are shown in Table 1. For measuring walking ability the subject was instructed to walk normally at a comfortable self-selected pace. Using two synchronized high-speed shutter video cameras, the side and frontal views of subjects were filmed at 30 fps, and anatomical landmarks on the selected joint axes including hip, knee, ankle, heel, and toe were recorded on magnetic tape. Biomechanical parameters were subsequently analyzed using a personal computer. Fitness testing consisted of grip strength, vertical jump, quick stepping in a sitting position, eye-closed foot balance, trunk flexion, and breath-holding time, which might represent (in order) strength, power, agility, flexibility, balance, and one aspect of endurance capacity.

Results

The biomechanical parameters measured in normal walking and the fitness test results are shown in Table 1. Percent changes in some selected walking items are drawn as a function of age in Figure 1.

Walking Speed

Walking speed (V) decreased from 1.4m/s at the age of about 50 (G-50) to 0.96m/s at G-80. Most of this decrease (76% of the total reduction) took place in the ages between G-60 and G-70 ($p < .01$). Stride length and stride rate also decreased with age, and signifi-

Table 1   Characteristics of Physique, Walking, and Fitness in Four Age Groups

Groups	G-50	G-60	G-70	G-80
Age (yr)	51.4 ± 3.1	59.9 ± 2.6	71.4 ± 2.2	77.0 ± 3.0
Height (m)	1.56 ± .06	1.52 ± .03*	1.48 ± .05**	1.46 ± .05**
Weight (kg)	55.0 ± 8.2	53.0 ± 6.4	44.3 ± 6.3**	45.4 ± 7.5*
Speed (m/s)	1.45 ± .12	1.38 ± .19	1.01 ± .17**	0.96 ± .23**
Stride length (m)	0.65 ± .05	0.61 ± .06	0.51 ± .07**	0.48 ± .08**
Stride rate (steps/s)	2.22 ± .15	2.28 ± .21	1.98 ± .19**	1.98 ± .21**
Step width (cm)	8.96 ± 3.45	8.50 ± 2.63	9.24 ± 3.59	16.0 ± 8.47*
Lateral hip D. (cm)	3.03 ± 0.93	2.60 ± 0.93	3.36 ± 1.21	3.86 ± 1.16
Toe height (swing) (cm)[a]	1.60 ± 0.58	2.09 ± 0.77	1.34 ± 0.56	1.42 ± 0.45
Toe height (front) (cm)[b]	8.98 ± 1.69	7.73 ± 2.07	6.44 ± 2.14**	5.97 ± 1.45**
Double support T. (s)	.069 ± .020	.072 ± .023	.112 ± .034**	.123 ± .033**
Swing support T. (s)	.383 ± .022	.367 ± .024	.398 ± .036	.388 ± .024
Fitness				
Grip strength (kg)	27.0 ± 4.3	22.2 ± 3.5**	18.1 ± 3.4**	17.9 ± 2.9**
Vertical jump (cm)	30.1 ± 5.8	22.8 ± 4.4**	17.7 ± 5.7**	13.4 ± 5.9**
Stepping (times/20s)[c]	32.6 ± 5.3	32.3 ± 4.4	29.7 ± 4.9	29.6 ± 3.1
Balance (s)[d]	16.8 ± 10.7	9.2 ± 6.2*	6.4 ± 5.6**	3.6 ± 2.3**
Trunk flexion (cm)	15.6 ± 7.0	9.9 ± 6.8	5.0 ± 8.0**	5.7 ± 7.8**
Breath hold (s)	41.9 ± 14.4	33.5 ± 8.8	34.1 ± 12.0	30.3 ± 9.0*

[a]The average toe height during the first half of forward foot swing. [b]The maximum toe height at the end of forward foot swing. [c]Open-close quick stepping by both feet in sitting position. [d]Standing time on one foot with closed eyes. $*p < .05$, $**p < .01$, compared to G-50. Mean ± SD.

86   Kaneko et al.

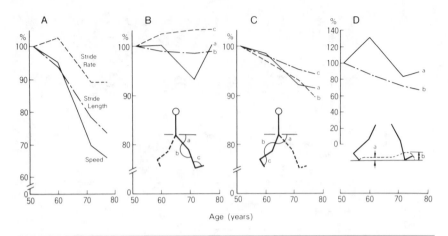

Figure 1. Relative changes (%) in four selected biomechanical parameters in walking.
A: walking speed, stride length, and stride rate. B and C: Angles in the hip, knee and ankle
joint at the end of forward foot swing (B) and at toe-off (C). D: the average height of toe during the first half period of forward foot swing (a) and the maximum height of toe just before
foot contact (b).

cant differences between age groups were quite similar to those observed in walking speed
(see Table 1). Percent decrements in Figure 1A suggest that a decrease in stride length
(30% reduction from G-50 to G-80) played a greater role in the speed reduction than it
did in stride rate reduction (−10%).

Leg Joint Movement

The maximum range of leg joint displacement during walking showed as much as a 10%
decrease with age in both the hip and knee, whereas twice the reduction (20%) took place
in the ankle joint. This reduction was attributable to progressively decreasing joint angles
at the instance of toe-off with advancing age, as the joint angles at the end of forward
foot swing did not show much decrease (Figure 1B and C). The angular velocity of ankle
plantar flexion during the kicking phase decreased from 4.22 to 2.57 rad/s ($p < .01$). This
reduction was twice as large as that seen at the hip or knee joints. Average height of the
toe during the first half of forward foot swing decreased slightly: 1.6 cm and 1.4 cm for
G-50 and G-80, respectively. On the other hand, the maximum height of toes at the end
of forward foot swing has shown a significant decrease between G-50 to G-80 ($p < .01$),
9.0-6.0 cm on the average (see Table 1 and Figure 1D).

Foot Movement

One complete step cycle can be divided into double support phase (DS) and single support
phase (SS). The duration of these two phases combined increased significantly ($p < .01$)
between G-60 and G-70, resulting in a slower stride rate. Percent of DS in one step cycle,
however, tended to increase linearly with age despite a concomitant decrease in SS (see
Figure 2).

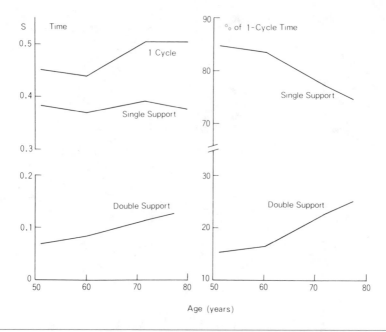

Figure 2. Changes in the duration (time) of one complete cycle, single support phase, and double support phase. Right frame indicates relative changes in percent of one complete cycle· in walking.

Lateral Movement

A three-dimensional film analysis of the frontal view revealed that the lateral distance between right and left toes (step width) did not change up to G-70 and increased significantly at the eldest age ($p < .05$). Lateral hip displacement tended to increase after G-60 but not significantly.

Fitness Level

As shown in Table 1, significant reductions with age were observed in grip strength, vertical jump, and foot balance ($p < .01$). The items related to neuromuscular functions showed high correlation with selected biomechanical parameters in walking such as speed, stride length, stride rate, and the height of toe at the end of foot swing forward (see Table 2). Double support time was also correlated negatively and significantly to most of the fitness items.

Discussion

Walking speed (V) showed a marked decline after about the age of 60, agreeing well with the results reported by Himann et al. (3), who demonstrated a curvilinear decline in a

88 Kaneko et al.

Table 2 Correlation Between Physical Fitness and Biomechanical Parameters in Walking

	Grip strength	Vertical jump	Stepping	Foot balance	Trunk flex.	Breath hold.
Speed	0.646***	0.712***	0.486***	0.546***	0.357**	0.264*
Stride length	0.659***	0.747***	0.458***	0.517***	0.413**	0.343**
Stride rate	0.377**	0.411**	0.351**	0.359**	0.182	0.040
Stride width	0.145	0.338*	0.103	0.239	0.229	0.264
Lateral hip D.	0.212	0.215	0.115	0.203	0.213	0.010
Toe height (swing)	0.437***	0.538***	0.311*	0.301*	0.419**	0.223
Toe height (front)	0.192	0.387**	0.153	0.143	0.178	0.021
Double support T.	−0.468***	−0.473***	−0.303***	−0.563***	−0.506***	−0.225
Single support T.	−0.076	−0.112	−0.038	−0.105	−0.151	−0.106

*$p < .05$, ** $p < .01$, *** $p < .001$.

cubic fashion and the existence of a "critical age" at 62 years. Stride length (SL) and stride rate (SR) decreased similarly to the reduction in V. However, the rate of reduction was greater in SL than in SR, suggesting that the V reduction might be affected more strongly by SL. Body height (H), which decreased significantly with age, might also affect V and SL reduction. However, significant decreases in the ratios of V/H and SL/H suggest that the speed reduction reflects not only an anatomical change but also a functional degeneration due to age.

Among possible factors to effect a reduction in SL, it should be particularly emphasized that the angles in the hip, knee, and ankle joints at toe-off decreased considerably. A marked decrease in the angular velocity of ankle planter flextion at toe-off should also be noted. Murray et al. (4) characterized aged men as having shorter double support times (DS) than young men. In the present study DS was less than single support time (SS) at every age examined, and the slowing down of SR was due to lengthened times of both DS and SS. However, an increase in the time of DS in advancing age implies that elderly people have more difficulty supporting the body on one foot in walking. This might be due to increased instability as indicated by the foot balance test (see Table 1). Bassey et al. (1) have shown a significant correlation between walking speed and standardized heart rate during bicycling in elderly men. Likewise, the fitness levels tested suggest that reduced neuromuscular function may account for the aging process in the various biomechanical parameters in normal walking, as most of the fitness items of the aged were found to be highly correlated with walking ability.

Conclusion

In the aging process, the speed of normal walking declines with a concomitant reduction of stride length and of stride rate. These changes are particularly remarkable after about the age of 60. A decrement in joint displacement and a lengthened single support time appear to be responsible for reducing stride length and stride rate. A close relationship between biomechanical parameters in walking and fitness level suggests that walking speed at one's self-selected pace may be a good measure of the aging process.

References

1. Bassey, E.J., Fentem, P.H., MacDonald, I.C., Scriven, P.M. Self-paced walking as a method for exercise testing in elderly and young men. Clin. Sci. Molec. Med. 51:609-612, 1976.

2. Cunningham, D.A., Rechnitzer, P.A., Pearce, M.E., Donner, A.P. Determinants of self-selected walking pace across ages 19-66. J. Gerontol. 37:560-564, 1982.

3. Himann, J.E., Cunningham, D.A., Rechnitzer, P.A., Paterson, D.H. Age-related changes in speed of walking. Med. Sci. Sports Exer. 20:161-166, 1988.

4. Murray, M.P., Kory, R.C., Clarkson, B.H. Walking patterns in healthy old men. J. Gerontol. 24:169-178, 1969.

5. Shephard, R.J. Physical activity and aging. Croom Helm: London & Sydney, 1987:1-15.

Physical Work Capacity and Body Composition of Japanese Females With Special Reference to Age

K. Iwanaga, T. Koba, and Y. Fukuba

Saga Research Institute, Otsuka Pharmaceutical Co., Ltd., Saga and Department of Biometrics, Research Institute for Nuclear Medicine and Biology, Hiroshima University, Hiroshima, Japan

In 1964, Wasserman and McIlroy (7) proposed the concept of anaerobic threshold (AT), and since then the adequacy of this parameter has been evaluated as an indicator of oxydation by the muscle. Although not yet fully elucidated, some works have suggested that AT falls with aging at a slower rate than does $\dot{V}O_2$max. In addition to these two important parameters regarding work performance, body fat is a reliable overall indicator of changing lifestyle of individuals reflecting current dietary and working or exercise habits. Body fat is also important in view of social problems of obesity. However, no standard value for fat content has been set for Japanese yet. This study was designed to evaluate age-related changes in physical work capacity and body composition of Japanese women in a cross-sectional manner.

Methods

Seventy-five Japanese females age 16-57 years participated as subjects in this study. No exclusion criteria, including histories of sports and other activities, were set in order to randomly recruit subjects. Exercise performance was determined by an incremental workload test using a bicycle ergometer. Workload was zero initially and then increased at 25 W every 2 min. The subjects received an explanation on the purpose and nature of the study prior to inclusion and were informed that they were able to voluntarily stop the test on exhaustion. The physiological monitoring utilized a mixing chamber method to determine variables including oxygen uptake ($\dot{V}O_2$), and heart rate (HR) on ECG at about 10-s intervals. The values obtained were used to calculate $\dot{V}O_2$max, maximum heart rate (HRmax), and ventilatory threshold (VT). VT was identified as the $\dot{V}O_2$ level corresponding to the minimum point on a statistical curve plotting $VE/\dot{V}O_2$ vs. $\dot{V}O_2$. VT data were obtained from 64 of 75 subjects tested. VT was not obtained in the other 11 because the $VE/\dot{V}O_2$ curve did not show a minimum. Body density was measured by an underwater weighing technique in all subjects, and the percent body fat (%Fat) was estimated according to Brožek et al. (2). Lung residual volume was determined with neon gas according to a closed circuit method at the time of underwater weighing. In addition, skinfold thickness was measured at the chest, rear upper arm, subscapla, iliac, abdomen, and front thigh.

Results and Findings

Table 1 lists mean and standard deviation (in parenthesis) of values obtained for each age group. Age group did not have an influence on the variables of height (Ht), lean body

Table 1   Physical Characteristics of Study Population

	Age (yr)					
	10-19	20-29	30-39	40-49	50-59	ANOVA
n	2	32	17	15	9	
Age (yr)	17.0	25.1	35.1	42.3	52.2	**
	(1.4)	(2.0)	(3.2)	(2.5)	(2.1)	
Wt (kg)	47.88	53.48	51.86	56.76	60.12	**
	(1.33)	(8.33)	(4.71)	(7.62)	(12.58)	
Ht (cm)	154.8	158.3	157.8	156.0	156.3	ns
	(1.1)	(4.5)	(5.5)	(4.1)	(5.5)	
%Fat	23.1	27.4	26.3	30.6	35.7	**
	(6.0)	(7.1)	(4.0)	(5.8)	(4.8)	
LBM (kg)	36.83	38.55	38.20	41.12	38.43	ns
	(1.85)	(4.90)	(4.01)	(8.21)	(7.01)	
$\dot{V}O_2$max	1.85	1.76	1.69	1.58	1.51	ns
(L $\cdot$ min^{-1})	(0.30)	(0.45)	(0.43)	(0.28)	(0.33)	
$\dot{V}O_2$max/Wt	38.7	33.1	32.6	28.0	25.7	**
(ml $\cdot$ kg^{-1} $\cdot$ min^{-1})	(7.3)	(7.9)	(7.8)	(4.8)	(6.2)	
HRmax	186.0	166.6	162.4	161.7	151.4	**
(beats $\cdot$ min^{-1})	(5.7)	(10.7)	(11.5)	(12.5)	(19.5)	
VT; $\dot{V}O_2$max	1.01	0.98[a]	1.00[b]	0.94[c]	0.87[d]	ns
(L $\cdot$ min^{-1})	(0.31)	(0.25)	(0.24)	(0.17)	(0.09)	
VT; $\dot{V}O_2$/Wt	21.2	18.6[a]	19.6[b]	16.3[c]	15.6[d]	ns
(ml $\cdot$ kg^{-1} $\cdot$ min^{-1})	(7.1)	(4.8)	(4.7)	(3.6)	(3.4)	
VT; %$\dot{V}O_2$max	54.1	56.0[a]	58.5[b]	56.3[c]	60.5[d]	ns
(%)	(8.2)	(9.1)	(9.7)	(7.1)	(15.1)	

[a]$n = 30$, [b]$n = 14$, [c]$n = 12$, [d]$n = 6$. **$p < .01$.

mean (LBM), and $\dot{V}O_2$max when determined by one-way analysis of variance. The HR max tended to be low, especially for 20- and 30-year-olds as compared to values in the literature (1). Possibly they stopped the test before reaching exhaustion; thus, $\dot{V}O_2$max might have been under the level estimated. It is, however, practically impossible to accurately determine the physiological limit in those who do not have a habit of daily physical exercise, and this may be particularly true in women and middle-aged or elderly individuals. Since this presents a problem in measurement from the clinical stand point, use of the data from this report as symptom-limiting maximums may be quite significant.

Table 2 shows correlation coefficients obtained between age and variables. The skin-fold thickness was expressed as a total of the six locations measured. Body weight (Wt) tended to increase with age as an intrinsic change, but regression was not statistically significant. Percent fat and skinfold thickness (SKF) showed a definite positive correlation with age (see Table 2 and Figure 1). These findings suggest that body fat increases even in cases in which body weight does not increase with age, and subcutaneous fat was a major contributory factor to the increase in %Fat. In fact, Forbes and Reina (4) presented longitudinal data on the decrease in LBM without body weight decrease in elderly people.

Table 2   Correlation Coefficients of Variables on Age

Ht	0.058	$\dot{V}O_2max$	−0.265*
Wt	0.223	$\dot{V}O_2max/Wt$	−0.378**
%Fat	0.381**	HRmax	−0.417**
LBM	−0.017	VT; $\dot{V}O_2$	−0.136
SKF	0.314**	VT; $\dot{V}O_2/Wt$	−0.212
		VT; $\%\dot{V}O_2max$	0.178

SKF = Skinfold thickness, *$p < .05$, **$p < .01$.

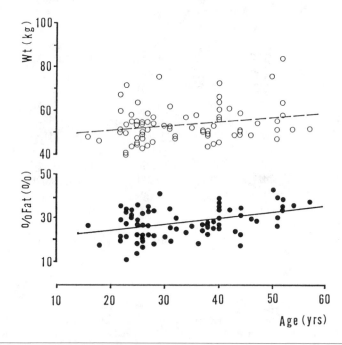

Figure 1. Body weight (Wt) and percent body fat (%Fat) to age ($n = 75$). Regression of Wt on age is described by the equation: Wt = 0.184 age + 48.181; $r = .223$, $p > .05$. Regression of %Fat on age is described by the equation: %Fat = 0.25 age + 20.21; $r = .381$, $p < .01$.

The aerobic work capacity index, $\dot{V}O_2max$ and HRmax, definitely fell with age, but VT changes were not dependent on age (see Table 2 and Figure 2). Posner et al. (6) investigated changes in $\dot{V}O_2max$ and VT in 68 male and 104 female subjects age 20-80 years and observed a significant age-related negative correlation. Reduction over a year in $\dot{V}O_2max$ was estimated to be 20.61 ml • min^{-1} and that in VT to be 4.98 ml • min^{-1}, indicating aging had less influence on VT than on $\dot{V}O_2max$. The reason for the different effect of aging has not been explained, but muscle fiber composition seems to change with age.

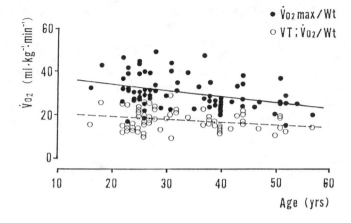

Figure 2. Maximum oxygen uptake ($\dot{V}O_2$max/Wt) and ventilatory threshold (VT;$\dot{V}O_2$/Wt) to age ($n = 64$). Regression of $\dot{V}O_2$max/Wt on age is described by the equation: $\dot{V}O_2$max/Wt$= -0.28$ age $+ 40.81$; $r = .378$, $p < .01$. Regression of VT on age is described by the equation: VT $= -0.101$ age $+ 21.490$, $r = -.212$, $p > .05$.

As aging proceeds, fast-twitch muscle fibers of skeletal muscle are lost, but aerobic slow-twitch muscle fibers do not decrease (5), and so VT as an indicator of oxidative capacity of muscle tissue might not have given age-related values.

Percent muscle fibers were not determined in the present study; however, the lack of correlation between LBM and age was thought to indicate that muscle amount remained essentially constant during the aging process, supporting insignificant alterations in VT. $\dot{V}O_2$max correlates with overall oxygen transporting capacity of the heart and other circulatory systems. When maximum cardiac output declines due to reduced HRmax or stroke volume, $\dot{V}O_2$max falls with age (6). Although the age–circulatory efficiency relationship has not been clarified yet, an obvious decrease in normal everyday activity after middle age could be one of the probable reasons for reduced function of the circulatory system (3).

Conclusion

Percent fat increases even in cases in which body weight does not increase with age, and subcutaneous fat is a major contributory factor for the increase in %Fat. $\dot{V}O_2$max and HRmax definitely fall with age, but VT changes are not dependent on age.

References

1. Åstrand, P.-O., Rodahl, K. Textbook of work physiology. New York: McGraw-Hill, 1970.

2. Brožek, J., Grande, F., Anderson, J.T., Keys, A. Densitometric analysis of body composition: revision of some quantitative assumptions. Ann. N.Y. Acad. Sci. 110:113-140, 1963.

3. Cunningham, D.A., Nancekievill, E.A., Paterson, D.H., Donner, A.P., Rechnitzer, P.A. Ventilation threshold and aging. J. Gerontol. 40:703-707, 1985.

4. Forbes, G.B., Reina, J.C. Adult lean body mass declines with age: some longitudinal observations. Metabolism 19:653-663, 1970.

5. Larsson, L. Morphological and functional characteristics of the aging skeletal muscle in man: a cross-sectional study. Acta Physiol. Scand. Suppl. 457, 1978

6. Posner, J.D., Gorman, K.M., Klein, H.S., Cline, C.J. Ventilatory threshold: measurement and variation with age. J. Appl. Physiol. 63:1519-1525, 1987.

7. Wasserman, K., McIlroy, M.B. Detecting the threshold of anaerobic metabolism in cardiac patients during exercise. Am. J. Cardiol. 14:844-852, 1964.

Effect of Habitual Exercise on Blood Pressure Response in Middle-Aged Women

A. Noji, R. Yanagibori, K. Aoki, Y. Suzuki, and A. Gunji

Department of Health Administration, Faculty of Medicine, University of Tokyo, Japan

For the prevention of aged men's cardiovascular disease, it is important to get a reliable predictor for the development of essential hypertension before one reaches middle age. In Japan, cardiovascular disease has been the number one factor in the death rate, which was 37% in 1985, and circulatory disease has been the highest in the prevalence rate. In both cases, hypertension is one of the main factors. And also, hypertension itself has been the most prevalent disease and also the most demanding on the medical budget.

Hypertension is thought to be caused when a person with a mediate hereditary disposition has been exposed to many harmful environmental factors (6, 9). However habitual physical exercise appears to possibly prevent and treat essential hypertension. Some recent reports have suggested that low intensity physical training lowers the level of blood pressure (4, 7, 8, 11, 12). But habitual physical exercise has still not been clearly proven to prevent the development of hypertension.

Classifying the response of blood pressure with increasing exercise intensity is one of the methods for predicting hypertension (5). In this study we have investigated the effect of habitual exercise on blood pressure response in normotensive middle-aged women.

Methods

Twenty-two normotensive women 34-50 years old, averaging 42 years old, were studied (see Table 1). They were divided into two groups: a high fitness group (Group HF) of 12 women who habitually engaged in sports such as swimming and jogging and a sedentary group (Group S) of 10 women. Each member of Group HF had been doing over 20 min of exercise more than three-times a week.

$\dot{V}O_2$max estimated (1) by means of substitution of HRmax in a regression equation between HR and $\dot{V}O_2$ during exercise with four different work intensities was 43.8ml/min/kg in Group HF and 35.2ml/min/kg in Group S, the difference of which was statistically significant ($p < .05$).

The variables measured are presented in Table 2. Height, weight, and skinfold (3, 10) were measured with all of the subjects at the beginning of the test. Family history, medical history, daily activity, and habitual exercise were recorded during interviews. Family history consists of the record of the disease or death of hypertension and/or cardiovascular disease in the second degree.

Exercise was performed with a Monark bicycle ergometer in an upright position. Pedal frequency was 50rpm continuously. Starting from 300kgm/min, exercise intensity was gradually increased with 75kgm/min every 4 min until it finally reached 525kgm/min in 16 min. Therefore, there were four different degrees of work intensity.

Table 1   Characteristics of Subjects

Variable	High fitness group	Sedentary group	t-test
n	12	10	
Age (yr)	43.1 ± 5.3	41.2 ± 5.5	ns
Height (cm)	157.8 ± 6.2	154.4 ± 5.2	ns
Weight (kg)	54.0 ± 4.2	52.4 ± 6.7	ns
%Fat (%)	28.3 ± 6.1	27.8 ± 6.5	ns
LBM (kg)	39.9 ± 4.8	37.5 ± 3.3	ns
$\dot{V}O_2$max/BW	43.8 ± 8.9	35.2 ± 4.5	$p < .05$
Rest			
SBP (mmHg)	115.7 ± 10.5	111.2 ± 9.2	ns
DBP_s (mmHg)	75.0 ± 8.7	72.2 ± 8.1	ns
HR (bpm)	65.8 ± 7.7	75.2 ± 13.8	ns

Table 2   Measurement Variables

Physique
  Height
  Weight
  Skinfold

Interview
  Family history
  Medical history
  Daily activity
  Habitual exercise

Rest and exercise
  Systolic blood pressure (SBP)
  Diastolic blood pressure (DBP)
  Heart rate (HR)
  Oxygen uptake ($\dot{V}O_2$)
  Max oxygen uptake ($\dot{V}O_2$max) (estimate)

Blood pressure was measured after 15 min rest in the upright position on the ergometer and during exercise (every 4 min) using the auscultation method with a Riva-Rocci mercury manometer. Diastolic pressure corresponds to Korotokoff Phase 4. All of the blood pressure measurements were carried out by the same investigator.

Heart rate was indicated continuously by electrocardiogram. And heart rate in the last 10 s of each work intensity degree was recorded to represent each degree. Expired gas was collected in a Douglas bag for 5 min in resting after 10 min rest and for 1 min during exercise at the last 1 min of each work intensity degree. Volume of the gas was measured by a standard dry gas meter. A sample of the gas was analyzed by a Shorunder microgas analyzer. Data were analyzed using the central computer of Tokyo University, HITAC M680 (VOS3).

Results

Blood pressure response to resting and four work loads in pedaling exercise is presented in Figure 1. In both Group HF and Group S, systolic blood pressure regularly increased with each intensity load, while diastolic blood pressure increased slightly during exercise. However, Group HF tended to have lower systolic and diastolic blood pressure during exercise than Group S.

The difference in systolic blood pressure increment was indicated by its increment ratio against the increment while resting. The difference of systolic blood pressure increment

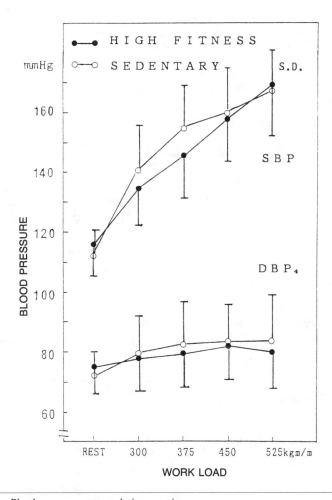

Figure 1. Blood pressure response during exercise.

ratio of the two groups is presented in Table 3. In Group HF, the systolic blood pressure increment ratio increased from 15.9% to 46.3%, while the ratio for Group S increased from 25.9% to 49.8%. At the lowest and second load, Group HF showed a significantly lower systolic blood pressure increment ratio than did Group S.

Coefficient variation of systolic blood pressure increment ratio at each work load with all subjects was 0.49, 0.35, 0.24, and 0.16 at each work load. An individual difference was distinguished at the lowest work load. Among 17 subjects who had a family history of hypertension and/or cardiovascular disease in second degree, 8 were in Group HF and 9 were in Group S. The systolic blood pressure increment ratio at the lowest work load shown just by the subjects with family history in each group was 15.8% in Group HF and 27.3% in Group S, the difference of which was statistically significant.

Analysis of variance test on systolic blood pressure increment ratio is presented in Table 4. Habitual exercise and family history were examined. Correlations between the systolic blood pressure increment ratio and habitual exercise were statistically significant. But there was no significant correlation between the systolic blood pressure increment ratio and family history.

Discussion

In this study, active women in their daily lives showed significantly higher $\dot{V}O_2$max compared with inactive women who have no exercise habit. The intensity of physical activities

Table 3   SBP Increment Ratio During Exercise

	%		
	High fitness	Sedentary	t-test
300 kgm/min	15.9 ± 6.4	25.9 ± 10.8	$p < .05$
375 kgm/min	25.5 ± 7.9	38.9 ± 10.2	$p < .05$
450 kgm/min	36.3 ± 8.6	43.5 ± 9.4	ns
525 kgm/min	46.3 ± 7.3	49.8 ± 8.3	ns

Table 4   Analysis of Variance Test on SBP Increment Ratio

Source of variation	Sum of squares	DF	Mean square	F	p
H. exercise ($\dot{V}O_1$)	547.8	1	547.8	7.4	$p < .05$
Family history ($\dot{V}O_2$)	42.2	1	42.2	0.5	ns
$\dot{V}O_1$ by $\dot{V}O_2$	136.9	1	136.9	1.9	ns
Within cells	1331.1	18	73.9		
Total	2058.0	21			

other than exercise they practice was almost same between the two groups. The higher $\dot{V}O_2$max in active women, therefore, can be attributable to their exercise habit. Hypertensive patients or normotensive persons with mediate hereditary disposition show an exaggerated rise of blood pressure during exercise (2, 5, 13).

In this study, the ratios of pressure rise against the resting pressure observed at rather lower work loads (300kgm/min and 375kgm/min) were significantly lower in active women than in inactive women. Examining 17 women (8 active women and 9 inactive women) who were defined to have a hereditary disposition of hypertension, the higher activity group showed a lower response of pressure rise ratio than the inactive group. These results suggest that habitual exercise is more influential in weakening the pressure rise caused by mild exercise than is a predisposition to hypertension as defined by family history.

Conclusion

1. Those who practiced habitual exercise more than three times a week showed higher $\dot{V}O_2$max than those who had no habit.
2. Active women showed a lower pressure response to mild exercise load than inactive women.
3. The effect of habitual exercise on mitigation of the pressure rise caused by a mild work load was greater than the hereditary predisposition to hypertension as defined by family history.
4. These results suggest that habitual exercise may contribute to preventing the development of hypertension among those who have a hereditary predisposition to hypertension.

References

1. American College of Sports Medicine. Guidelines for graded exercise testing and exercise prescription. Philadelphia: Lea & Febiger, 1980.

2. Amery, A., et al. Influence of hypertension on the hemodynamic response to exercise. Circulation 36:231, 1967.

3. Brozek, J., et al. Densitometric analysis of body composition: revision of some quantitative assumptions. Ann. N.Y. Acad. Sci. 110:113, 1963.

4. Choquette, G., Ferguson, R.J. Blood pressure reduction in borderline hypertensives following physical training. Can. Med. Assoc. J. 108:699, 1973.

5. Dlin, R.A., et al. Follow-up of normotensive men with exaggerated blood pressure response to exercise. Am. Heart J. 106:316, 1983.

6. Gross, F., et al. Management of arterial hypertension. Geneva: WHO, 1984.

7. Hanson, J.S., Nedde, W.H. Preliminary observations on physical training for hypertensive males. Cir. Res. 27(Suppl. 1):49, 1970.

8. Krotkiewski, M., et al. Effects of long-term physical training on body fat, metabolism and blood pressure in obesity. Metabolism 28:650, 1979.

9. Mcilhany, M.L., et al. The heritability of blood pressure: an investigation of 200 pairs of twins using the cold pressor test. Johns Hopkins Med. J. 136:57, 1975.

10. Nagamine, S., Suzuki, S. Anthropometry and body composition of Japanese young men and women. Human Biol. 36:8, 1964.

11. Ressl, J., et al. Hemodynamic effects of physical training in essential hypertension. Acta Cardiol. 32:121, 1977.

12. Roman, O., et al. Physical training program in arterial hypertension: a long-term prospective follow-up. Cardiology 67:230, 1981.

13. Sannersteds, R. Hemodynamic response to exercise in patients with arterial hypertension. Acta Med. Scand. 458(Suppl.):7, 1966.

Relationship Between Physical Fitness and Body Composition in Aging of Japanese Women

S. Torikoshi, K. Yokozawa, and Y. Sato

Tokyo Women's Christian University and Ochanomizu Women's University, Tokyo, Japan

As aging advances, habitual physical activity—and thus physical fitness—decreases; for example, maximum oxygen uptake ($\dot{V}O_2$max) would be associated with a diminished rate of activity. Results of inactivity include a deterioration of body composition as body fat increases and a decrease in muscle mass despite increasing body weight. Increased body fat would also become one of the risk factors of adult diseases. In the present study, Japanese women in a wide range were investigated for relationship between physical fitness, body composition, arterial pressure, and aging. The results given stimulate interest in body fat as a factor influencing $\dot{V}O_2$max and arterial pressure.

Methods

Ninety-two Japanese women who were randomly selected and who volunteered were studied. Items of measurement are shown in Table 1. Average ages and body sizes of the subjects are shown in Table 2. On questioning they described their daily lifestyles and we recorded their positive physical exercise frequency. Body composition was estimated by means of the body density determined from body weight in water (4) and functional residual air volume calculated depending on vital capacity (7). Skinfolds of 12 points measured by a caliper were averaged and their value was termed as mean skinfold (MSF) (see Figure 1). General fitness tests were performed by sufficient methods standardized by the Japanese Education Ministry. $\dot{V}O_2$max was directly measured by the Douglas bag method in treadmill running with increasing work loads. However, for some subjects over 50 years old who were not accustomed to positive physical activity or who had near hypertension, a direct measurement of $\dot{V}O_2$max was avoided. An indirect method to determine

Table 1 Measurement Items

Lifestyle	Daily physical activity, dietary habits, and habitual exercise (frequency)
Physique	Height, weight, body composition (fat volume, lean body mass), skinfold (12 points), and circumference (11 points)
Physical fitness	Maximum oxygen uptake, blood pressure, side step, back and grip strength, vertical jump, and standing trunk flexion

$\dot{V}O_2$max was applied to them so they performed 3-4 work loads of submaximal treadmill running. During exercise, oxygen uptake ($\dot{V}O_2$) and heart rate (HR) were measured and then a regression equation was taken out from a relationship between the $\dot{V}O_2$ and HR. Further, maximal HR (HRmax) estimated by a regression, HRmax $= 220 -$ Age (1), was substituted for the regression equation, and the value of $\dot{V}O_2$ calculated was concluded as $\dot{V}O_2$max. Systolic (SAP) and diastolic blood pressures (DAP) were taken by the auscultatory method.

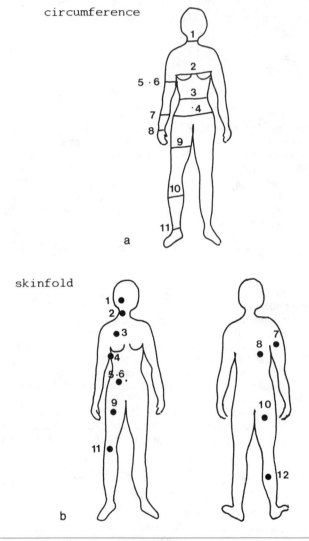

Figure 1. Anthropometric measurements: (a) circumference—neck (1), chest (2), abdominal (3), hip (4), upper arm extention (5), upper arm flexion (6), forearm (7), wrist (8), thigh (9), calf (10), ankle (11). (b) skinfold—cheek (1), neck (2), chest (3), side chest (4), abdominal-vertical (5), abdominal-horizontal (6), upper arm (7), back (8), thigh front (9), thigh back (10), knee (11), calf (12).

Table 2   Results of Physical Characteristics

Age (yr)	n	Height (cm)		Weight (kg)		Fat (%)		LBM (kg)		Mean of skinfold (mm)	
10-14	5	152.3	6.85	47.3	5.81	22.7	1.95	36.6	4.07	18.2	2.37
15-19	10	160.0	4.46	53.2	9.01	24.2	4.87	40.0	4.87	19.0	3.27
20-24	9	159.8	4.26	50.4	4.81	22.3	3.99	39.2	3.88	16.8	4.33
25-29	10	160.7	4.41	54.8	5.19	25.9	5.92	40.5	4.84	15.5	3.66
30-34	7	160.8	6.76	54.6	5.71	28.6	4.09	39.1	4.47	16.1	4.09
35-39	6	154.7	2.59	50.5	5.83	31.7	6.20	34.5	3.23	18.3	3.50
40-44	14	157.2	3.88	51.5	4.52	28.6	4.21	36.7	3.11	18.1	3.49
45-49	8	156.6	7.35	55.2	4.13	31.9	3.73	37.0	2.52	16.8	2.62
50-54	10	155.6	4.88	51.7	7.27	32.9	3.89	34.8	4.35	17.9	5.84
55-59	8	155.7	4.61	54.0	3.76	35.1	3.80	35.4	1.19	20.9	3.43
60-64	5	155.5	5.71	59.4	10.82	39.3	2.66	36.1	7.21	23.2	8.07

Age (yr)	n	Chest (cm)		Abdominal (cm)		Hip (cm)		Upper arm (cm)		Thigh (cm)	
10-14	5	78.3	5.27	67.9	4.32	80.7	3.41	23.5	1.48	49.8	2.98
15-19	10	82.5	6.63	64.4	6.99	80.5	8.22	25.5	2.22	51.5	3.37
20-24	9	80.5	4.78	62.1	3.03	81.6	5.70	23.4	1.38	50.3	4.01
25-29	10	82.1	4.19	65.8	4.92	84.5	2.99	25.9	1.99	50.4	9.60
30-34	7	83.2	4.94	65.8	4.50	81.6	3.28	25.7	2.38	53.9	3.36
35-39	6	80.9	6.67	65.4	3.02	81.8	5.07	24.6	1.15	50.5	3.98
40-44	14	83.6	4.08	67.1	4.62	83.0	5.67	25.7	1.86	49.0	4.26
45-49	8	84.8	5.10	69.6	5.68	86.1	5.31	26.8	1.45	51.6	2.90
50-54	10	83.0	7.21	69.4	7.38	84.9	6.10	25.9	2.88	49.4	3.66
55-59	8	87.4	2.02	71.1	4.80	88.0	3.82	26.2	1.31	49.6	2.59
60-64	5	91.2	16.31	78.1	13.82	93.6	12.92	28.1	4.81	53.5	5.48

Note. Mean ± *SD*.

Results and Discussion

At each age, body height (Ht) and weight (Wt) were little bit greater in the present subjects than in average Japanese women, but not significantly different. As shown in Table 3, exercise frequency in their lifestyle was relatively higher, because about 64% had exercise habits, and performed positive exercise more than one time per week. Further, while persons

Table 3   Exercise Frequency

Age (yr)	n	Frequency				
		0	M1	W1	W2	W3
10-14	5	0	0	1	0	4
15-19	10	1	0	5	4	0
20-24	9	4	1	2	0	2
25-29	10	5	0	1	0	4
30-34	7	4	0	1	1	1
35-39	6	1	1	2	1	1
40-44	14	2	2	3	0	7
45-49	8	4	0	2	1	1
50-54	10	2	1	5	0	2
55-59	8	1	2	3	1	1
60-64	5	2	0	1	1	1
Total	92	26	7	26	9	24
Ratio	100%	28.3%	7.6%	28.3%	9.8%	26.0%

without exercise habits were about 28%, 26% of the subjects had performed exercise over three times per week. The percentage of body fat (%F) was found to average between 22 and 25% for subjects in their teens and 20s, which were almost the same results as those for the previous study (5). As age was increased, %F gradually increased to more than 30% at over 45 years old. In contrast to %F, lean body mass (LBM) had a decreasing tendency with age over 35 years old. MSF showed the bottom value in the 20s and then increased to reach the highest in the 60s. This tendency was almost the same as that of %F. Circumferences combined with skinfold clearly increased in the chest, abdominal, and hip with increasing age over 45 years old. These facts indicate that increasing body fat in middle-aged women is mainly stored in the trunk part of the body.

In a general fitness test, muscle strength was observed by back (BS) and hand grip strength (HGS) (see Table 4). Developing BS reached the peak at the first half of the 20s, and it showed a gradually decreasing tendency as age increased. Vertical jump (VJ), which indicated the power of the lower limbs, lowered from the peak given during the first half of the teens as age increased. HGS developed until the first half of the 40s with aging and then decreased, but the changing rate was within about +10%. The results suggest that the combined muscle strength of trunk part and lower limb decreases above middle age, but the upper limb strength is mostly maintained even in middle age.

$\dot{V}O_2$max per Wt showed the peak at the first half of the teens, 50.4 ml/kg/min, and then gradually decreased to below 50% of the peak, 21.2 ml/kg/min, during the 60s. At each stage of age, the averaged $\dot{V}O_2$max/wt presented was a little bit higher than it was in Japanese women reported by the previous study (6), but the values were almost the same as those in Swedish (3) and American women (2). Probably, because over 70% of our subjects were active women, the $\dot{V}O_2$max given should be higher than for sedentary Japanese women. $\dot{V}O_2$max/LBM was not so different between the range of age from the latter half of the teens to the first half of the 50s, while the peak, 65.2 ml/LBM kg/min,

Table 4 Results of Physical Fitness

Age (yr)	n	VO₂max L/min		ml/Wtkg/min		ml/LBMkg/min		SAP (mmHg)		DAP (mmHg)	
10-14	5	2.39	0.33	50.4	1.4	65.2	2.3	99	12	60	6
15-19	10	2.13	0.21	40.1	3.7	53.5	4.5	103	7	63	8
20-24	9	2.05	0.24	40.6	4.0	53.2	5.5	101	9	66	11
25-29	10	2.16	0.32	39.4	4.3	53.4	4.5	104	6	67	9
30-34	7	2.02	0.31	37.3	6.9	52.3	7.9	103	14	61	13
35-39	6	1.83	0.26	36.2	6.1	53.0	8.2	99	8	68	5
40-44	14	1.90	0.25	36.8	4.5	51.7	4.7	108	7	72	11
45-49	8	2.01	0.29	36.8	5.6	54.2	6.9	113	7	70	5
50-54	10	1.80	0.23	35.3	5.8	52.9	7.1	128	22	82	12
55-59	8	1.58	0.19	28.7	4.1	46.6	5.4	107	18	76	14
60-64	5	1.26	0.29	21.2	4.7	34.9	8.6	144	53	88	25

Age (yr)	n	Vital capacity (cc)		Back strength (kg)		Grip strength (kg)		Vertical jump (cm)	
10-14	5	2808	491	82.0	24.9	25.0	2.1	51.6	8.6
15-19	10	2808	406	89.7	18.7	27.4	3.9	45.5	9.7
20-24	9	3457	509	92.7	23.2	29.3	5.5	41.3	4.8
25-29	10	3112	537	98.8	23.9	30.8	5.0	44.8	5.2
30-34	7	3297	474	82.7	11.4	30.0	2.9	39.9	6.7
35-39	6	2633	497	86.3	14.2	29.7	5.2	36.0	5.4
40-44	14	2784	279	87.7	14.3	31.5	4.2	37.2	6.9
45-49	8	2790	254	89.8	16.3	31.9	3.7	37.1	6.5
50-54	10	2606	474	88.8	19.8	31.1	3.7	32.3	4.9
55-59	8	2662	392	74.6	14.8	26.9	4.1	32.9	4.4
60-64	5	2200	271	74.2	15.5	27.7	5.8	24.0	4.7

Note. Mean ± SD.

was given during the first half of the teens (see Table 4). These results suggest that $\dot{V}O_2max$/wt decreased as age increased depending on the increase in body fat. Both SAP and DAP increased with age and they increased significantly during the late 30s (see Table 4). As using all of the data given, %F and fat volume (FV) were significantly correlated to MSF, $\dot{V}O_2max$, $\dot{V}O_2max$/wt, SAP, and DAP, respectively (see Table 5). It is very important that $\dot{V}O_2max$/wt was inversely correlated to %F and FV with high correlation coefficients. Also, it is a very significant finding that $\dot{V}O_2max$/wt, SAP, and DAP were more significantly correlated to FV compared with %F.

Table 5   Correlation Coefficients

v.s.	Mean of skinfold	$\dot{V}O_2$max (ml/wt)	SAP	DAP
%Fat	0.524	−0.729	0.421	0.423
Fat	0.620	−0.766	0.562	0.544

$p < .001.$

Conclusion

From the above results, we conclude that the high FV and %F are very important risk factors related to positive physical activity, because aerobic power is decreased and blood pressure is increased by increasing FV and %F with increasing age. Further, FV is a more important risk factor compared with %F.

References

1. American College of Sports Medicine. Guidelines for graded exercise testing and exercise prescription. 2nd ed. Lea & Febiger, 1980.

2. American Heart Association, Committee on Exercise. Exercise testing and training of apparently healthy individuals: a handbook for physicians. Chicago: AMA, 1972.

3. Åstrand, I. Aerobic work capacity in men and women with special reference to age. Acta Physiol. Scand. 49(Suppl.):169, 1960.

4. Brozek, J.F., Grand, J.T., Anderson, J.T., Keya, A. Densitometric analysis of body composition revision of some quantitative assumptions. Ann. N.Y. Acad. Sci. 110:113-140, 1963.

5. Kitagawa, K. Body composition of Japanese male and female. J. Phys. Fit. Sports Med. 28:199-202, 1979. (in Japanese)

6. Kobayashi, K. Aerobic power of the Japanese. Tokyo: Kyorin Shoin Press, 1982. (in Japanese)

7. Wilmore, J.H. The use of actual, predicted and constant residual volumes in the assessment of body composition by underwater weighting. Med. Sci. Sports Exer., 1:87-90, 1969.

Responses to a Submaximal–Maximal Stress Test in the Elderly

N. Takeshima, F. Kobayashi, T. Watanabe, K. Sumi, K. Tanaka, and T. Kato

College of General Education, Nagoya City University, Mizuho, Nagoya; Department of Hygiene, Aichi Medical University; Institute of Health and Sports Sciences, University of Tsukuba; and Department of Public Health, Aichi Medical University, Japan

A profound decline in the maximal capacity of the aerobic system has been reported with advancing age in the elderly. However, the submaximal capacity of that system in the elderly has not yet been extensively studied in comparison with young individuals. The present study was undertaken to determine to what extent the submaximal and maximal capacities of the aerobic system in the elderly differ from those in their younger counterparts.

Methods

Fourteen healthy males (6 elderly men and 8 young men) and 12 healthy females (5 elderly women and 7 young women) completed this study after the risks and discomfort associated with each procedure had been explained to them in detail. The mean values ($\pm$ SD) of the anthropometric variables made on elderly men (Group EM), elderly women (Group EW), young men (Group YM), and young women (Group YW) are tabulated in Table 1.

Table 1 Anthropometric and Body Composition Measurements

Variable	Elderly men	Young men	Elderly women	Young women
Age, yr	71.8 $\pm$ 2.4	21.1 $\pm$ 0.6*	66.8 $\pm$ 1.6	18.6 $\pm$ 0.8*
Height, cm	163.2 $\pm$ 3.3	172.4 $\pm$ 2.3*	154.2 $\pm$ 5.6	158.8 $\pm$ 4.0
Weight, kg	60.8 $\pm$ 6.9	63.1 $\pm$ 7.3	50.4 $\pm$ 7.1	51.6 $\pm$ 6.1
Triceps, mm	10.3 $\pm$ 1.9	9.2 $\pm$ 3.7	13.1 $\pm$ 4.4	12.5 $\pm$ 4.3
Subscapular, mm	18.3 $\pm$ 4.3	11.0 $\pm$ 2.8*	16.9 $\pm$ 6.6	13.0 $\pm$ 2.4
Fat, %	15.7 $\pm$ 2.4	12.1 $\pm$ 2.6*	18.9 $\pm$ 5.1	14.0 $\pm$ 2.5
Fat, kg	9.6 $\pm$ 2.1	7.7 $\pm$ 2.4	9.8 $\pm$ 3.6	8.7 $\pm$ 2.1
LBM, kg	51.2 $\pm$ 5.3	55.4 $\pm$ 5.4	40.6 $\pm$ 3.8	42.9 $\pm$ 4.7
Katura index	1.07 $\pm$ 0.11	0.97 $\pm$ 0.11	1.04 $\pm$ 0.14	0.97 $\pm$ 0.07

*$p < .05$.

Anthropometric Measurement

Anthropometric measurements included height, weight, triceps skinfold, and subscapular skinfold. Skinfold thicknesses were measured on the right side of the body using an Eiken-type caliper at the triceps and subscapular. The sum of thicknesses at the two sites was used for estimation of body density (5). The percentage of body fat (1) was then estimated.

Physiological Measurement

Prior to the cardiovascular-respiratory assessment during submaximal and maximal cycling exercise, the subject was required to sit on a chair for approximately 15-20 min for the measurement of resting condition. At this time, pulmonary ventilation ($\dot{V}E$), oxygen uptake ($\dot{V}O_2$), heart rate (HR), systolic blood pressure (SBP), and diastolic blood pressure (DBP) were measured.

$\dot{V}O_2$, $\dot{V}E$, HR, SBP, and DBP corresponding to lactate threshold (LT) and their maximal values were measured by a cycling exercise test on a Monark bicycle ergometer. The test was initiated with 2 min of unloaded warm-up cycling. Following the 2-min warm-up cycling, a work load of 15 W was administered and thereafter increased 15 W every minute until voluntary exhaustion. The pedal rate, paced by an auditory-visual metronome, was kept at 60 rpm.

Metabolic measurements of expiratory gases were determined by standard techniques of open-circuit spirometry, using a Nihondenki San-ei Aerobic Processor (type 391). LT was defined as the level of work intensity at which lactate accumulates in the blood and $\dot{V}E$ increases disproportionately with respect to $\dot{V}O_2$ during the incremental cycling test. Maximal oxygen uptake ($\dot{V}O_2$max) was defined as the highest mean value of the sum of two successive 30-s $\dot{V}O_2$ values recorded during the cycling test.

Blood pressure recordings were made from the left arm with Nippon Colin Stress Test Blood Pressure Monitor (STBP-680) at the end of each exercise bout. HR was continuously monitored via a CCr-lead electrocardiogram. Blood samples for determination of blood lactate concentration were drawn from the antecubital vein of the right arm every minute during exercise. The samples were immediately deproteinized in chilled perchloric acid and kept refrigerated until assayed.

Data Treatment

Differences between elderly and young groups on selected variables were evaluated using the Student's t test. The Pearson product-moment correlational technique was used in all correlational analyses. A probability level of less than 5% was taken as indicating statistical significance. Values were expressed as means $\pm$ SD.

Results

No statistically significant differences were observed in HRrest, SBPrest, DBPrest, and %$\dot{V}O_2$max @ LT between Groups EM and YM nor in HRrest, $\dot{V}E$ @ LT, DBP @ LT, DBPmax, and %$\dot{V}O_2$max @ LT between Groups EW and YW (see Tables 2 and 3). There were statistically significant differences in $\dot{V}O_2$ @ LT, $\dot{V}O_2$max, $\dot{V}E$ @ LT, $\dot{V}E$max, HR @ LT, HRmax, SBP @ LT, SBPmax, DBP @ LT, and DBPmax between Groups EM and YM and in SBPrest, DBPrest, $\dot{V}O_2$ @ LT, $\dot{V}O_2$max, $\dot{V}E$max, HR @ LT, HRmax, SBP @ LT, and SBPmax between Groups EW and YW. $\dot{V}O_2$ @ LT of Group EM corresponded to only 57% of that of Group YM, while $\dot{V}O$ @ LT of Group EW averaged 75% of that of Group YW. $\dot{V}O_2$max of Groups EM and EW corresponded to 51% and 65% of that of Groups YM and YW, respectively. Likewise, differences in $\dot{V}E$ @ LT, $\dot{V}E$max, HR @ LT, and HRmax between male groups (EM versus YM) were about 7-18% larger than those observed between female groups (EW versus YW). Figure 1 shows a close association between $\dot{V}O_2$ @ LT and $\dot{V}O_2$max. When the data of all four groups were pooled, a significant correlation ($r = .882$) was obtained.

Table 2   Resting Heart Rate and Blood Pressure

Variable	Elderly men	Young men	Elderly women	Young women
HR, b/min	66.5 ± 11.1	66.5 ± 13.5	72.8 ± 9.0	76.0 ± 13.0
SBP, mmHg	120.3 ± 9.9	128.6 ± 11.1	144.2 ± 26.0	114.4 ± 14.8*
DBP, mmHg	73.2 ± 9.8	69.6 ± 5.8	86.8 ± 11.6	70.7 ± 7.3*

*$p < .05$.

Table 3   Submaximal and Maximal Cardiovascular-Respiratory Responses to Cycling Exercise

Variable	Elderly men	Young men	Elderly women	Young women
$\dot{V}O_2$ @ LT, ml/kg/min	14.2 ± 2.5	25.0 ± 3.6*	13.6 ± 3.2	18.2 ± 3.7*
$\dot{V}O_2$max, ml/kg/min	24.2 ± 6.1	47.5 ± 5.8*	22.7 ± 0.7	35.1 ± 6.0*
$\dot{V}E$ @ LT, l/min	30.2 ± 0.8	42.3 ± 7.3*	22.3 ± 3.8	26.4 ± 3.2
$\dot{V}E$max, l/min	68.8 ± 10.4	112.2 ± 20.0*	49.2 ± 10.6	72.3 ± 13.0*
HR @ LT, b/min	99.0 ± 11.3	128.9 ± 20.0*	111.0 ± 17.2	130.0 ± 5.7*
HRmax, b/min	144.5 ± 16.0	192.6 ± 10.0*	155.4 ± 14.5	183.3 ± 11.6*
SBP @ LT, mmHg	150.8 ± 23.0	173.9 ± 12.9*	178.4 ± 24.3	138.1 ± 13.1*
SBPmax, mmHg	201.0 ± 13.9	226.0 ± 28.4*	206.4 ± 17.8	173.6 ± 12.9*
DBP @ LT, mmHg	89.2 ± 18.9	77.0 ± 8.2*	88.4 ± 20.7	77.4 ± 11.2
DBPmax, mmHg	103.0 ± 18.5	72.3 ± 15.6*	105.6 ± 15.5	89.1 ± 12.3
%$\dot{V}O_2$max @ LT, %	59.6 ± 7.6	52.9 ± 7.3	59.3 ± 12.8	53.8 ± 8.0
%$\dot{V}E$max @ LT, %	44.7 ± 6.8	38.5 ± 7.6	46.2 ± 8.3	37.7 ± 8.7
%HRmax @ LT, %	68.9 ± 9.0	66.7 ± 8.5	71.4 ± 8.7	71.1 ± 3.8
%SBPmax @ LT, %	74.9 ± 9.7	77.5 ± 7.2	86.6 ± 11.3	79.8 ± 7.6
%DBPmax @ LT, %	87.0 ± 14.0	111.1 ± 23.2*	82.9 ± 7.9	89.2 ± 23.9

*$p < .05$.

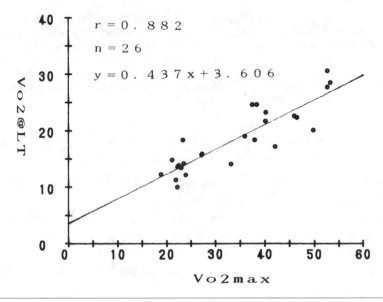

Figure 1.   Relationship between maximal oxygen uptake and oxygen intake corresponding to lactate threshold.

Discussion

It has been well recognized that $\dot{V}O_2$max and HRmax decrease with aging in both sexes (2, 9, 11). Previous studies (3, 6, 7) have dealt with assessment of maximal aerobic power in the elderly. Seals et al. (6) have, for instance, reported 25.4 ± 4.6 ml/kg/min for 24 elderly persons (age 63 ± 2 years), 27.4 ± 3.7 ml/kg/min for seven elderly men out of the 24 subjects, and 21.9 ± 4.1 ml/kg/min for four elderly women out of the 24 subjects. Typical $\dot{V}O_2$max values for the general population at retirement have been reported to be about 27 ml/kg/min in a man and 24 ml/kg/min in a woman (7).

In the present study, $\dot{V}O_2$max averaged 24.2 ml/kg/min for Group EM and 22.7 ml/kg/min for Group EW. These values are considered representative for the elderly, since our subjects were 5-10 years older than the general population at retirement. Hossack and Bruce (3) have reported the annual rate of decline of $\dot{V}O_2$max is -0.46 ml/kg/min/year for men and -0.33 ml/kg/min/year for women. Mean differences in $\dot{V}O_2$max between Groups EM and EW (7%) and Groups YM and YW (35%) were similar to those in $\dot{V}O_2$ @ LT between Groups EM and EW (5%) and Groups YM and YW (37%).

Interestingly however, a 96% or 76% greater mean difference was found in $\dot{V}O_2$max or $\dot{V}O_2$ @ LT between Groups EM and YM, while the percentage difference between EW and YW was much smaller (55% or 34%). Thus, these findings indicate that gender differences in $\dot{V}O_2$ @ LT as well as in $\dot{V}O_2$max are much smaller in elderly individuals than in young individuals and that both $\dot{V}O_2$max and $\dot{V}O_2$ @ LT decrease with aging to a greater extent in men than in women. Relatively smaller mean differences in $\dot{V}O_2$ @ LT as compared with $\dot{V}O_2$max in both sexes may partly be accounted for by an increase in percent slow-twitch (Type I) fibers with advancing age (4).

Despite the fact that Group EW subjects were only 5 years younger than Group EM subjects, HR @ LT and HRmax for this group were on the average 12 b/min and 11 b/min higher, although differences were not significant. These findings suggest that a more profound decline of both HR @ LT and HRmax with aging is also found in men than in women. On $\dot{V}E$ @ LT and $\dot{V}Emax$, a similar trend was seen. The reason for such trends should be a matter worthy of additional interesting research. Mean values of $\%\dot{V}O_2max$ @ LT were $59.6 \pm 7.6\%$ and $59.3 \pm 12.8\%$ in Groups EM and EW, respectively. These values are in agreement with values ($60 \pm 2\%$ and $58 \pm 2\%$) reported by Thomas et al. (10) for 44 retired males (age 61.8 ± 0.5 years) and 45 retired females (age 62.5 ± 0.5 years), respectively, although $\dot{V}O_2max$ and ventilatory threshold were slightly higher in their subjects than in our male subjects.

Another interesting finding was that both SBP @ LT and SBPmax were significantly higher in Group EW than in Group YW, whereas in Group EM both were significantly lower than in Group YM. This may be attributed to a relatively smaller augmentation in submaximal-maximal SBP for Group YW. Hossack and Bruce (3) have also found that mean systolic arterial pressure is consistently higher in women than in men from rest to maximal exercise, although the absolute increase from rest to maximal exercise is similar in both sexes. In women and particularly in elderly women, submaximal and maximal cardiac outputs seem to be maintained predominantly by an increase in cardiac rate rather than by an increase in stroke volume. It is therefore indicated that the optimum training intensity in terms of HR would be slightly higher in women than in men, regardless of age.

The relationship between $\dot{V}O_2$ @ LT and $\dot{V}O_2max$ was, as shown in Figure 1, $r = .882$ for the total subjects ($n = 26$), indicating that approximately 78% of the variance in the $\dot{V}O_2$ @ LT can be accounted for by $\dot{V}O_2max$ alone. The magnitude of the correlation is in agreement with previous investigations (8, 12, 13). Since the maximal or supramaximal exercise stress testing is not necessarily safe and requires an excessive amount of time, it appears that a convenient equation to predict $\dot{V}O_2max$ of the elderly would be highly advantageous in applied situations. The present study suggests that such a useful prediction equation with relatively high accuracy could be formulated in future studies.

In conclusion, we emphasize the gender difference in the capacity of the aerobic system during submaximal and maximal exercise. In elderly women the relative decline in $\dot{V}O_2$ @ LT, $\dot{V}O_2max$, $\dot{V}E$ @ LT, $\dot{V}Emax$, HR @ LT, and HRmax appears to be much smaller as compared with elderly men. Our findings suggest that the cardiac and ventilatory responses to submaximal and maximal exercise would be relatively higher in elderly women than in elderly men, when considering the significant differences in those responses found between young men and young women.

References

1. Brozek, J., Grande, F., Anderson, J.T., Keys, A. Densitometric analysis of body composition: revision of some quantitative assumptions. Ann. N.Y. Acad. Sci. 110:113-140, 1963.

2. Bruce, R.A., Fisher, L.D., Cooper, M.N., Gey, G.O. Separation of effects of cardiovascular disease and age on ventricular function with maximal exercise. Am. J. Cardiol. 34:757-763, 1974.

3. Hossack, K.F., Bruce, R.A. Maximal cardiac function in sedentary normal men and women: comparison of age-related changes. J. Appl. Physiol. 53:798-804, 1982.

4. Larsson, L., Karlsson, J. Isometric and dynamic endurance as a function of age and skeletal muscle characteristics. Acta Physiol. Scand. 104:129-136, 1978.

5. Nagamine, S., Suzuki, S. Anthropometry and body composition of Japanese young men and women. Human Biol. 36:8-15, 1964.

6. Seals, D.R., Hagberg, J.M., Hurley, B.F., Ehsani, A.A., Hollszy, J.O. Endurance training in older men and women: I. Cardiovascular responses to exercise. J. Appl. Physiol. 57:1024-1029, 1984.

7. Shephard, R.J. Physical activity and aging. 2nd ed. London: Croom Helm, 1978.

8. Tanaka, K., Matsuura, Y., Matsuzaka, A., Hirakoba, K., Kumagai, S., Sun-O.S., Asano, K. A longitudinal assessment of anaerobic threshold and distance-running performance. Med. Sci. Sports Exerc. 16:278-282, 1984.

9. Tanaka, K., Nobuta, Y., Hasegawa, Y. A simplified method for the assessment of cardiorespiratory fitness. Kyoiku Igaku 33:212-219, 1988. (in Japanese)

10. Thomas, S.G., Cunningham, D.A., Thompson, J., Rechnitzer, P.A. Exercise training and "ventilation threshold" in elderly. J. Appl. Physiol. 59:1472-1476, 1985.

11. Voigt, A.E., Bruce, R.A., Kusumi, F., Pettet, G., Neilson, K., Whitkanack, S., Japia, J. Longitudinal variations in maximal-exercise performance of healthy sedentary middle aged women. J. Sports Med. 15:323-327, 1975.

12. Withers, R.T., Sherman, W.M., Miller, J.M., Costill, D.L. Specificity of the anaerobic threshold in endurance trained cyclist and runners. Eur. J. Appl. Physiol. 47:93-104, 1981.

13. Yamabe, H., Kobayashi, K., Fujii, H., Kado, T., Fukuzaki, H. Cardiorespiratory response during exercise in effort angina pectoris. Jpn. J. Chest Dis. 21:631-638, 1983.

Physiological Responses During Exercise in Older Male Runners

M. Higuchi, K. Iwaoka, T. Fuchi, S. Matsuo, and S. Kobayashi
Division of Health Promotion, National Institute of Nutrition, Shinjuku-ku, Tokyo, Japan

We examined the physiological profiles of older endurance runners (OR) by comparing them with those of young runners (YR) using the incremental treadmill running test of Saltin and Åstrand (12). In the first experiment (2), physiological responses during maximal exercise were compared in OR ($n = 11$, age 64 ± 3 years, body fat $12 \pm 2\%$; mean $\pm$ SD) and YR ($n = 7$, 35 ± 2 years, $12 \pm 2\%$) to clarify the relative roles of cardiovascular parameters accounting for the decrease of maximal oxygen uptake ($\dot{V}O_2$max) with aging in runners. The parameters examined include maximal heart rate (HRmax), maximal stroke volume (SVmax), and arteriovenous oxygen difference (a-$\bar{v}O_2$ diff). OR and YR were selected so as to have an identical weekly training distance of 50 km. The 10-km race records in the latest year of OR and YR were 43 ± 4 and 38 ± 3 min, respectively. To determine $\dot{V}O_2$max, subjects completed the treadmill test. The expired gases were collected in Douglas bags during the last 2-3 min of the test. Heart rate (HR) was monitored continuously by ECG throughout the test.

A noninvasive CO_2 rebreathing method based on the Fick principle was used to determine cardiac output (Q) immediately after the exercise test. We calculated a-$\bar{v}O_2$ diff at $\dot{V}O_2$max by dividing the $\dot{V}O_2$max by the Q at $\dot{V}O_2$max (Qmax). SVmax was calculated by dividing the Qmax by the HRmax. Table 1 shows the physiological profiles at maximal exercise in OR by comparing with those of YR. All parameters in OR except a-$\bar{v}O_2$ diff were significantly lower than those in YR. The decrease of $\dot{V}O_2$max in OR was associated with the

Table 1 Physiological Responses During Maximal Exercise in Young and Older Runners

	Older runners		Young runners	
n	11		7	
$\dot{V}O_2$ (ml/kg/min)	50	$\pm$ 4 *	61	$\pm$ 3
Heart rate (beats/min)	172	$\pm$ 6 *	186	$\pm$ 11
Cardiac output (ml/kg/min)	291	$\pm$ 40 *	356	$\pm$ 31
Stroke volume (ml/kg)	1.69	$\pm$ 0.24*	1.96	$\pm$ 0.16
a-$\bar{v}O_2$ difference (ml/100 ml)	16.8	$\pm$ 1.4	17.0	$\pm$ 2.7

Note. Values are means $\pm$ SD. *$p < .05$ compared to young runners.

reductions of HRmax and SVmax. The decrease of HRmax with aging is well known even in master athletes (4, 5, 11). This decrease of HRmax appears to be the result of an inevitable deterioration of the cardiovascular functions with aging. The age-associated reduction of SVmax may be accounted for by an increased peripheral resistance and a decreased myocardial contractility. We found that only the a-$\bar{v}O_2$ diff could be maintained with endurance training in spite of aging. This could be explained by the marked adaptability of muscle to the increased use, such as the pronounced augmentation of the enzyme activities and the capillarization in the exercised muscle (3, 10). We concluded that the decreases of $\dot{V}O_2$max, HR$_{max}$, and SVmax are inevitable with aging even in highly trained older athletes and that the decrease of $\dot{V}O_2$max with aging seems to be explained by the decrease of the central circulatory functions such as HRmax and SVmax, while a-$\dot{V}O_2$ diff, one of the factors that represents the capacity of peripheral functions, could be maintained by vigorous regular exercise.

In the second study (7), the possible age-related difference in blood lactate accumulation during submaximal exercise and its relations to endurance performance were examined. Physiological characteristics and 5-km run times of OR and YR are summarized in the upper part of Table 2. The two age groups were matched as closely as possible on the basis of training distance (61-66 km/wk) and percent body fat. Treadmill grade was level during the first 3 min and thereafter increased gradually every 3 min until exhaustion with a constant velocity. Blood samples were drawn from a fingertip at the end of each stage and analyzed for lactate concentration. $\dot{V}O_2$ at the onset of blood lactate accumulation (OBLA-$\dot{V}O_2$), which means the $\dot{V}O_2$ corresponding to 4 mM of blood lactate, was determined using a log-log transformation. Several variables related to blood lactate accumulation are listed in the lower part of Table 2. No significant difference was found in peak blood lactate between OR and YR. Although OR's OBLA-$\dot{V}O_2$ was significantly lower than YR, this difference remarkably reduced when the values were expressed on %$\dot{V}O_2$max basis. Table 3 shows the results of correlation analysis between $\dot{V}O_2$max, OBLA-$\dot{V}O_2$, and 5-km run time. Both $\dot{V}O_2$max and OBLA-$\dot{V}O_2$ were strongly correlated to 5-km run time in each group.

Table 2   Physiological Characteristics, Peak Blood Lactate, and Onset of Blood Lactate Accumulation (OBLA) in Older and Young Runners

	Older runners	Young runners
n	9	10
$\dot{V}O_2$max (ml/kg/min)	49 ± 5**	64 ± 6
$\dot{V}$Emax (L/kg/min)	1.80 ± 0.23*	2.11 ± 0.26
HRmax (beats/min)	173 ± 6**	184 ± 6
5-km run time (min)	20.7 ± 2.0**	17.0 ± 1.1
Peak LA (mM)	7.7 ± 1.0	8.5 ± 2.8
OBLA		
$\quad\dot{V}O_2$ (ml/kg/min)	42 ± 4**	54 ± 9
$\quad\dot{V}O_2$max (%)	86 ± 6	84 ± 10

Note. Values are means ± SD. *$p < .05$, **$p < .01$, compared to young runners.

Table 3   Correlation Coefficients Between 5-km Run Time (min) and $\dot{V}O_2$max, OBLA-$\dot{V}O_2$(ml/kg/min)

	Older runners	Young runners
$\dot{V}O_2$max	−0.803**	−0.802**
OBLA-$\dot{V}O_2$	−0.680*	−0.648*

$*p < .05, **p < .01.$

The figures of OBLA expressed as %$\dot{V}O_2$max in the study coincide well with those of previous studies reported for young runners (8, 13). According to the study of Örlander et al. that focused the effects of training on skeletal muscle metabolism and the ultrastructure (10), the aging muscle remained trainable and the training response was almost similar to that seen in younger age group. Consequently, these adaptations of muscle to endurance training could reduce lactate production and thus raise lactate threshold (LT) or OBLA even in older individuals. Another finding in the second study was a significant correlation between OBLA-$\dot{V}O_2$ and 5-km run time in OR as well as in YR. This finding is similar to the previous studies demonstrated a strong correlation between distance running performance and LT or OBLA in trained young runners (1, 8, 13). These results indicate that there is no remarkable difference in the peripheral physiological function during exercise between OR and YR.

The third study (6) concerned the facts that plasma levels of norepinephrine (NE) gradually increase with age in resting subjects and older subjects have a greater increase in NE levels in response to a uniform stress (14). However, there is one report in which age-associated changes of exercise-induced NE responses were taken into consideration (9). Sympatho-adrenergic function involved in HR responses during graded exercise between OR ($n = 9$, age 67 ± 5 years, 5-km run time 20.5 ± 1.6 min, training distance 67 ± 30 km/week), and YR ($n = 9$, 24 ± 3 years, 16.0 ± 0.5 min, 90 ± 32 km/week) was compared. Testing started with a submaximal work load and increased every 3 min until exhaustion. HR and $\dot{V}O_2$ were measured during final 1 min of each work load, and blood samples were taken from a venous catheter immediately after each exercise stage for the determination of NE. NE was analyzed electrochemically after separating by HPLC method. Table 4 shows the results of the responses of $\dot{V}O_2$ and HR at the same relative work rates in OR and YR. Table 5 demonstrates NE concentrations at rest and during exercise. Although OR had a similar HR to YR at rest, NE was significantly higher in OR than in YR. At 60 and 70% of $\dot{V}O_2$max OR had a lower HR by 17 and 14% than YR, respectively, whereas NE was remarkably higher in OR than that in YR. Although OR had a substantially lower HR at $\dot{V}O_2$max level than YR, no significant difference in NE was observed between the age groups. These results suggest the possibility that older men had lower HR associated with the age-related deterioration of adrenoceptor function during exercise.

We concluded that the age-related deterioration of aerobic capacity in well-trained older runners might be induced mainly by the reduction of central circulatory function such as HR and stroke volume rather than peripheral one and that this alteration of the central function seems to be related to the lowered adrenoceptor function in older runners.

Table 4 Responses of $\dot{V}O_2$ and Heart Rate at the Same Relative Work Rates

	% $\dot{V}O_2$max	Older runners	Young runners
$\dot{V}O_2$ (ml/kg/min)	−60	31 ± 1* (4)	42 ± 2 (6)
	−70	35 ± 2* (7)	48 ± 3 (8)
	−80	38 ± 3* (9)	54 ± 3 (9)
	−90	42 ± 4* (9)	59 ± 3 (8)
	Max	48 ± 4* (9)	67 ± 4 (9)
Heart rate (beats/min)	Rest	59 ± 8 (9)	59 ± 9 (9)
	−60	117 ± 7* (4)	141 ± 8 (6)
	−70	132 ± 8* (7)	153 ± 8 (8)
	−80	138 ± 9* (9)	165 ± 6 (9)
	−90	148 ± 8* (9)	178 ± 5 (8)
	Max	166 ± 7* (9)	191 ± 7 (9)

Note. Values are means ± *SD*. Numbers in parentheses are sample sizes. *$p < .01$ compared to young runners.

Table 5 Plasma Norepinephrine Concentrations at Rest and During Exercise (ng/ml)

% $\dot{V}O_2$max	Older runners	Young runners
Rest	0.31 ± 0.13 (8)*	0.17 ± 0.11 (8)
−60	0.97 ± 0.26 (4)**	0.46 ± 0.19 (6)
−70	1.33 ± 0.39 (7)**	0.78 ± 0.22 (7)
−80	1.75 ± 0.54 (9)	1.58 ± 0.31 (8)
−90	2.62 ± 1.02 (9)	2.99 ± 0.95 (6)
Max	8.30 ± 1.89 (9)	7.25 ± 2.89 (9)

Note. Values are means ± *SD*. Numbers in parentheses are sample sizes. *$p < .05$, **$p < .01$ compared to young runners.

Acknowledgments

The present studies were supported partly by grants from the Foundation of Life Sciences in Kyoto, the Meiji Life Foundation of Health and Welfare, and Research Grant on Aging and Health, Ministry of Health and Welfare, Japan. We thank Dr. Yoko Nakashima for analyzing NE.

References

1. Farrell, P.A., Wilmore, J.H., Coyle, E.F., Billing, J.E., Costill, D.L. Plasma lactate accumulation and distance running performance. Med. Sci. Sports Exer. 11:338-344, 1979.

2. Fuchi, T., Iwaoka, K., Higuchi, M., Kobayashi, S. Cardiovascular changes for deterioration of aerobic capacity with aging in distance runners. Med. Sci. Sports Exer. 19(Suppl.):S61, 1987.

3. Grimby, G., Danneskiold-Samsœ, B., Hvid, K., Saltin, B. Morphology and enzymatic capacity in arm and leg muscles in 78-81 year old men and women. Acta Physiol. Scand. 115:125-134, 1982.

4. Hagberg, J.M., Allen, W.K., Seals, D.R., Hurley, B.F., Ehsani, A.A., Holloszy, J.O. A hemodynamic comparison of young and older endurance athletes during exercise. J. Appl. Physiol. 58:2041-2046, 1985.

5. Heath, G.W., Hagberg, J.M., Ehsani, A.A., Holloszy, J.O. A physiological comparison of young and older endurance athletes. J. Appl. Physiol. 51:634-640, 1981.

6. Higuchi, M., Iwaoka, K., Matsuo, S., Nakashima, Y., Kobayashi, S. Age-related changes of sympathoadrenergic function on heart rate responses during exercise. Can. J. Sport Sci. 13(Suppl.):16P, 1988.

7. Iwaoka, K., Fuchi, T., Higuchi, M., Kobayashi, S. Blood lactate accumulation during exercise in older endurance runners. Int. J. Sports Med. 9:-253-256, 1988.

8. Kindermann, W., Schramm, M., Kiel, J. Aerobic performance diagnostics with different experimental settings. Int. J. Sports Med. 1:110-114, 1980.

9. Lehmann, M., Kiel, J. Age-associated changes of exercise-induced plasma catecholamine responses. Europ. J. Appl. Physiol. 55:302-306, 1986.

10. Örlander, J., Kiessling, K.H., Larsson, L., Karlsson, J., Aniansson, A. Skeletal muscle metabolism and ultrastructure in relation to age in sedentary men. Acta Physiol. Scand. 104:249-261, 1978.

11. Pollock, M.L., Miller, H.S., Wilmore, J.H. Physiological characteristics of champion American track athletes 40 to 75 years of age. J. Geront. 29:645-649, 1974.

12. Saltin, B., Åstrand, P.-O. Oxygen uptake in athletes. J. Appl. Physiol. 23:353-358, 1967.

13. Sjödin, B., Jacobs, I., Svedenhag, J. Changes in onset of blood lactate accumulation (OBLA) and muscle enzyme after training at OBLA. Europ. J. Appl. Physiol. 49:45-57, 1982.

14. Ziegler, M.G., Lake, C.R., Kopin, I.J. Plasma norepinephrine increases with age. Nature 261:333-334, 1976.

The Starting Age of Training and Its Effect on Reduction in Physical Performance Capability With Aging

Y. Aoyagi and S. Katsuta

School of Physical Education, Fukuoka University and Institute of Health and Sport Sciences, University of Tsukuba, Japan

⌐An inevitable consequence of aging is a reduction in physical performance capabilities. Numerous cross-sectional and longitudinal studies are generally consistent in describing declines in maximal static and dynamic strength, maximal speed of movement in muscles, and maximal oxygen consumption ($\dot{V}O_2$max) (4, 5). Recently published data indicate that continued exercise training can slow the rate of reduction in these functional indices as a person ages (5, 7).⌐

⌐Although it is of interest that a lifelong program of physical activity may slow the rate of decline of muscle and cardiovascular functions with aging, a more important question for the general population is whether exercise training initiated at earlier ages can be more effective against these age-related functional impairments. The purpose of this investigation is to test the hypothesis that older persons can minimize the reduction in muscle strength, speed of contraction, and $\dot{V}O_2$max that occurs with age if they start training before the age of approximately 50 years, above which a decline in strength has been reported to become more pronounced (6).

Methods

The 31 male athletes and 8 untrained men who participated in the study were selected for their similar age range (60-68 years) and occupational activity. The athletes were divided into three groups based on the starting age of training. The first group, designated T_{26} ($n = 10$), had been training since before their mid-30s (mean 26 years); the second group, designated T_{45} ($n = 10$), since their 40s (mean 45 years); and the third group, designated T_{56} ($n = 11$), since their 50s (mean 56 years). The three groups were matched as closely as possible on the basis of (a) age, (b) types of activities included in their training regimen (e.g., jogging), (c) kilometers run per week, and (d) level of competitiveness. All athletes did some distance training on a regular basis (minimum of 5 km continuously, 3 days per week). Height, weight, circumferences (upper arm and thigh), percent body fat (two skinfolds) (8), and body mass index (weight [kg]/height [m]$_2$) were obtained or calculated for all subjects.

Isometric and isokinetic elbow flexion (EF) and knee extension (KE) torques were measured on the dominant side of the body separately using a Cybex II (Lumex Inc., New York) dynamometer. Isometric testing was performed at a joint angle of 90° for EF and 60° for KE. The isokinetic velocities used in the test were 30, 90, and 180° $\cdot$ s^{-1}. The measurements were made in sequence from slow to fast speeds within each muscle group.

Peak torque was recorded during three isometric contractions and on two isokinetic contractions at each of the three velocities. A 1-min rest was allowed between each contraction.

Maximal isometric back-lift strength was tested at a hip angle of 150° (i.e., back 30° from vertical). Back-lift strength measures involved the use of a spring back-lift dynamometer and bar (Takei Co., Tokyo). During isometric testing, the subjects, with mixed grip, lifted straight up and extended their backs maximally while keeping their legs straight. Three contractions were administered and took approximately 3 s each with a 1-min rest interval between contractions.

Maximal elbow flexion (MFV) and knee extension velocities (MEV) were assessed by means of a special, very light lever arm with essentially no inertia at the center of rotation (i.e., no torque produced). In the same postural positions (sitting) as used for strength measurements, the subjects were instructed to flex the arm as quickly as possible starting from an elbow angle of 0° or to extend the leg from a knee angle of 90°. The subjects performed five subsequent flexions of extensions with a 20-s rest in between. The time required to flex from 15 to 75° or to extend from 75 to 15° was measured electronically with photoelectric cells and the highest angular velocity attained during the five trials was used as a value for MFV or MEV, respectively.

Aerobic fitness ($\dot{V}O_2$max) was assessed by the Åstrand indirect test (2), beginning at a level of 50 W on a Monark bicycle ergometer. The pedaling frequency was 50 complete pedal turns per minute. Heart rates were recorded from a bipolar chest lead on an electrocardiograph during the last 20 s of every minute. The subject pedaled at this work level until a steady state was attained between 120-170 beats • min^{-1}. The two heart rate values that delimited the steady state were then averaged, and this value was applied to the Åstrand nomogram and the predicted maximal oxygen uptake corrected for age. The data were analyzed for means ± SD for the groups. A one-way analysis of variance was used to determine significant differences between groups. A p value < .05 was accepted as statistically significant.

Results and Discussion

As shown in Tables 1 and 2, there were no significant differences between the T_{26}, T_{45}, and T_{56} groups in the type (long slow distance) and amount (km • wk^{-1}) of exercise to which they habitually subjected themselves nor in physical characteristics. It was only the starting age of training that differed between these trained groups. Therefore, our assessment of three trained groups used in this study is that these groups were adequate to determine the effect of the starting age of training on the reduction in physical performance capability with aging.

As the velocities of measurement were increased, the T_{26} and T_{45} groups, which at all velocities did not differ from each other, had significantly greater torques for EF than the untrained group (see Figure 1). In contrast, torque differences in KE between any of the three trained groups, which produced values that were greater than the untrained group, were not detected at any angular velocity tested (see Figure 1). The discrepancy between EF and KE in the magnitude of intergroup differences in muscle strength at the different velocities could be explained on the basis of the manner that the master athletes trained. It is well known that the training mode has a significant, specific effect on the training results (7). That is, arm training more specifically affects the arms, and leg training affects the legs. Thus, the leg muscle that was most active during running showed larger torque differences between the trained and untrained groups and smaller torque differences between the trained groups than the arm or back muscles (see Figure 2), providing evidence for a marked effect of training on the quadriceps muscle. Therefore, it appears that the rate of decline of strength that occurs with age can be reduced even in older

Table 1   Starting Age and Consecutive Years of Training, Training Frequency per Week, and Distance Trained per Day and per Week for Master Athletes

Groups	n	Starting age (yrs)	Consecutive years	Frequency (days $\cdot$ wk^{-1})	Distance trained (km $\cdot$ day^{-1})	(km $\cdot$ wk^{-1})
T_{26}	10	25.6 $\pm$ 9.0	37.0 $\pm$ 10.9	4.8 $\pm$ 1.7	10.7 $\pm$ 4.8	51.7 $\pm$ 30.9
T_{45}	10	45.1 $\pm$ 3.2	17.7 $\pm$ 2.1	5.1 $\pm$ 1.4	9.1 $\pm$ 3.2	48.7 $\pm$ 27.1
T_{56}	11	55.5 $\pm$ 3.7	7.7 $\pm$ 2.9	5.6 $\pm$ 1.2	8.8 $\pm$ 3.3	50.4 $\pm$ 25.5

Note. Values are means $\pm$ *SD*. n = number of subjects.

Table 2   Physical Characteristics and Body Composition of Subjects

Variables	T_{26}	T_{45}	T_{56}	Untrained
Age, yrs	62.5 $\pm$ 2.7	62.8 $\pm$ 2.2	63.3 $\pm$ 2.0	62.5 $\pm$ 1.1
Height, cm	163.5 $\pm$ 7.3	161.4 $\pm$ 4.6	161.5 $\pm$ 6.5	158.2 $\pm$ 5.1
Weight, kg	56.2 $\pm$ 5.2	54.3 $\pm$ 7.3	53.8 $\pm$ 4.7	56.1 $\pm$ 7.8
BMI, kg $\cdot$ m^{-2}	21.1 $\pm$ 1.9	20.8 $\pm$ 2.2	20.7 $\pm$ 1.8	22.5 $\pm$ 3.3
Fat, %	10.9 $\pm$ 3.2	11.2 $\pm$ 4.9	11.4 $\pm$ 5.3	16.9 $\pm$ 7.7
Arm girth, cm	26.1 $\pm$ 1.8	26.5 $\pm$ 2.3	25.3 $\pm$ 1.8	26.2 $\pm$ 2.4
Thigh girth, cm	49.6 $\pm$ 2.7	48.4 $\pm$ 2.6	48.2 $\pm$ 2.2	48.3 $\pm$ 5.0

Note. Values are means $\pm$ *SD*. n no. of subjects) = 10 for T_{26}, 10 for T_{45}, 11 for T_{56}, and 8 for untrained. BMI = body mass index.

persons who began to train in their mid-50s, although to what extent the rate can be reduced may be related to the type of training performed.

The relationship between MFV or MEV and the starting age of training was similar to the relationship between strength and the starting age of training (see Figure 3). However, the relative differences in MFV or MEV between the T_{56} and untrained groups were smaller compared to the differences in strength. The present finding is confirmed by Aniansson and Gustafsson (1), who failed to show changes in MEV with training, despite an increase in muscle strength in the quadriceps of men aged 69-74 years. Thus, it might be suggested that elderly persons can hardly decrease the rate of decline of maximal shortening velocity that occurs with aging (6) even if they begin training in their mid-50s.

Numerous cross-sectional and lnogitudinal studies have presented data indicating that as sedentary men age, their maximal oxygen consumption ($\dot{V}O_2$max) decreases at a rate of approximately 0.45 ml $\cdot$ kg^{-1} $\cdot$ min^{-1} $\cdot$ year^{-1} (5). Inasmuch as $\dot{V}O_2$max averages approximately 45 ml $\cdot$ kg^{-1} $\cdot$ min^{-1} at age 25, this rate of decline amounts to approximately 10% per decade after the age of 25 (5). Recently published data appear to indicate that the rate of loss of $\dot{V}O_2$max as a person ages can be reduced by means of a high level of physical activity (5, 7). The rate of decline in $\dot{V}O_2$max with age in these studies appears to be approximately 5% per decade, which is only half the rate generally found in sedentary persons

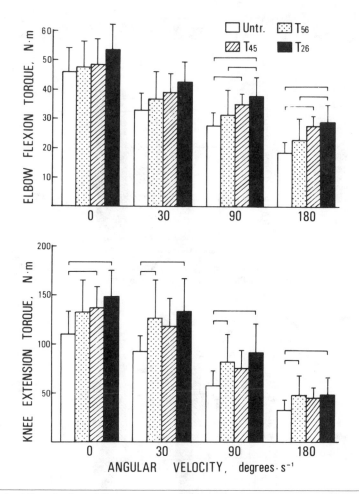

Figure 1.   Elbow flexion and knee extension torques at angular velocities of 0 to 180° • s⁻¹ for the different groups of subjects. ⌐‾‾‾‾‾‾‾‾⌐ = significant difference between groups (*p* < .05).

(5). On the other hand, it is commonly suggested that maximal aerobic power will easily increase 10-20% under the influence of a good aerobic training program (3). Recent data indicate that individuals over the age of 60 can increase their $\dot{V}O_2$max in response to training and that their adaptive capacity, at least on a relative basis, is similar to that of younger persons (5).

Assuming that these general trends in previous literature hold true in the present case, Figure 4 describes a simplified model of $\dot{V}O_2$max decline with age in sedentary and physically trained men with the three different starting ages (26, 45, and 56 years) of endurance activities. Note that in this model, all conditions are identical for all trained groups. The trainability in any of the trained groups is 20% of each initial value that falls to the line representing sedentary men, which was drawn with the assumption that $\dot{V}O_2$max declines at a rate of 10% per decade from a value at age 25 of 45 ml • kg⁻¹ • min⁻¹. Also, the

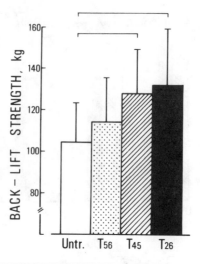

Figure 2. Back-lift strength for the different groups of subjects. ⌐————⌐ = significant difference between groups ($p < .05$).

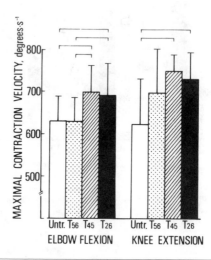

Figure 3. Maximal elbow flexion and knee extension velocities for the different groups of subjects. ⌐————⌐ = significant difference between groups ($p < .05$).

rate of decline in $\dot{V}O_2$max with age in any trained group is 5% per decade from a value at the age when the endurance athletes started training.

Indeed, although it might be claimed that these are very critical assumptions that are not completely met in the present study, the $\dot{V}O_2$max at age 63 for each trained group in this model seems compatible with the present data (see Figure 5). However, there were no significant differences in $\dot{V}O_2$max, whether expressed as L • min^{-1} or ml • kg^{-1} • min^{-1}, between the T_{26} and T_{45} groups. Thus, it might be suggested that there is a turning point in age (50 years) until which $\dot{V}O_2$max decreases slowly or imperceptibly and above which the

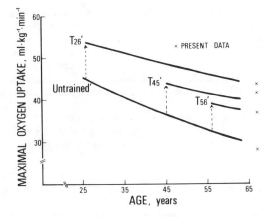

Figure 4. Model of decline in maximal oxygen uptake with age in groups of sedentary and physically trained men. Curves for the three groups of athletes and untrained subjects are from reports in the literature (3, 5, 7). The T_{26}', T_{45}', T_{56}' and untrained' groups in this model correspond to the T_{26}, T_{45}, T_{56}, and untrained groups in the present study.

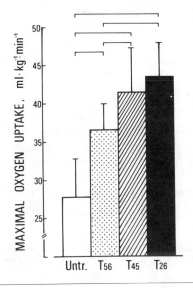

Figure 5. Maximal oxygen uptake for the different groups of subjects. ⌐‾‾‾‾‾‾¬ = significant difference between groups ($p < .05$).

decline is accelerated, as reported on muscle strength (6). It is, however, well documented that the decline of $\dot{V}O_2$max becomes manifested as early as the third decade well before there is any apparent change in the muscle fiber cross-sectional area, the total fiber number and size, and the aerobic metabolic potential of the cell (4), supporting the notion that aerobic power is limited by central factors, most notably the reduction in maximal cardiac output and maximal heart rate (5).

It is interesting to note that Skinner and Riddell (9) have presented data suggesting that formerly active men who had been inactive for at least 10 years were more trainable in terms of maximal aerobic power than their never-active contemporaries. In this study, four athletes in each of the trained groups were such formerly active persons, who had competed earlier in sports at least three times • week^{-1} for a minimum of 2 years. In contrast, the number of never-active athletes, with no history of regular participation in physical activities in the past, was 1 in 10 (10%) in the T_{26} group, 3 in 10 (30%) in the T_{45} group, and 7 in 11 (64%) in the T_{56} group. Thus, the differences in $\dot{V}O_2$max between trained groups may be associated with the previous training experience of subjects. More research concerning the contribution of prior endurance training experience to the sensitivity of the organism to training is necessary before a more definitive statement can be made.

Conclusion

We found much support for a relationship between the starting age of training and the age-related decline of physical performance capability. Thus, the hypothesis that older persons can minimize the reduction in muscle strength, speed of contraction, and $\dot{V}O_2$max that occurs with age if they start training before the age of approximately 50 years is accepted. However, although the men ran an average of 50 km • week^{-1}, it is not clear whether training was constant across their respective training year time span. Furthermore, whether this hypothesis can be verified after additional years is not known. A longitudinal study using the same athletes will be necessary to give a more definitive interpretation of the present findings.

References

1. Aniansson, A., Gustafsson, E. Physical training in elderly men with special reference to quadriceps muscle strength and morphology. Clin. Physiol. 1:87-98, 1981.

2. Åstrand, P.-O., Rodahl, K. Textbook of work physiology: physiological bases of exercise. 3rd ed. New York: McGraw-Hill, 1986.

3. Bouchard, C., Lortie, G. Heredity and endurance performance. Sports Med. 1:38-64, 1984.

4. Grimby, B., Saltin, B. Mini-review: the ageing muscle. Clin. Physiol. 3:209-218, 1983.

5. Hagberg, J.M. Effect of training on the decline of $\dot{V}O_2$max with aging. Fed. Proc. 46:1830-1833, 1987.

6. Larsson, L. Morphological and functional characteristics of the ageing skeletal muscle in man: a cross-sectional study. Acta Physiol. Scand. 457(Suppl.):1-36, 1978.

7. Pollock, M.L., Foster, C., Knapp, D., Rod, J.L., Schmidt, D.H. Effect of age and training on aerobic capacity and body composition of master athletes. J. Appl. Physiol. 62:725-731, 1987.

8. Sato, K. Studies on the body fat mass of the Japanese: on the body fat mass at adolescence. J. Phys. Fit. Jpn. 24:134-150, 1975.

9. Skinner, J.S., Riddell, J. Trainability of formerly-active (10 years or more before) vs. never-active males aged 30-39 years. Med. Sci. Sports Exerc. 15:133, 1983.

PART II

HEALTH AND FITNESS OF THE DISABLED

Functional Neuromuscular Stimulation for Physical Fitness Training of the Disabled

R.M. Glaser

Department of Physiology and Biophysics, Wright State University School of Medicine, Dayton, Ohio, U.S.A.

Muscle paralysis limits one's ability to voluntarily exercise and can result in marked loss of physical fitness. A major goal of our research effort is to develop and evaluate the effectiveness of specialized exercise techniques by which individuals with various neuromuscular disorders (e.g., spinal cord injury, head trauma, stroke, and multiple sclerosis) can improve their physical fitness. Additionally, it appears that appropriate exercise can potentially reduce health complications of sedentary lifestyles (e.g., cardiovascular diseases, muscle atrophy, osteoporosis, and decubitus ulcers) and enhance rehabilitation outcome. Two recent reports from our laboratory have thoroughly reviewed the area of arm exercise training for wheelchair users (6, 10). This paper presents current research data related to using functional neuromuscular stimulation (FNS) of paralyzed leg muscles for improving the physical fitness of disabled individuals.

Individuals with paralyzed legs typically make compensatory use of the functional arms. Thus, the upper-body musculature is used for manual wheelchair locomotion, exercise training, and sports activities. However, arm exercise capability is inherently limited (to about 2/3 of leg exercise capability for able-bodied individuals) by the relatively small muscle mass involved (1, 19). Therefore, the ability of paraplegics to develop high levels of physical fitness (e.g., cardiopulmonary or aerobic) is also limited. This is due to the fact that the upper-body muscles tend to fatigue (because of peripheral factors) prior to the cardiopulmonary system being driven to sufficiently high output levels for long enough durations to enable substantial central training effects to take place (2, 3). Quadriplegics have even lower exercise and fitness development capabilities because of the paralyzed upper-body musculature. It is also doubtful that arm exercise has any effect on alleviating the deterioration of the lower body.

During the past several years, the use of FNS-induced contractions to exercise paralyzed lower-limb muscles has received increasing attention. This technique has the potential for improving physical fitness of disabled individuals to higher levels than can be achieved through voluntary arm exercise alone. This is due in part to the activation of muscles that are usually dormant, greater muscle mass that can be utilized, and improved circulation of blood (7, 12). Quadriplegics may may find this involuntary exercise mode to be especially beneficial. However, it should be emphasized that FNS exercise is not known to (and probably does not) cure neuromuscular disorders. It should also be realized that any health and physical fitness benefits that are derived from participating in FNS exercise programs will most likely be lost within several weeks after the exercise is discontinued. Therefore, if FNS exercise is found to be beneficial, it should become part of one's lifestyle.

Some of the FNS exercise techniques to be described are currently experimental and require specially constructed equipment. However, commercial electrical neuromuscular stimulator systems have recently become available to permit FNS exercise in a clinical or home setting. Disabled individuals with an interest in this form of exercise training should consult with their physician or therapist.

Requirements and Precautions for FNS Use

A major requirement for FNS use is that the motor units of the paralyzed muscles are intact and functional (i.e., the damage to the central nervous system is upper motor neuron in nature). Individuals who will most likely respond favorably to FNS typically exhibit reflex contractions and spasms in the affected muscles. Muscles may be tested for FNS response using a small single-channel electrical stimulator and skin surface electrodes placed over motor points (where motor nerves enter the muscle). The location of motor points is determined by placing a stationary electrode over the muscle and moving an exploratory electrode around the muscle while stimulating at an intensity that causes slight contractions. At motor points, greater contraction force will be obtained for a given stimulation level (i.e., threshold level will be lower). With individuals who respond well to FNS, as stimulation intensity is gradually increased, more motor units will be recruited and contraction force will increase.

A physical examination is prudent prior to using FNS for exercise training. This exam should include an electrocardiogram, radiographs of the paralyzed limbs, and range-of-motion testing. To prevent injuries to the deteriorated muscles, bones, and joints, FNS-induced contractions should be smooth and limited with respect to maximal force development. In some individuals, FNS may trigger spasms and reflex contractions in the stimulated and other muscles. Thus, it is important to closely observe the activity to be certain that it is not hazardous. As a precaution, it is advisable to monitor heart rate and blood pressure, especially during initial FNS exercise sessions. Some individuals may exhibit autonomic dysreflexia with excessively high blood pressure (>175 mmHg) during FNS use. As with any mode of exercise, activity should be discontinued immediately if abnormal responses occur that place the user at risk.

FNS-Induced Weight-Lifting Exercise

Early FNS exercise training studies used either static (isometric) contractions or dynamic (movement through a range of motion) contractions without external load resistance (15, 16). Periodic on-off patterns of muscle stimulation were utilized. There were gains in strength and resistance to fatigue reported for training with these exercise modes. However, recent studies that incorporated well-established weight-training principles (i.e., progressive overload, low number of repetitions at relatively high resistance, 2-3 sets of exercise, and exercise frequency of 2-4 times per week) in conjunction with FNS of gradually ramped intensity levels have provided more dramatic results (14, 17).

An example of this resistance exercise technique is knee extension weight lifting induced by FNS of the paralyzed quadriceps muscles (14, 17). This can be performed at a rate of 3-5 lifts per minute for each leg in a reciprocal pattern, and 10-30 lifts per set can be used. With improvements in performance, a load weight progression of 0.5 kg appears to be suitable. Although specially designed stimulators and weight-lifting devices can be constructed to enable this exercise (8, 9), small commercial stimulators (that provide gradually ramped output intensity) and ankle weights could also be used. Results indicated that by gradually increasing load resistance on the muscles (over a several week period) as well as the number of repetitions, quadriceps strength and resistance to fatigue could be markedly increased. Figure 1 illustrates the load weight progression used to train 6 spinal cord-injured (SCI) subjects with knee extension exercise that took place three times per week for 12 weeks (14). After the training program, 4 of the subjects were able to lift over 10 kg with each leg (in a reciprocal pattern) during two consecutive 10-min, 20-contraction (with each leg) sets. It is likely that similar techniques and protocols could be used to FNS train other muscles. Although this weight-lifting exercise can result in peripheral adaptations to increase muscle strength and resistance to fatigue, the aerobic

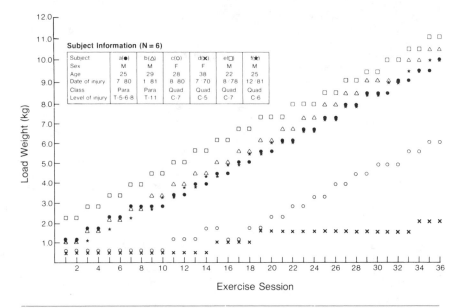

Figure 1. Subject load weight progression data (right leg) during 12 weeks (3X/wk) of FNS-induced knee extension exercise training. (Modified from Gruner et al., 1983).

metabolic and cardiopulmonary responses are not of sufficient magnitudes and durations to permit cardiopulmonary (central circulatory) training to occur (4).

There is currently no compelling evidence that this FNS exercise, or any other form of FNS exercise, can reverse osteoporosis (Glaser, 1986). It is therefore plausible that FNS weight training can ultimately make the muscles stronger than the bones and that forceful contractions can result in fractures. Osteoporosis is difficult to precisely evaluate, because at least a 30-50% change in bone mass can occur before it is detected by standard radiographs. Thus, it is advisable to set reasonable upper limits to the maximal resistance that is used for training (e.g., 10-15 kg for knee extension exercise). The number of repetitions and sets may be increased when maximal permissible loading has been achieved.

FNS-Induced Cycle Ergometer Exercise

In 1982, a Monark cycle ergometer was modified to permit paraplegics and quadriplegics to exercise via computer-controlled, FNS-induced contractions of the quadriceps, hamstring, and gluteus maximus muscles (18). Subsequently, highly sophisticated versions of this device became available for clinical and home use (Therapeutic Technologies Inc., Ft. Lauderdale, FL). These FNS cycle ergometers can be pedaled up to 50 rpm, at which rate there are 50 contractions of the contralateral muscle groups each minute. Thus, this exercise brings in more muscle mass than the above described FNS weight-lifting exercise, and the muscles are stimulated to contract at a considerably higher rate. FNS cycle ergometer exercise appears to be well suited for endurance (rather than strength) training as many users can maintain continuous pedaling for 30-min periods. Improvements in cardiopulmonary fitness may be derived from this FNS exercise training.

Initially, individuals pedal this FNS cycle ergometer with no load resistance (0 watts). When 30 min of continuous pedaling can be achieved, subsequent exercise sessions use added load resistance to increase the power output (PO) to 6 W. When 30 min of continu-

130   Glaser

ous pedaling can be achieved at this higher PO, the PO is further increased by a 6-W increment. This progressive intensity protocol is repeated with gains in fitness up to a maximum PO of 42 W for this device.

A recent study evaluated metabolic and cardiopulmonary responses of 12 SCI subjects to this mode of FNS exercise to better understand potential training effects (11). PO levels ranged from 0 to 30 W depending upon the capability of the individual. Figure 2 provides

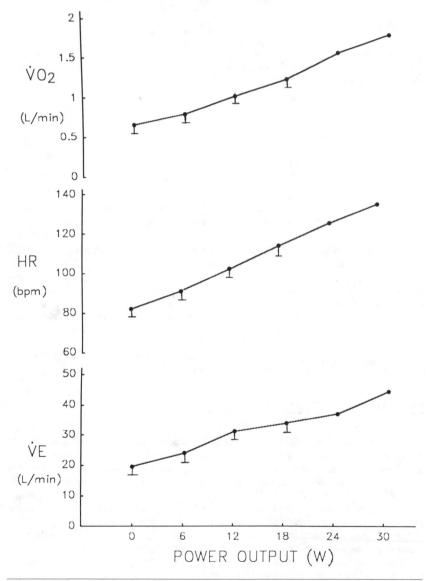

Figure 2. Steady state oxygen uptake ($\dot{V}O_2$), pulmonary ventilation ($\dot{V}E$), and heart rate (HR) responses of spinal cord injured subjects in relation to power output for FNS cycle ergometry. (Modified from Glaser et al., 1988).

the steady state oxygen uptake ($\dot{V}O_2$), pulmonary ventilation ($\dot{V}E$), and heart rate (HR) data obtained for 5 min of exercise at each PO level. Twelve subjects completed exercise at 0 W, 10 at 6 W, 9 at 12 W, 4 at 18 W, and 1 at 24 and 30 W. $\dot{V}O_2$, $\dot{V}E$ and HR responses tended to be linear with PO, indicating appropriate metabolic and cardiopulmonary adjustments. The one subject that pedaled at 30 W had a peak $\dot{V}O_2$ of 1.77 L/min, $\dot{V}E$ of 45 L/min, and HR of 135 beats/min.

Since this cycle ergometer has a maximal PO capability of 42 W, it appears that well-trained SCI individuals who can achieve this PO may reach a $\dot{V}O_2$ of about 2 L/min (with concomitant $\dot{V}E$ and HR responses). When considering that aerobic training is typically conducted at about 50-60% of maximal $\dot{V}O_2$ (maximal $\dot{V}O_2$ may be about 3-4 L/min for leg exercise by able-bodied individuals, and it is probably much lower for arm exercise by SCI individuals), FNS cycling offers a potential means to achieve this training metabolic rate. Indeed, able-bodied individuals usually jog at $\dot{V}O_2$ levels of 1.5-2.0 L/min. It is not likely that such high $\dot{V}O_2$ levels can be elicited by arm exercise for sufficient periods of time (e.g., 30 min) for substantial cardiopulmonary training due to the small muscle mass utilized.

In another study, six C6-C7 quadriplegic men performed (at separate times) FNS cycle ergometer exercise at a mean PO of 11 W and arm crank ergometer exercise at a mean PO of 38 W (5). Although both of these exercise modes elicited almost identical $\dot{V}O_2$ levels of 1.0 L/min, FNS cycling produced a 59% greater ventricular stroke volume (92 vs 58 ml/beat) and 20% greater cardiac output (8.01 vs 6.66 L/min). Superior venous return of the blood to the heart during FNS cycling may have been due in part to activation of the venous muscle pump via induced contractions of the lower-extremity muscles and the cycling motion. In addition, a 25% lower heart rate (87 vs 116 beats/min) and 19% lower rate-pressure product for FNS cycling indicated that the higher cardiac volume-load was accomplished with lower myocardial O_2 demands. These data suggest that FNS cycle ergometer pedaling may be a more efficient and safer (with respect to cardiovascular risks) mode of exercise than arm cranking for the purpose of aerobic conditioning in quadriplegics.

Hybrid Exercise

A hybrid form of exercise, where FNS-induced leg exercise is performed simultaneously with voluntary arm exercise, may provide a greater aerobic training capability than either mode of exercise performed separately (13). This is potentially due to (a) greater muscle mass that can be utilized, (b) greater magnitudes of metabolic and cardiopulmonary responses that can be achieved, and (c) improved circulation of blood to the active muscles, which can enhance their performance (i.e., FNS leg exercise may elevate venous return and cardiac output to increase blood flow to the arm muscles, and voluntary arm exercise may induce sympathetically mediated cardiovascular responses to increase blood flow to the leg muscles).

The concept of hybrid exercise was first tested on six high-level SCI individuals using combined FNS-induced knee extension and voluntary arm cranking exercise (13). Higher magnitudes of peak $\dot{V}O_2$, $\dot{V}E$, and HR responses were obtained during this exercise, which indicated the possibility of obtaining additive physiologic effects. In addition, the FNS-activated quadriceps muscles exhibited greater resistance to fatigue during arm cranking (20).

Recent laboratory experiments (20) using combined FNS-induced leg cycling and voluntary arm cranking produced much more dramatic results. Figure 3 shows the $\dot{V}O_2$ achieved by a paraplegic subject at rest and during FNS leg cycling at 6.1 W, voluntary arm cranking at 25 W, and hybrid exercise at a total of 31.1 W. Separately, both modes of exercise increased $\dot{V}O_2$ to about 0.5 L/min above the resting level of about 0.25 L/min. However, when performed simultaneously, the $\dot{V}O_2$ increased to 1.25 L/min indicating an additional 0.5 L/min increment. Thus, it appears possible that SCI individuals performing this hybrid exercise can achieve higher $\dot{V}O_2$ levels during exercise training periods to enhance aerobic conditioning capability, while deriving training benefits for both the upper- and lower-body musculature. This technique has elicited peak $\dot{V}O_2$ levels of over 1.5 L/min in some quadriplegics and over 2.0 L/min in some paraplegics who were not highly trained. Considering that most studies of maximal effort arm exercise for highly trained elite wheel-chair athletes (paraplegics) have reported peak $\dot{V}O_2$ values of slightly above 2.0 L/min (6), the hybrid exercise mode appears to be quite advantageous in that this high VO_2 magnitude can be elicited from nonathletic SCI individuals from the general population.

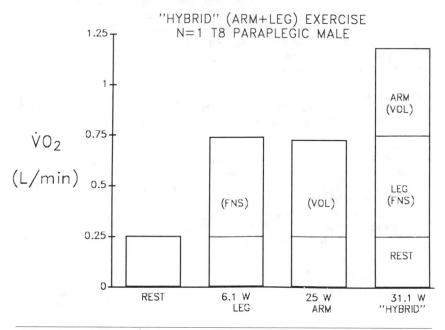

Figure 3. Oxygen uptake ($\dot{V}O_2$) of a T8 paraplegic male subject at rest, during FNS cycle ergometry at 6.1 watts, during voluntary arm cranking at 25 watts, and during hybrid exercise (simultaneous FNS leg cycling and voluntary arm cranking) at a total power output of 31.1 W. Note the additive effect upon $\dot{V}O_2$.

Conclusions

The purpose of this paper is to acquaint the reader with techniques that are being researched to permit exercise of paralyzed leg muscles via FNS. It seems clear that FNS-induced weight-lifting exercise can markedly improve the strength and resistance to fatigue of paralyzed muscles for this exercise mode. Evidence also suggests that FNS-induced cycle ergometer exercise can elicit aerobic metabolic and cardiopulmonary responses of sufficient magnitudes and for long enough durations to elicit central cardiopulmonary training effects. However, it is my opinion that FNS exercise should be used in conjunction with arm exercise (separately and combined) when possible to obtain optimal levels of total body fitness. In this regard, hybrid-type exercise appears to be most promising for enabling effective and efficient development of aerobic fitness in paraplegic and quadriplegic individuals.

It appears that FNS exercise may ultimately contribute to improved health, physical fitness, and rehabilitation potential of paralyzed individuals. More research is needed to develop safe and effective FNS exercise techniques and protocols as well as to document the physiologic responses and training benefits.

Acknowledgment

Most of the research projects described in this paper were supported by the Rehabilitation Research and Development Service of the U.S. Department of Veterans Affairs.

References

1. Åstrand, P.-O., Saltin, B. Maximal oxygen uptake and heart rate in various types of muscular activity. J. Appl. Physiol. 16:977-981, 1961.

2. Bar-Or, O., Zwiren, L.D. Maximal oxygen consumption test during arm exercise—reliability and validity. J. Appl. Physiol. 38:424-426, 1975.

3. Clausen, J.P., Klausen, K., Rasmussen, B., Trap-Jensen, J. Central and peripheral circulatory changes after training of the arms and legs. Am. J. Physiol. 225:675-682, 1973.

4. Collins, S.R., Glaser, R.M. Comparison of aerobic metabolism and cardiopulmonary responses for electrically induced and voluntary exercise. Proceedings of the Eighth Annual Conference on Rehabilitation Technology. Washington, D.C.: Rehabilitation Engineering Society of North America, 1985:391-393.

5. Figoni, S.F., Glaser, R.M., Hendershot, D.M., Gupta, S.C., Suryaprasad, A.G., Rodgers, M.M., Ezenwa, B.N. Hemodynamic responses of quadriplegics to maximal arm-cranking and FNS leg cycling exercise. Proceedings of the Tenth Annual Conference of the Engineering in Medicine and Biology Society. Piscataway, NJ: Institute of Electrical and Electronics Engineers, 1988: 1636-1637.

6. Glaser, R.M. Exercise and locomotion for the spinal cord injured. In: Terjung, R.L., ed. Exercise and sport sciences reviews. Volume 13. New York: Macmillan, 1985:263-303.

7. Glaser, R.M. Physiologic aspects of spinal cord injury and functional neuromuscular stimulation. Central Nervous System Trauma 3:49-61, 1986.

8. Glaser, R.M., Collins, S.R., Horgan, H.R. An electrical stimulator for exercising paralyzed muscles. Proceedings of the Tenth Annual Conference on Rehabilitation Technology. Washington, D.C.: Rehabilitation Engineering Society of North America, 1987:597-599.

9. Glaser, R.M., Collins, S.R., Strayer, J.R., Glaser, M. A closed-loop stimulator for exercising paralyzed muscles. Proceedings of the Eighth Annual Conference on Rehabilitation Technology. Washington, D.C.: Rehabilitation Engineering Society of North America, 1985:388-390.

10. Glaser, R.M., Davis, G.M. Wheelchair-dependent individuals. In: Franklin, B.A., Gordon, S., Timmis, G.C., eds. Exercise in modern medicine: testing and prescription in health and disease. Baltimore: Williams & Wilkins, 1988:237-267.

11. Glaser, R.M., Figoni, S.F., Collins, S.R., Rodgers, M.M., Suryaprasad, A.G., Gupta, S.C., Mathews, T. Physiologic responses of SCI subjects to electrically induced leg cycle ergometry. Proceedings of the Tenth Annual Conference of the Engineering in

Medicine and Biology Society. Piscataway, N.J.: Institute of Electrical and Electronics Engineers, 1988:1638-1640.

12. Glaser, R.M., Rattan, S.N., Davis, G.M., Servedio, F.J., Gupta, S.C., Suryaprasad, A.G. Central hemodynamic responses to lower-limb FNS. Proceedings of the Ninth Annual Conference of the Engineering in Medicine and Biology Society. Piscataway, N.J.: Institute of Electrical and Electronics Engineers, 1987:615-617.

13. Glaser, R.M., Strayer, J.R., May, K.P. Combined FES leg and voluntary arm exercise of SCI patients. Proceedings of the Seventh Annual Conference of the Engineering in Medicine and Biology Society. Piscataway, N.J.: Institute of Electrical and Electronics Engineers, 1985:308-313.

14. Gruner, J.A., Glaser, R.M., Feinberg, S.D., Collins, S.R., Nussbaum, N.S. A system for evaluation and exercise-conditioning of paralyzed leg muscles. J. Rehab. Res. Dev. 20:21-30, 1983.

15. Kralj, A., Bajd, T., Turk, R. Electrical stimulation providing functional use of paraplegic patient muscles. Med. Prog. Tech. 7:3-9, 1980.

16. Peckham, P.H., Mortimer, J.T., Marsolais, E.B. Alteration in the force and fatigability of skeletal muscle in quadriplegic humans following exercise induced by chronic electrical stimulation. Clin. Orthop. Rel. Res. 114:326-334, 1976.

17. Petrofsky, J.S., Phillips, C.A. Active physical therapy: a modern approach to rehabilitation therapy. J. Neurol. Orthop. Med. Surg. 4:165-173, 1983.

18. Petrofsky, J.S., Phillips, C.A., Heaton, H.H., III, Glaser, R.M. Bicycle ergometer for paralyzed muscles. J. Clin. Eng. 9:13-19, 1984.

19. Zwiren, L.D., Bar-Or, O. Responses to exercise of paraplegics who differ in conditioning level. Med. Sci. Sports 7:94-98, 1975.

20. Glaser, R.M. Central and peripheral etiology of fatigue for the disabled. 1988 AAEE Didactic Program: Muscle Fatigue. Rochester, Minnesota: American Association of Electromyography and Electrodiagnosis, 1988: 21-26.

Factors That Limit the Maximal Aerobic Power of Children With a Chronic Disease

O. Bar-Or

Children's Exercise and Nutrition Centre, McMaster University, Hamilton, Ontario, Canada

Many children with diseases have reduced fitness. In some, it may reflect a sedentary lifestyle and a resulting detraining effect. In others, it results from a specific pathophysiologic process that limits their exercise capacity. For a more detailed review, see Bar-Or (3, 4), Godfrey (18), Haller and Lewis (23), and Wasserman and Whip (51). Among all the fitness components that may be affected by disease, there are five that have drawn the most attention. These are maximal aerobic power, the metabolic cost of performing submaximal activities, muscle strength, peak muscle power, and muscle endurance (4). It is important to emphasize, however, that such a division is somewhat artificial due to the interrelationships among fitness components. For example, there is sometimes a close link between the reduction of muscle strength, muscle power, and local muscle endurance in patients with muscular dystrophy, muscular atrophy, or joint disease.

The reduction in maximal aerobic power, whether measured as maximal oxygen uptake ($\dot{V}O_2$max), mechanical power at a heart rate (HR) of 170 beats/min (32), mean power during a progressive test (20), highest mechanical power on the cycle ergometer (26), the highest stage reached during a multistage treadmill test (11), or the anaerobic threshold (38), is the most quoted disease-related effect on fitness.

Most of the pediatric literature on the relationship between disease and low aerobic fitness is related to congenital heart defects. While some authors (e.g., 20) have suggested that the degree of reduction in maximal aerobic power depends on the specific defect, others (11, 15, 32) have shown that such a reduction in fitness is not specific to any particular defect. Thus, one cannot distinguish among defects merely by performing a maximal aerobic power test.

Usually the subnormal maximal aerobic power that accompanies a pediatric disease can be explained by a specific deficiency in the oxygen transport chain, whether at the respiratory, cardiovascular, blood, or muscular level. The purpose of this review is to outline briefly those pediatric conditions that specifically affect one or more of the components of the oxygen transport system. The understanding of such specific pathophysiologic processes is a prerequisite for any intelligent intervention that is meant to increase the child's fitness and well-being.

Table 1 summarizes those diseases that induce a reduction in maximal aerobic power in pediatric populations. The table also points out the specific components within the oxygen transport system that may be affected by each disease. Most of the information upon which this table is constructed was derived from experimental findings. Some of it, however, is based on common sense and deduction and still needs experimental confirmation.

Table 1 Effect of Pediatric Disease on Maximal Aerobic Power of Children

Disease	Low $\dot{V}$Emax	Low DL	Low SVmax	Low HRmax	Low CaO$_2$max	High CvO$_2$max
Anemia					X	
Anorexia nervosa (severe)				X		X
Aortic stenosis			X			
Arthritis						X
Asthma (severe)	X					
Atrial septal defect (severe)					X	
Cerebral palsy						X
Congenital complete heart block				X		
Cystic fibrosis	X	X			X	
Hypohydration (severe)			X			
Malnutrition (severe)					X	X
Muscular atrophy						X
Muscular dystrophy						X
Obesity (marked)	X					
Paraplegia (traumatic)	X					X
Pulmonary stenosis			X			
Quadriplegia	X					X
Right-to-left shunt					X	
Scoliosis (severe)	X					X
Sickle-cell anemia			X		X	
Spina bifida	X					X
Tetralogy of Fallot			X		X	
Thalassemia			X		X	
Ventricular septal defect					X	

Note. SV = stroke volume, CaO$_2$ = oxygen content in the arterial blood, CvO$_2$ = oxygen content in the mixed-venous blood, $\dot{V}$E = minute ventilation, DL = lung diffusion capacity.

Maximal Minute Ventilation ($\dot{V}$Emax)

$\dot{V}$Emax has not been considered a limiting factor in the maximal aerobic power of healthy people, unless they are highly trained endurance athletes (14). It does, however, limit the performance of children with diseases such as cystic fibrosis (8), advanced kyphoscoliosis (42), and obesity (13, 53). A low $\dot{V}$Emax is also likely to occur in children who are bound to a wheelchair (e.g., with spina bifida, traumatic paraplegia, or quadriplegia) probably resulting from a high position of the diaphragm muscle, which reduces the vital capacity.

It has been shown (21) that children with asthma respond to maximal exercise with normal $\dot{V}E$. Their alveolar ventilation is sometimes even above normal. One can assume, however, that when the asthma is severe and inadequately treated, the very prolonged expiratory phase due to bronchoconstriction will induce a subnormal $\dot{V}Emax$ and low $\dot{V}O_2max$.

Lung Diffusing Capacity

Seldom is the rate of gas diffusion between the alveoli and the pulmonary capillaries a limiting factor during exercise. While this occurs in several adulthood pulmonary diseases (27, 51), the only pediatric disease in which a subnormal lung diffusion capacity during exercise has been documented and confirmed is cystic fibrosis (19, 54). An imbalance between the alveolar ventilation and perfusion at the pulmonary capillaries, which results in an exaggerated gradient of oxygen pressure between the alveoli and the arterial blood, has been shown in children with cystic fibrosis (19) and advanced scoliosis (43). In contrast, children with asthma respond to exercise with a decrease in their alveolo-arterial oxygen pressure gradient (17, 21).

Maximal Stroke Volume (SVmax)

Several congenital cardiac diseases are accompanied by a low SVmax, which results in a low maximal cardiac output and $\dot{V}O_2max$. For recent reviews see Mocellin (31, 32) and Driscoll (15). A low SVmax will occur primarily when there is an obstruction to the outflow tract of the left or right ventricle, as in aortic stenosis (10, 46) and pulmonary stenosis (25, 34), respectively. Pulmonary valve stenosis is one component of the tetralogy of Fallot, which also causes a low SVmax (33, 52). Other conditions that are accompanied by low stroke volume and low maximal aerobic power include Mustard's operation for d-transposition of the great arteries (30) and Fontan's operation for tricuspid atresia or single ventricle (16). A left-to-right shunt, as in atrial or ventricular septal defects, causes some of the left ventricular SV to be shunted to the right heart. The end result is a functionally low systemic stroke volume, which may explain the reported (11, 20) low aerobic fitness in some children with these conditions. This hemodynamic change depends, however, on the size of the shunt. An opposite process may take place whenever the shunt (mostly in a large ventricular septal defect) induces a rise in pulmonary blood pressure, which ultimately may reverse the direction of the shunt. Advanced dehydration is accompanied by a reduction in SV, which may be one reason for the low aerobic performance in dehydrated people (1, 41).

Maximal Heart Rate (HRmax)

A low HR is another reason for a low cardiac output. While a compensatory increase in stroke volume and a resulting normal cardiac output may take place at rest and submaximal exercise, a normal cardiac output during intense activities cannot be maintained. The end result is low maximal cardiac output and $\dot{V}O_2max$. Conditions in which a low HRmax in children is the primary cause of their low maximal cardiac output include congenital complete atrioventricular block (49) and treatment with beta adrenergic blocking agents (47). Intracardiac surgery, such as in the Mustard or Senning procedures, sometimes affects the sinoatrial node, which induces a low HRmax (24). Low HRmax has also been described in such diseases as anorexia nervosa (36, 48), although it is unlikely to be the primary cause of low maximal aerobic power.

Oxygen-Carrying Capacity by the Arterial Blood

A low arterial content of oxygen (CaO_2) may become a limiting factor in aerobic exercise of high intensity. At rest and at low-to-moderate intensities, oxygen supply to the exercising muscles may still be adequate due to a compensatory rise in cardiac output, a "shift to the right" in the oxygen dissociation curve (as in iron-deficiency anemia [45]), or a decrease in the mixed-venous oxygen content. Such compensatory mechanisms become inadequate, however, during intense activities. This results in an insufficient extraction of oxygen in the periphery (as manifested by a low arterio-mixed venous difference in oxygen content) and a low $\dot{V}O_2$max.

There are respiratory, cardiac, and hematological causes of low CaO_2. Cystic fibrosis is the most common respiratory disease that may limit the lung diffusing capacity. This, in high-intensity exercise, is manifested by arterial oxygen desaturation (8). Among cardiac conditions, a right-to-left shunt would cause a venous admixture of blood and a low arterial oxygen saturation. In some of the congenital cardiac defects, such as the tetralogy of Fallot (32), this is manifested more so during exercise than at rest. The child often becomes cyanotic, and her or his $\dot{V}O_2$max is markedly low.

The most obvious hematological cause of low oxygen content in the arterial blood is a low concentration of functional hemoglobin, as in iron-deficiency anemia (12, 37), sickle-cell anemia (2), thalassemia major (9), or chronic renal failure (5). However, as has been described in recent years, many endurance athletes including adolescents may incur a reduction in their performance and maximal aerobic power due to iron deficiency that is not accompanied by low hemoglobin concentration.

Rowland et al. (40), for example, who studied adolescent cross-country runners, found low concentration of serum ferritin (<12 mg ml^{-1}) with normal hemoglobin levels in 45% of the females and 17% of the males studied. A similar prevalence has been described by Nickerson and Tripp (35) among high school female runners. This so called nonanemic iron deficiency becomes more pronounced with an increase in the intensity and duration of endurance training. Its etiology is not entirely clear, but it probably reflects a hematopoietic disturbance in the bone marrow as well as enhanced iron losses in the active athlete. Nor is it entirely clear how this condition affects aerobic performance. For a recent review on nonanemic iron deficiency in adolescents and its management, see Rowland (39). More research is needed in this area as it affects many more young athletes than does iron-deficiency anemia.

Utilization of Oxygen by the Tissues

Even when sufficient amounts of oxygen reach the exercising muscles, maximal aerobic power will be low if the muscles do not utilize the oxygen at their disposal or if the mass of the muscle tissue is abnormally low. An example for the former is spastic cerebral palsy (5, 6, 29), in which muscle movement is limited by the spasticity and its maximal metabolic requirements are less than normal. It should be stressed that during submaximal exercise these muscles require above normal $\dot{V}O_2$ (28), which increases the fatigue of the child (3). Such a child will be working at a higher than normal percentage of his or her $\dot{V}O_2$max compared with healthy children who perform identical tasks.

Pediatric conditions in which muscle mass (or the mass of the healthy, functional muscle tissue) is small and $\dot{V}O_2$max is low include Duchenne or Becker muscular dystrophy (7, 44), central core myopathy (22), spinal muscular atrophy, spina bifida, other paraplegias, quadriplegia, advanced rheumatoid arthritis, cystic fibrosis, and extreme malnutrition (as in anorexia nervosa). The degree of the aerobic deficiency usually depends on the severity of the muscle disease. It should be realized however that low aerobic fitness in some of these conditions depends also on factors other than the skeletal muscles. For example,

Duchenne muscular dystrophy can affect the myocardium, which in turn may cause a decrease in cardiac output. For a further review on the effects of muscle disease on exercise performance, see Haller and Lewis (23).

Summary and Conclusions

Many pediatric diseases and illnesses are accompanied by a sedentary lifestyle and the resulting detraining and low maximal aerobic power. However, as seen from this review, such diseases can be accompanied also by specific pathophysiologic changes that affect oxygen transport and its utilization in the exercising child. These can take place at the respiratory, cardiovascular, blood, and metabolic levels of the oxygen transport chain. Zeroing in on the specific deficiency in this chain is important for a basic understanding of the pathophysiologic processes. It can also help in designing specific rehabilitation programs through exercise. However, a certain disease can often affect more than one link in the oxygen transport chain. An example is cystic fibrosis, in which deficiencies occur simultaneously at the ventilatory, lung diffusion, and skeletal muscle levels. One should further realize that several fitness components other than maximal aerobic power alone may be affected in the same child. A rehabilitation program will need to address some or all of them.

References

1. Allen, T.E., Smith, D.P., Miller, D.K. Hemodynamic response to submaximal exercise after dehydration and rehydration in high school wrestlers. Med. Sci. Sports 9:159-163, 1977.

2. Alpert, B.S., Dover, V., Strong, W.S., Covitz, W. Longitudinal exercise hemodynamics in children with sickle cell anemia. Am. J. Diseases of Children 138:1021-1024, 1984.

3. Bar-Or, O. Exercise in pediatric assessment and diagnosis. Scand. J. Sports Sci. 7:34-38, 1985.

4. Bar-Or, O. Pathophysiological factors which limit the exercise capacity of the sick child. Med. Sci. Sports Exer. 18:276-282, 1986.

5. Bar-Or, O., Inbar, O., Spira, R. Physiological effects of a sports rehabilitation program on cerebral palsied and post-poliomyelitic adolescents. Med. Sci. Sports 8:157-161, 1976.

6. Berg, K. Effects of physical training of school children with cerebral palsy. Acta Paediatr. Scand. 204(Suppl.):27-33, 1970.

7. Carroll, J.E., Hagberg, J.M., Brooke, M.H., Shumate, J.B. Bicycle ergometry and gas exchange measurements in neuromuscular diseases. Arch. Neurol. 36:457-461, 1979.

8. Cerny, F.J., Pullano, T.P., Cropp, G.J.A. Cardiorespiratory adaptations to exercise in cystic fibrosis. Am. Rev. Respir. Dis. 126:217-220, 1982.

9. Cooper, D.M., Hyman, C.B., Weiler-Ravell, D., Noble, N.A., Agnes, C.L., Wasserman, K. Gas exchange during exercise in children with thalassemia major and Diamond-Blackfan anemia. Pediatr. Res. 19:1215-1219, 1985.

10. Cueto, L., Moller, J.H. Haemodynamics of exercise in children with isolated aortic valvular disease. Br. Heart J. 35:93-98, 1973.

11. Cumming, G.R. Maximal exercise capacity of children with heart defects. Am. J. Cardiol. 42:613-619, 1978.

12. Davies, C.T.M. The physiologic effects of iron deficiency anemia and malnutrition on exercise performance in East African school children. Acta Paediatr. Belgica Suppl. 28:253-256, 1974.

13. DeMeersman, R.E., Stone, S., Schaefer, D.C., Miller, W.W. Maximal work capacity in prepubescent obese and nonobese females. Clin. Pediatr. 24:199-200, 1985.

14. Dempsey, J.A. Is the lung built for exercise? Med. Sci. Sports Exer. 18:143-155, 1986.

15. Driscoll, D.J. Diagnostic use of exercise testing in pediatric cardiology: the non-invasive approach. In: Bar-Or, O., ed. Advances in pediatric sport sciences, Vol. 3. Champaign, IL: Human Kinetics, 1988.

16. Driscoll, D.J., Danielson, G.K., Puja, F.J., Schaff, H.V., Hsie, C.T., Staats, B.A. Exercise tolerance and cardiorespiratory response to exercise after Fontan operation for Tricuspid atresia or functional single ventricle. J. Am. Coll. Cardiol. 7:1087, 1986.

17. Geubelle, F., Dechange, J., Louis, I., Beyer, M. Respiratory function, energetic metabolism, and work capacity in boys with asthma syndrome. Acta Paediatr. Belgica 31:79-86, 1978.

18. Godfrey, S. Exercise testing in children: applications to health and disease. Philadelphia: Saunders, 1973.

19. Godfrey, S., Mearns, M. Pulmonary function and response to exercise in cystic fibrosis. Arch. Diseases of Childhood 46:144-151, 1971.

20. Goldberg, S.J., Mendes, F., Hurwitz, R. Maximal exercise capability of children as a function of specific cardiac defects. Am. J. Cardiol. 41:349-353, 1969.

21. Graff-Lonnevig, V. Cardio-respiratory function, aerobic capacity and effect of physical activity in asthmatic boys. Stockholm: Karolinska Institute, 1978. Thesis.

22. Hagberg, J.M., Carroll, J.E., Brooke, M.H. Endurance exercise training in a patient with central core disease. Neurology 30:1242-1244, 1980.

23. Haller, R.G., Lewis, S.F. Pathophysiology of exercise performance in muscle disease. Med. Sci. Sports Exer. 16:456-459, 1984.

24. Hesslein, P.S., Gutsgesell, H.P., Gillette, P.C. Exercise assessment of sinoatrial node function in children after Mustard's operation (abstract). Pediatr. Res. 14:445, 1980.

25. Howitt, G. Hemodynamic effects of exercise in pulmonary stenosis. Br. Heart J. 28:152-160, 1966.

26. James, F.W. Exercise testing in children and young adults: an overview. Cardiovascular Clinics 9:187-203, 1978.

27. Jones, N.L., Campbell, E.J.M. Clinical exercise testing. Philadelphia: Saunders, 1982.

28. Lundberg, A. Oxygen consumption in relation to work load in students with cerebral palsy. J. Appl. Physiol. 40:873-875, 1976.

29. Lundberg, A. Maximal aerobic capacity of young people with spastic cerebral palsy. Dev. Med. Child Neurol. 20:205-210, 1978.

30. Mathews, R.A., Fricker, F.J., Beerman, L.B., Stephenson, R.J., Fischer, D.R., Neches, W.H., Parh, S.C., Lenox, C.C., Zuberbuhler, J.R. Exercise studies after the Mustard operation in the transposition of the great arteries. Am. J. Cardiol. 51:1526-1529, 1983.

31. Mocellin, R. Children with cardiac disease and exercise. In: Binkhorst, R.A., Kemper, H.C.G., Saris, W.H.M. Children and exercise XI. Champaign, IL: Human Kinetics, 1985:26-41.

32. Mocellin, R. Exercise testing in children with congenital heart disease. Pediatrician 13:18-25, 1986.

33. Mocellin, R., Bastanier, C., Hofacker, W., Buhlmeyer, K. Exercise performance in children and adolescents after surgical repair of tetralogy of Fallot. Europ. J. Cardiol. 4:367-374, 1976.

34. Moller, J.H., Rao, S., Lucas, R.V. Exercise hemodynamics of pulmonary valvular stenosis (study of 64 children). Circulation 46:1018-1026, 1972.

35. Nickerson, H.J., Tripp, A.D. Iron deficiency in adolescent cross country runners. Physician and Sportsmed. 11:60-66, 1983.

36. Nudel, D.B., Gootman, N., Nussbaum, M.P. Altered exercise performance and abnormal sympathetic response to exercise in patients with anorexia nervosa. J. Pediatr. 105:34-37, 1984.

37. Parsons, E.C., Wright, F.H. Circulatory functions in the anemias of children: I. Effect of anemia on exercise tolerance and vital capacity. Am. J. Diseases of Children 57:15-28, 1939.

38. Reybrouck, T.M. The use of the "anaerobic threshold" in pediatric exercise testing. In: Bar-Or, O., ed. Advances in pediatric sports sciences, Vol. 3. Champaign, IL: Human Kinetics, 1988.

39. Rowland, T.W. Iron deficiency and supplementation in the young endurance athlete. In: Bar-Or, O., ed. Advances in pediatric sports sciences, Vol. 3. Champaign, IL: Human Kinetics, 1988.

40. Rowland, T.W., Black, S.A., Kelleher, J.F. Iron deficiency in adolescent endurance runners. J. Adol. Health Care 8:322-326, 1987.

41. Saltin, B. Aerobic and anaerobic work capacity after dehydration. J. Appl. Physiol. 19:1114-1118, 1964.

42. Shneerson, J.M. The cardiorespiratory response to exercise in thoracic scoliosis. Thorax 33:457-463, 1978.

43. Shneerson, J.M. Pulmonary artery pressure in thoracic scoliosis during and after exercise while breathing air and pure oxygen. Thorax 33:747-754, 1978.

44. Sockolov, R., Irwin, B., Dressendorfer, R.H., Bernauer, E.M. Exercise performance in 6- to 11-year-old boys with Duchenne muscular dystrophy. Arch. Phys. Med. Rehab. 58:195-201, 1975.

45. Sproule, B.J., Mitchell, J.H., Miller, W.F. Cardiopulmonary physiological responses to heavy exercise in patients with anemia. J. Clin. Invest. 39:378-388, 1960.

46. Taylor, M.R.H. The response to exercise of children with congenital heart disease. London: University of London, 1972. Thesis.

47. Thoren, C. Effects of B-adrenergic blockade on heart rate and blood lactate in children during maximal and submaximal exercise. Acta Paediatr. Scand. 177(Suppl.):123-125, 1967.

48. Thoren, C. Working capacity in anorexia nervosa. In: Borms, J., Hebbelinck, M., eds. Pediatric work physiology. Basel: Karger, 1978:89-95.

49. Thoren, C., Herin, P., Vavra, J. Studies of submaximal and maximal exercise in congenital complete heart block. Acta Paediatr. Belgica 28(Suppl.):132-143, 1974.

50. Ulmer, H.E., Griener, H., Schuler, H.W., Scharer, K. Cardiovascular impairment and physical working capacity in children with chronic renal failure. Acta Paediatr. Scand. 67:43-48, 1978.

51. Wasserman, K., Whipp, B.J. Exercise physiology in health and disease. Am. Rev. Respir. Dis. 112:219-249, 1975.

52. Wessel, H.U., Cunningham, W.J., Paul, M.H., Bastanier, C.K., Muster, A.J., Idriss, F.S. Exercise performance in tetralogy of Fallot after intracardiac repair. J. Thoracic and Cardiovascular Surg. 80:582-593, 1980.

53. Whipp, B.J., Davis, J.A. The ventilatory stress of exercise in obesity. Am. Rev. Respir. Dis. 129(Suppl.):S90-S92, 1984.

54. Zelkowitz, P.S., Giammona, S.T. Effects of gravity and exercise on the pulmonary diffusing capacity in children with cystic fibrosis. J. Pediatr. 74:393-398, 1969.

Somatic Growth, Biological Maturation, and Physical Performance of Mentally Retarded Boys

G. Beunen, K. Breugelmans, J. Lefevre, H. Maes, D. De Corte, and A. Claessens

Research Unit Developmental and Differential Kinanthropology, Institute of Physical Education, KU Leuven, Belgium

In 1936, Flory (2) published an extensive monograph on the physical growth of mentally retarded boys. In general, mentally retarded children tend to lag behind the growth and development of their average peers except for fat mass and skinfolds, for which mentally retarded children obtain higher values: the more serious the handicap, the more the deviation from the average population. Furthermore, some differentiation has been observed based on the cause of the mental retardation (4). Whether the same mechanisms cause the mental retardation and the delay in growth and maturation has yet to be determined.

The well-documented studies of Rarick (4, 5, 6) have shown that mentally retarded children perform, on the average, well below the performance level of intellectually normal children of the same chronological age and sex. However, the basic structure of the performance capacities of mentally retarded children is remarkably similar to the factor structure of intellectually normal children. In the present study an attempt was made to obtain an overall picture of the somatic growth, biological maturation, and performance capacities of mildly to moderately mentally retarded boys.

Methods

The sample consisted of 55 boys from the same special education school situated 30 km north of Antwerp. Only 13- and 14-year-old boys with no physical handicap were selected. Their IQs ranged from 50-80 and averaged 72.

The measurement and tests selected were those examined in a nationwide physical fitness study on Belgian boys (3). The advantage was that Belgian reference data were available for all the measurements and tests. Furthermore, the test team had extensive experience with all the measurements and tests and were instructed by the same principal investigators who conducted the nationwide study.

Fifteen anthropometric dimensions were taken: two lengths, weight, five breadths, three circumferences, and four skinfolds. The Leuven Physical Fitness test battery was administered, and an X ray of the left hand and wrist was taken for an assessment of skeletal maturity. Skeletal maturity was assessed according to the Tanner-Whitehouse system (TW2) (7). All the ratings were made by the same observer who had rated the 20,000 X rays for the nationwide study. High intra- and interobserver reliability has been ascertained even over a period of more than 6 years (1). Age-specific comparisons were made between the mean somatic and motor characteristics of the mentally retarded boys and the national reference values (3).

Results

With the exception of biiliac breadth, biepicondylar femur breadth, thigh circumference, and calf skinfold, all the anthropometric dimensions of the 13-year-old mentally retarded boys correspond closely to those of an average population (see Figure 1). For breadths, the mentally retarded boys had higher values. Mentally retarded boys were also advanced in the biological maturity of the carpals. At 14 years of age the differences were more

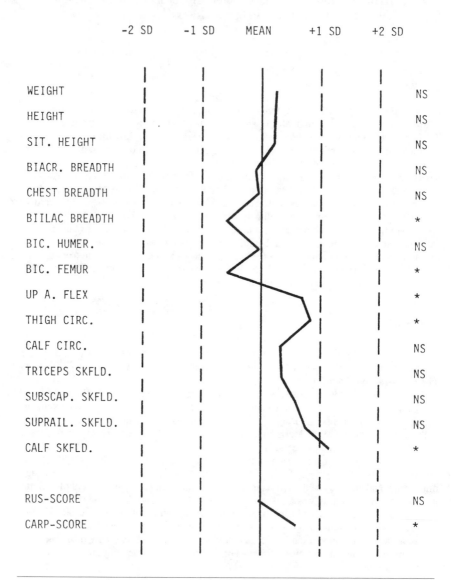

Figure 1. Mean somatic characteristics of 13-year-old mentally retarded boys ($n = 23$) in comparison with national reference values (Ostyn et al., 1980).

pronounced. The mentally retarded boys were retarded in their biological maturity status, especially for the radius-ulna and short bones. They also showed smaller body dimensions for most measurements with the exception of skinfolds, for which they obtained higher means (see Figure 2).

For motor performance capacities, the differences were more striking. At both ages the mentally retarded boys did not perform as well in most motor tests. The most striking differences were found in speed factors (see Figure 3).

Discussion

The small differences in somatic growth for the 13-year-olds are somewhat in contrast to what is generally observed in the literature. However, it has been reported that mongoloid

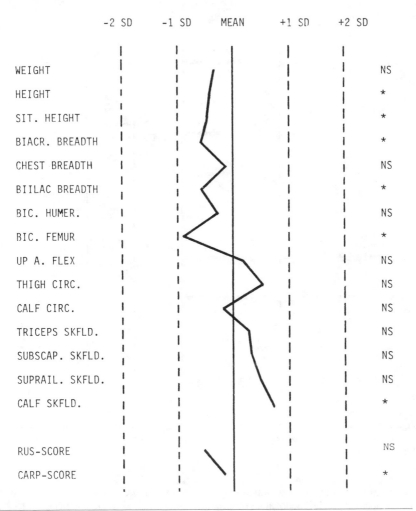

Figure 2.   Mean somatic characteristics of 14-year-old mentally retarded boys ($n = 32$) in comparison with national reference values (Ostyn et al., 1980).

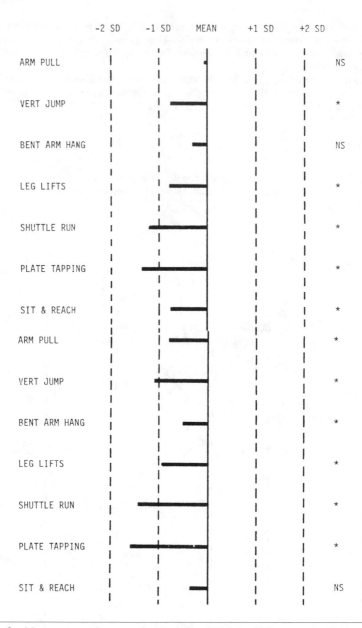

Figure 3. Mean motor performance characteristics of 13-year-old (upper part) and 14-year-old (lower part) mentally retarded boys in comparison with national reference values (Ostyn et al., 1980).

and metabolically abnormal children in particular show more severe growth retardation than nonpathological (functional and cultural familial) retarded children (4). The observations in the sample of 14-year-olds in the present study correspond more closely with the general findings: smaller body dimensions for lengths and breadths and higher subcutaneous fat in mentally retarded boys. In addition, a delay in the biological maturation process was observed for the radius-ulna and short bones.

In motor performance the mentally retarded boys perform less well than boys of normal intelligence, which is in agreement with what was previously reported. The advantage of this study is that exactly the same testing procedures were used by test leaders who were instructed by the investigators who also conducted the nationwide study. Differences in test protocol, measurement techniques, instruments, and observer bias are thus kept at a minimum. The differences between the mentally retarded boys and boys of normal intelligence were quite large. The mean performance on the seven tests of the mentally retarded boys was located at about 0.9 SD below the mean of the reference group.

One might ask if the retardation in motor performance is mainly a function of intellectual inadequacy or a reflection of environmental circumstances. Research findings indicate that both play a role (4). These boys can, with adequate help, acquire reasonable levels of performance. Furthermore, their body fat can be reduced by more intense training programs. One important conclusion is that these boys need more adequate adapted physical education programs in which attention is given to their fitness levels.

References

1. Beunen, G., Cameron, N. The reproducibility of TW2 skeletal age assessments by a self-taught assessor. Ann. Human Biol. 7:155-162, 1980.

2. Flory, C.D. The physical growth of mentally deficient boys. Monographs of the Society for Research in Child Development (serial no. 6), 1936.

3. Ostyn, M., Simons, J., Beunen, G., Renson, R., Van Gerven, D. Somatic and motor development of Belgian secondary schoolboys: norms and standards. Leuven: Leuven University Press, 1980.

4. Rarick, G.L. Motor performance of mentally retarded children. In: Rarick, G.L., ed. Physical activity human growth and development. New York: Academic Press, 1973:225-256 (Chapt. 10).

5. Rarick, G.L. The factor structure of the motor domain of mentally retarded children and adolescents. In: Ostyn, M., Beunen, G., Simons, J., eds. Kinanthropometry II. Baltimore: University Park Press, 1980:149-160.

6. Rarick, G.L., Dobbins, D.A., Broadhead, G.D. The motor domain and its correlates in educationally handicapped children. Englewood Cliffs: Prentice Hall, 1976.

7. Tanner, J.M., Whitehouse, R.H., Cameron, N., Marshall, W.A., Healy, M.J.R., Goldstein, H. Assessment of skeletal maturity and prediction of adult height (TW2 method). London: Academic Press, 1983.

Development of Auditory Reaction Times, Using Fine and Gross Motor Movements in Visually Impaired Children

H. Nakata

Institute of Special Education, University of Tsukuba, Tsukuba, Ibaraki, Japan

Studies of visually impaired children have suggested that their motor performance is poorly developed. Developmental lags of motor performance have been observed in self-initiated mobility and locomotion (1) and in gross motor performance tests (3, 4, 14, 15). Physical work capacity has been reported to be much lower than in sighted children and adults (5, 8, 16, 13, 7). In addition, Lee et al. (10) and Shindo et al. (13) have described that mild endurance training is effective in improving cardiorespiratory fitness of the visually impaired. It has been suggested that delayed motor development in the blind is due to lack of vision, to parental overprotection (3), and to their educational environment (15).

Little research has been reported on fine motor development of visually impaired children, although considerable attention has been paid to gross motor development (6). The present experiment was designed to clarify the influence of visual impairment on fine and gross motor performance.

Auditory reaction time task was chosen as one index of motor performance. Reaction time (RT) measures were used to study the nature of mental process and the reaction process with fine motor movements (12). However, the reaction in human movements is sometimes more generalized, involving several large muscle groups, as in running, jumping (17), and removing the foot from a footplate (9). In the experiment, a button press by the index finger of the preferred hand was selected as the fine motor reaction and a forward jump of the whole body as the gross one. The purpose of this study was to cross-sectionally examine the development of auditory RTs of visually impaired children and adolescents using fine and gross motor movements.

Method

The subjects were 134 partially sighted, 78 totally blind, and 290 sighted boys 6-17 years old. Partially sighted subjects were those with a visual acuity of more than 0.02 but less than 0.3 with best correction. Totally blind subjects were those with a visual acuity of 0 or light perception. Furthermore, visually impaired subjects were free of significant multiple handicapping conditions; visually impaired subjects were not mentally retarded nor did they exhibit any obvious physical disabilities that may have influenced the experiment.

RTs were measured using a 1000 Hz pure tone as a stimulus. The apparatus was a Takei-Kiki chronometer model 11, which was mounted on a table out of the subjects' view. The sound source was placed at a distance of 1 m away from the subject at eye level. The subjects were asked to press a button to a sound stimulus (finger-press RT) and to jump forward about 40 cm from a footplate (forward-jumping RT). Five different foreperiod times ranging 2-6 s were randomly assigned among trials. A warning signal was given orally by the experimenter 2-6 s before the stimulus.

Each subject had a total of 20 responses, 10 each for the finger-press and forward-jumping RTs. For each subject, mean RTs were determined for both RT tasks.

Results and Discussion

Figure 1 shows developmental trends of finger-press and forward-jumping RTs for partially sighted, totally blind, and sighted subjects. For the sighted the mean times of finger-press reaction decreased gradually with increasing age until approximately 11 years and were fairly constant from 11 to 17 years. The performance of partially sighted and totally blind subjects exhibited a similar development to that of the sighted. The results support Bernard (2), who compared sighted and nonsighted subjects of mean age 13 years. On the other hand, it was observed that partially sighted and totally blind subjects showed slower RTs in forward jumping of whole body than those of the sighted. Values of forward-jumping RT were widely scattered in the visually impaired. These results suggest that the lack of vision exerts a greater influence on the development of the gross motor RT in visually impaired children and adolescents.

The effects of visual impairment on the gross motor RT are quite clear in Figure 2. Means of RTs for the visually impaired subjects as a group were obtained for each age. In the forward jumping RT task, the differences between sighted and visually impaired subjects became larger and little difference was found in a finger-press RT task between the two groups.

Figure 3 shows a comparison of RTs of the partially sighted with those of the totally blind. Visually impaired subjects were divided into four groups with respect to age: 6-8, 9-11, 12-14, and 15-17 age ranges. As a result of a two-way ANOVA (RTs x subjects), significant main effects were found between partially sighted and totally blind subjects at 6-8 age ranges ($F = 4.579$, $df = 1/34$, $p < .05$), and interaction was not significant.

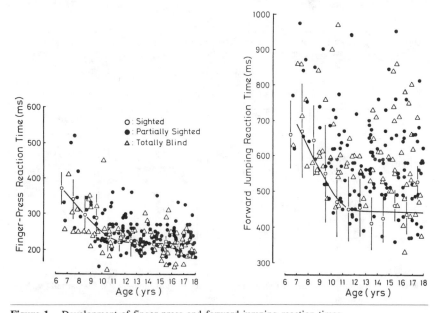

Figure 1. Development of finger-press and forward-jumping reaction times.

There were not significant main effects between the two groups in the other three age ranges and interactions were not significant. From these results, it can be concluded that there is no difference in the fine and gross motor RTs between partially sighted and totally blind groups.

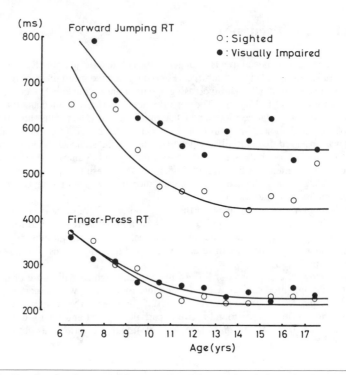

Figure 2.   Developmental curves of finger-press and forward-jumping reaction times.

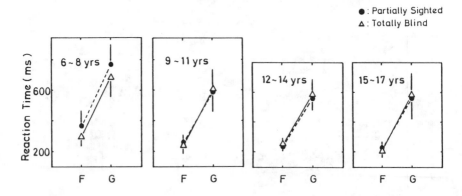

Figure 3.   Relationships between finger-press (F) and forward-jumping (G) for partially sighted and totally blind subjects with respect to age ranges.

Figure 4 presents a comparison of fine and gross motor RTs between sighted and visually impaired subjects. As a result of a two-way ANOVA, significant interactions were obtained at 7, 9, 10, 11, 13, 14, 15, and 16 years of age. In these age groups, significant differences were found in the gross motor RT task between sighted and visually impaired subjects. This was evident as a slower gross motor RT in visually impaired subjects.

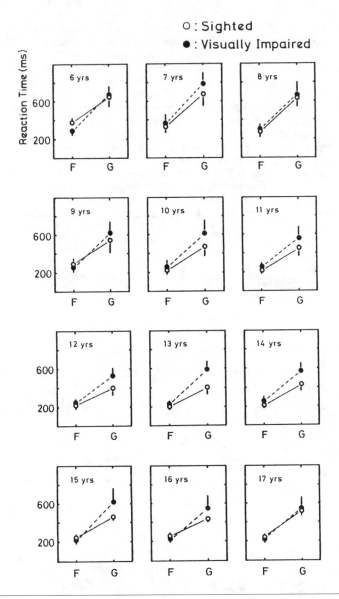

Figure 4. Relationships between finger-press (F) and forward-jumping (G) for sighted and visually impaired subjects.

In Figure 5, relative frequency distributions of RTs are presented with respect to two age groups: 6-10 and 11-17 age ranges. There was no definite pattern of distributions in finger-press RTs between sighted and visually impaired subjects. However, visually impaired subjects in the 11-17 age group showed wider distribution in forward-jumping RT than that of the sighted. Results of this study suggest that, in general, visually impaired children and adolescents are neurologically intact, as the difference between sighted and visually impaired subjects were not found in the finger-press RT task, which involves several small muscle groups. The results suggest also that visually impaired children and adolescents have acquired fine motor skills through nonvisual motor learning, and the severity of the visual impairment is not a significant factor on the fine motor RT task. On the other hand, the forward-jumping RT task requires several large muscle groups to control whole body movement. Visually impaired children and adolescents may have difficulty in acquiring gross motor skills because of the lack of mobility, which is attributed to the lack of vision. Some of visually impaired children and adolescents, however, surpassed the performance of the sighted in the jumping-forward RT task, as shown in Figure 1. It seems unlikely that visual impairment restricts physical activity and thus acquisition of motor skills.

In conclusion, visually impaired children and adolescents showed a similar development to that of the sighted on the fine motor RT task. On the gross motor RT task, in general, they exhibited slower RTs over the age ranges. However, superior performance was obtained by some of the visually impaired on the gross motor RT task. These results suggest that low levels of gross motor performance are not an inevitable consequence of the visual handicap (11), and that well-designed adapted physical education programs or educational environment (15) should be provided for visually impaired children.

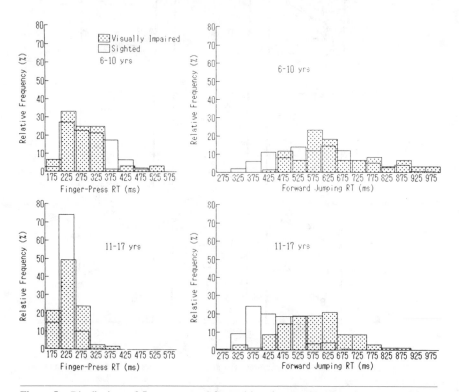

Figure 5. Distributions of finger-press and forward-jumping reaction times for the sighted and visually impaired.

References

1. Adelsen, E., Fairberg, S. Gross motor development in infants blind from birth. Child Development 45:114-126, 1974.

2. Bernard, J. Simple auditory reaction time in blind and sighted adolescents. Percept. and Mot. Skills 48:465-466, 1979.

3. Buell, C. Motor performance of visually handicapped children. Exceptional Children 17:69-72, 1950.

4. Case, S., Dawson, Y., Schartner, J., Donaway, D. Comparison of levels of fundamental skill and cardio-respiratory fitness of blind, deaf, and non-handicapped high school age boys. Percept. and Mot. Skills 36:1291-1294, 1973.

5. Cumming, G.R., Goulding, D., Baggley, G. Working capacity of deaf and visually and mentally handicapped children. Arch. Disease in Childhood 46:490-495, 1971.

6. Depauw, K.P. Physical education for the visually impaired: a review of the literature. J. Visual Impairment and Blindness 75:162-164, 1981.

7. Hopkins, W.G., Gaeta, H., Thomas, A.C., Hill, P. McN. Physical fitness of blind and sighted children. Europ. J. Appl. Physiol. 56:69-73, 1987.

8. Jankowski, L.W., Evanse, J.K. The exercise capacity of blind children. J. Visual Impairment and Blindness 75:248-251, 1981.

9. Kelly, R.L., Barton, J.R. III, Abernathy, L. Reaction times, using fine and gross motor movements of moderately and severely mentally handicapped adults to auditory and visual stimuli. Percept. and Mot. Skills 65:219-222, 1987.

10. Lee, M., Ward, G., Shephard, R.J. Physical capacities of sightless acolescents. Dev. Med. Child Neurol. 27:767-774, 1985.

11. Natale, J. di, Lee, M., Ward, G., Shephard, R.J. Loss of physical condition in sightless adolescents during a summer vacation. Adapted Phys. Activity Q. 2:144-150, 1985.

12. Niemi, P., Naatanen, R. Foreperiod and simple reaction time. Psychol. Bull. 89:133-162, 1981.

13. Shindo, M., Kumagai, S., Tanaka, H. Physical work capacity and effect of endurance training in visually handicapped boys and young male adults. Europ. J. Physiol. 56:501-507, 1987.

14. Short, F.X., Winnick, J.P. The influence of visual impairment on physical fitness test performance. J. Visual Impairment and Blindness 80:729-731, 1986.

15. Short, F.X., Winnick, J.P. Adolescent physical fitness: a comparative study. J. Visual Impairment and Blindness 82:237-239, 1988.

16. Sundberg, S. Maximal oxygen uptake in relation to age in blind and normal boys and girls. Acta Paediatr. Scand. 71:603-608, 1982.

17. Yabe, K., Tsukahara, R., Mita, K., Aoki, H. Developmental trends of jumping reaction time by means of EMG in mentally retarded children. J. Mental Deficiency Res. 29:137-145, 1985.

Muscular Exercises for Myoelectric Control of Artificial Limbs

Y.Z. Luo

Shanghai Institute of Physiology, Chinese Academy of Sciences, Shanghai, China

When myoelectric signals from some muscles of an amputee's stump are used to control an artificial limb, two conditions must be satisfied. First, the intensities of these signals must be large enough so that they can be picked out from background noise and disturbances. Second, each muscle used as a signal source must be contracted and relaxed properly under the control of the amputee, so that the EMG patterns necessary for controlling an artificial limb can be generated reliably. Before exercise, these conditions are usually not satisfied for many amputees. The EMG signals of some stump muscles are very small because of prolonged disuse of these muscles. When some amputees contract a stump muscle, its antagonist can not be relaxed and therefore the EMG pattern will be confused. Some amputees have even forgotten how to contract their muscle in the stump. To solve these problems, exercises of stump muscles are prescribed for amputees. After practicing the exercises, most of the amputees satisfy the above-mentioned two conditions. Now more than 200 disabled persons amputated from the wrist to the shoulder have been fitted with suitable artificial limbs after such muscular exercises.

Method of Exercises

Selection of Muscles

Before the beginning of the exercises, the muscles to serve as signal sources for controlling an artificial limb are selected. As many amputees' muscles have been lost, the muscles in the stumps are very limited; therefore, controlling the artificial limbs with one to three degrees of freedom only requires a pair of antagonists as signal sources (1, 2). For forearm amputees, one flexor and one extensor that can record the strongest EMG are selected. For the above-the-elbow amputees, only biceps and triceps are used. For the whole-arm amputees, one muscle is the pectoralis and the other is the infraspinatus or teres minor. The electrodes should be positioned on the strongest signal position for each muscle.

Measurement of EMG

During the measuring of EMG, the average peak-to-peak EMG values of the two muscles are displayed on two needle voltmeters. Amputees can observe the amplitudes and changes of their own EMG. The amputees can correct their actions with the help of visual feedback. The measurements are taken once a week.

Bilateral Training Method

During the training we let the amputee's amputated limb and contralateral health limb perform the same movements. This method is very helpful for regaining ability to control muscles in the stump.

Daily Exercises

After the first training and measuring of EMG, amputees begin to do exercises by themselves every day. Following the training, amputees perform exercises for at least 2 hr every day, 1 hr in the morning and 1 hr in the afternoon. During the 2 hr they do as much exercise as they can. Electromotor stimulation is also used as a supplemental method of treatment.

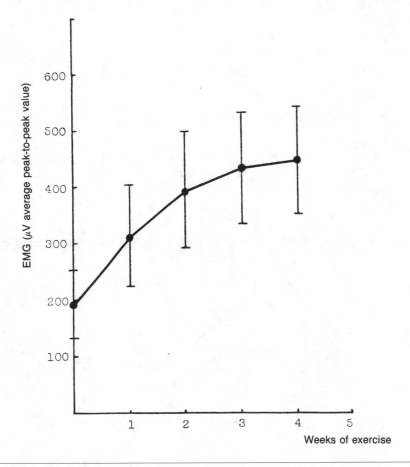

Figure 1.   The change of average EMG intensity along with the time of exercises of 30 muscles.

Results

Significant effects were observed both in increasing EMG intensity and improving EMG patterns. The changes of EMG intensity along with the time of exercises are shown in Figure 1. The results were derived from 30 muscles of 15 amputees (15 pairs of antagonists). Their ages ranged from 19 to 44: males numbered 11, females 4. The subjects included 3 whole-arm amputees, 8 above-the-elbow emputees, and 4 forearm amputees. From Figure 1 it is shown that the average EMG intensity of the 30 muscles increased rapidly during the first 2 weeks, and the rising slope gradually decreased with the time of exercises.

Improvement of EMG Patterns

When a muscle is contracted to generate one EMG signal pattern, the ratio of EMG amplitudes of this muscle to its antagonist is used to measure the quality of this EMG pattern,

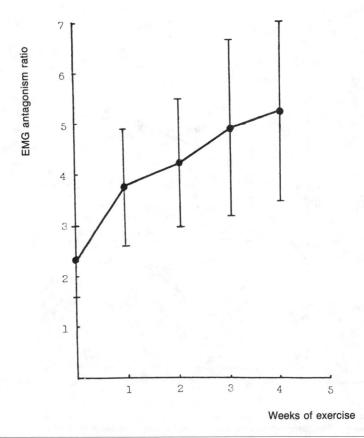

Figure 2. The change of average EMG antagonism ratio of 30 muscles along with the time of exercises.

reflecting the ability of the amputee to control the stump muscles. In the following description, this ratio will be called the EMG antagonism ratio of a muscle. Figure 2 shows the EMG antagonism ratio of the 30 muscles during 4 weeks of exercise. The ratio rose very fast in the first week, then slowed down.

Results of Long-Term Exercises

Figures 3 and 4 show the results of long-term exercises. These results were recorded from a bilateral arm amputee's four stump muscles. The amputee was a 25-year-old man. These results showed that if the exercise term continued long enough, the increase of the EMG intensities and the EMG antagonism ratios of these muscles would become very slow and almost stop.

Results of Bilateral Training

There was an example for the effect of this training method: a left above-the-elbow amputee who was 18 years old. He could not make the triceps in the stump contract. After 1 week of training, the EMG of this muscle was still zero. Then the bilateral training method was used for one week. The EMG of his triceps reached 600 μV, and the EMG antagonism ratio reached 6.

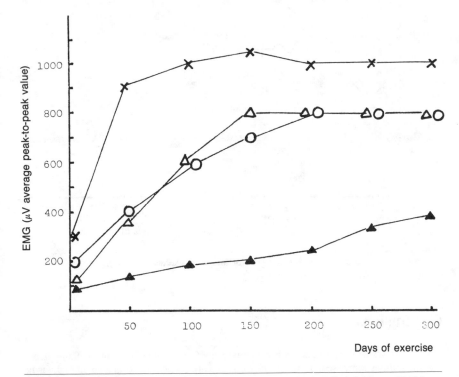

Figure 3.   EMG of four muscles for long-term exercises: left biceps, X; left triceps O; right biceps, ▲; right triceps, △.

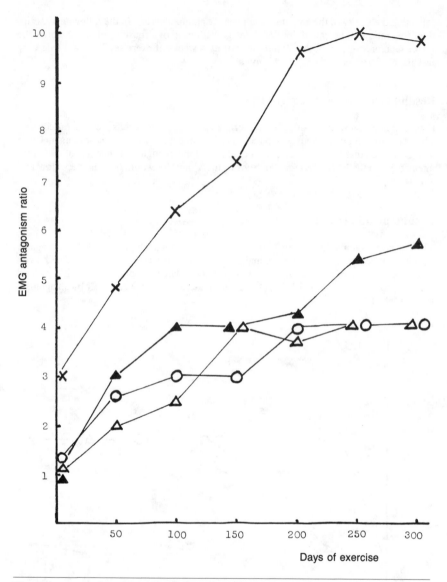

Figure 4. Antagonism ratio of four muscles for long-term exercises: left biceps, X; left triceps O; right biceps, ▲; right triceps, △.

Conclusions

1. Exercises of stump muscles can increase EMG intensities and improve amputees' control abilities for these muscles. If the exercises are carried out for a long enough term, the EMG of muscles will tend to reach their maximal values. If the exercises are continued, these maximal values can be kept up.

2. At the beginning of exercises, the EMG intensities and the EMG antagonism ratios increase rapidly. These results further support the concept of the neural factor (3).

3. The visual feedback and the bilateral training method are very helpful for getting the better results and improving the EMG patterns.

References

1. Luo, Y.Z. et al. Arm protheses with multiple degrees of freedom controlled by two channels of myoelectric signals. Chinese J. Biomed. Eng. 2(1):16-22, 1983.

2. Luo, Y.Z. Research and application of myoelectrically controlled artificial limbs in our institute. Proceedings of 2nd China-Japan International Symposium on Biomedical and Rehabilitation Engineering, Shanghai Jiao Tong University, China, Chinese Association of Rehabilitation Medicine, Life Support Technology Society, Japan. 1986.

3. Moritani, T., deVries, H.A. Neural factors versus hypertrophy in the time course of muscle strength gain. Am. J. Phys. Med. 58(3):115-130, 1979.

Evaluation of Physical Fitness in Paraplegic Wheelchair Basketball Players

M. Kobayashi, T. Hirano, and T. Fukunaga

Faculty of Social Welfare, Nihon Fukushi University, Okuda, Mihama-cho, Aichi, and Department of Sports Science, College of Arts and Science, University of Tokyo, Komaba, Tokyo, Japan

Various studies on the maximal and submaximal exercise responses of wheelchair-dependent subjects who have only upper limb function due to spinal cord injuries have recently been reported (1, 2, 3). Manual wheelchair exercises require use of the relatively small upper-body muscles for propulsion. Glaser et al. (2) reported a comparison of the submaximal physiological responses taken during wheelchair ergometer and bicycle exercise. They found that mechanical efficiency of arm exercise was significantly lower than leg exercise at the same power output level. Wicks et al. (1983) investigated the cardiorespiratory responses to progressive incremental arm cranking in physically disabled athletes.

The purpose of this study is to measure maximal physiological responses during progressive incremental wheelchair exercise and to consider physical fitness in relation to the level of injury of wheelchair basketball players who are paraplegic.

Methods

The subjects were 12 male wheelchair basketball players with paraplegia due to spinal cord injuries and poliomyelitis (age [mean $\pm$ SD] = 27.9 $\pm$ 6.3 years; class point = 2.2 $\pm$ 0.9 point; athletic experience = 4.6 $\pm$ 4.7 years). They had consistently participated in wheelchair sports (e.g., basketball, tennis, or marathon races) year round, and they were athletes of average skill for Japan. All subjects were classified into three groups (Class 1, Class 2, and Class 3) according to the level of injury and physical performance capacity during wheelchair sports activities based on the International Stoke Mandeville Games Classification Guide.

Each subject participated in anthropometric tests, strength tests, and maximal $\dot{V}O_2$ tests during maximal wheelchair exercise, using his wheelchair on the motor drive treadmill belt. All subjects were familiarized with the wheelchair exercise on the treadmill prior to the tests. The subjects were asked to perform the wheelchair exercise while the load was gradually increased until exhaustion. The subjects had started with progressive incremental surface grades of 2, 4, and 6% every 3 min at a constant velocity of 50 m/min. Then, treadmill velocity was increased by 20 m/min every 1 min at constant grade of 6% until exhaustion.

Heart rate was determined from an electrocardiogram recording during the last 15 s of each minute of exercise, and respiratory rate was determined by means of a thermostat method during same time. O_2 uptake was measured during the resting period and maximal wheelchair exercise test. Expired gas was collected each minute during exercise and for 5 min during the rest period using the Douglas bag method. Oxygen and carbon dioxide concentrations were analyzed by a Fukuda Respilyzer (BM-10) system.

The data from each minute of submaximal and maximal exercise, which included O_2 uptake ($\dot{V}O_2$), heart rate (HR), respiratory rate (RR), ventilation ($\dot{V}E$), respiratory exchange ratio (R), ventilatory equivalent for O_2, and pulse were calculated for each group and all subjects. The $<.05$ or $<.01$ level was used to note significant differences in all analyses.

Results

Table 1 presents the basic data of $N = 12$ wheelchair basketball athletes. The mean values of anthropometric tests for weight, height, horizontal reach, sitting height, forearm girth, upper arm girth, chest girth, and percent body fat were 56.6 ± 9.1 kg, 165.8 ± 11.1 cm, 172.1 ± 8.1 cm, 85.9 ± 6.1 cm, 28.4 ± 1.7 cm, 33.7 ± 3.2 cm, 95.3 ± 7.6 cm, and $14.3 \pm 5.5\%$, respectively. These means are significantly lower than those for West German wheelchair basketball players for body weight, height, horizontal reach, and sitting height; however, the values for horizontal reach, forearm girth, upper arm girth, and chest girth were significantly higher than those for normal healthy subjects in Japan. In all subjects muscle strength and muscle power were 54.0 ± 7.2 kg (grip strength), 23.8 ± 4.9 kg (elbow flexion strength), 18.3 ± 3.5 kg (elbow extension strength), and 5.6 ± 2.3 w/kg (arm power per body weight), respectively.

The results of the present study in relation to muscle functions were significantly different, from 56.9% to 97.3%, compared with West German players. Vital capacity, $\dot{V}O_2$max, $\dot{V}E$max, and HRmax were 3.63 ± 0.93 L, 35.3 ± 9.3 ml/kg.min, 94.3 ± 27.2 L/min, and 190.1 ± 9.7 b/min, respectively. These figures were significantly lower than those for normal healthy adults in Japan, but there were no differences compared with All-Japan

Table 1   Basic Data of $N = 12$ Wheelchair Athletes

Subject	Age (yr)	Body weight (kg)	Sitting height (cm)	Class point	Athletic experience (yr)	Disability
1	23.8	48.0	75.2	1.0	1.0	Paraplegia TH4
2	32.0	53.0	87.0	1.0	5.0	Paraplegia TH8
3	38.1	64.5	88.2	1.0	15.0	Paraplegia TH9
4	18.9	51.0	76.9	1.5	1.0	Paraplegia TH3
5	30.3	63.0	84.4	2.0	1.5	Paraplegia TH11
6	26.5	65.5	89.5	2.0	2.5	Paraplegia TH11
7	36.6	48.0	88.1	2.0	11.0	Poliomyelitis
8	22.1	53.0	81.1	2.5	1.0	Paraplegia TH12
9	34.3	72.0	98.1	3.0	4.0	Poliomyelitis
10	28.1	44.0	88.6	3.0	10.0	Poliomyelitis
11	21.9	66.5	86.0	3.5	1.0	Paraplegia TH12
12	22.6	50.5	87.2	3.5	2.0	A/K amputation
Mean	27.9	56.6	85.9	2.2	4.6	
SD	6.3	9.1	6.1	0.9	4.7	

Sports Convention players of wheelchair basketball, using the same parameters. The mean ratio among determined data of this study and the West German study was 93.7% (range: 82.7-106.5%) with anthropometric tests and 69.6% (range: 56.9-97.3%) with muscle function tests. Therefore, the mean ratio between paraplegics and nonhandicapped subjects was 101.4% with anthropometric tests, 107.8% with muscle function tests, and 91.8% with cardiorespiratory responses in maximal exercise.

Figure 1 shows the relationship between the level of injury for paraplegia (class point) and elbow flexion strength, maximal arm power, HRmax, and $\dot{V}O_2$max of 12 subjects. No significant correlation coefficients were obtained between elbow flexion strength, maximal arm power output, and class point. HR max and $\dot{V}O_2$max, however, were significantly correlated (HR: $r = .554$, $\dot{V}O_2$: $r = .605$) with class points. Thus in paraplegic subjects significant correlation coefficients were observed between the level of injury and cardiorespiratory functions. There were no differences with anthropometric characteristics or muscle functions in relation to three class groups. However, vital capacity, $\dot{V}O_2$max, HRmax, and $\dot{V}E$max of Class 3 groups were significantly higher than with other class groups. It is clear that exercise training and wheelchair sports in paraplegics can elicit an increase in cardiorespiratory functions and muscle power output of the upper limbs.

References

1. Coutts, K.D., Rhodes, E.C., McKenzie, D.C. Maximal exercise responses of tetraplegics and paraplegics. J. Appl. Physiol. 55:479-482, 1983.

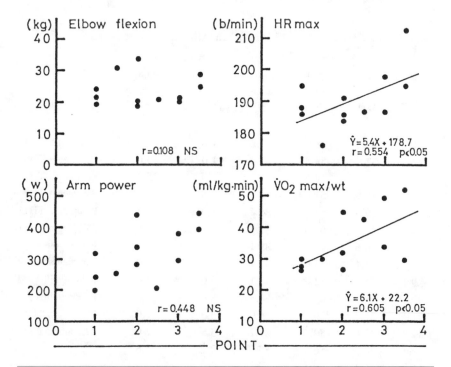

Figure 1.   The relationship between the level of injury for paraplegia and physical fitness parameters ($N = 12$).

2. Glaser, R.M., Sawka, M.N., Laubach, L.L., Suryaprasad, A.G. Metabolic and cardiopulmonary responses to wheelchair and bicycle ergometry. J. Appl. Physiol. 46:1066-1070, 1979.

3. Van Der Woude, L.H.V., Hendrich, K.M.M., Veeger, H.E.J., Can Ingen Schenau, G.J., Rozendal, R.H., De Groot, G., Hollander, A.P. Manual wheelchair propulsion: effects of power output on physiology and technique. Med. Sci. Sports Exer. 20:70-78, 1988.

Physiological Characteristics of Wheelchair Basketball Players

T. Ibusuki, T. Kondo, H. Soya, and H. Yagi

College of Medical Care and Technology, Gunma University, Japan

Sports for the disabled in Japan are modeled after British and European models and after the Tokyo Paralympics in 1964, which has played the most important role in sports for disabled. As a result, the All-Japan SPorts Convention for the disabled was held in 1965, using the same facility that was used for the Tokyo Paralympics. The 23rd convention was held in 1987, and the number of participants was 1,957. Recently, local sports conventions for the disabled have become more popular, and federations of sports associations have formed, such as associations for wheelchair basketball, archery, table tennis, swimming, skiing, wheelchair marathon, and tennis.

Heidebrandt et al. (2) have indicated that the normal daily locomotion patterns of wheelchair-dependent individuals are insufficient to maintain or improve their fitness levels. Furthermore, extended periods of inactivity, due to fatigue of the upper body musculature resulting from wheelchair propulsion, contribute to decreases in physical work capacity. More commonly, the maximal uptake of sedentary disabled adults is low. Contributing factors include postmorbid muscle wasting and body fat accumulation and possibly an unnecessary restriction of the patient's physical activity level during or subsequent to rehabilitation. Significant differences of muscle strength and cardiorespiratory fitness between individuals differing in habitual activity have indicated the probable benefits from sports participation and other forms of fitness conditioning. The purpose of this study was to describe some of the pulmonary functions and the physiological responses to maximal arm-cranking exercises of wheelchair basketball players. For comparison purposes a group of male college students was also studied.

Materials and Methods

Seven disabled male wheelchair basketball players (WCBP) and seven untrained male college students (AB) were studied. Their characteristics are given in Tables 1 and 2. Disabled subjects had completed the initial rehabilitation phase of their treatment and had been using a wheelchair as a normal means of locomotion for at least 17 months. One had a high medullary lesion, five had low medullary lesions, and one had polio. All disabled subjects were paraplegics. Disabled subjects were active and participated in sports events 4-6 hours per week. Able-bodied subjects were not active.

Measurements of Pulmonary Function

A respirator (Auto-spiro DISCOM-21, Chest) was used to measure vital capacity (VC), inspiratory reserve volume (IRV), expiratory reserve volume (ERV), forced expiratory volume (FEV 1.0), maximal voluntary ventilation (MVV), maximal midexpiratory flow

Table 1   Physical Characteristics of the Subjects

Subject	Age (years)	Diagnosis	Level of lesion	Time since injury (years)	International classification of disability
WCBP: male (N = 7)					
1	18.9	Traumatic	T7	1.5	2
2	26.5	Spinal	T10	7.8	1
3	27.6	Injury	T12	15.6	2
4	33.5		T12	9.3	2
5	29.9		T12	9.3	2
6	26.3		L.1	8.2	3
7	26.0	Polio		25.6	2

Note. AB: College students, male (N = 7) 19-23 years (mean 20.9 years).

Table 2   Anthropometric Characteristics of the Subjects

Variables	WCBP (N = 7)		AB (N = 7)	
	$\overline{X}$	SD	$\overline{X}$	SD
Height, cm	166.5	6.2	172.3	5.5**
Weight, kg	56.3	2.7	66.0	9.7**
Chest, cm	93.9	6.8	90.2	4.0
Arm, cm	33.7	2.7	31.3	3.3
Forearm, cm	29.0	1.8	26.0	1.6**
Grip strength, kg	56.6	5.0	47.5	6.9**

** $p < .05$.

(MMF), and peak expiratory flow rate (PEFR). All spirometry was performed in the sitting position with noseclip and corrected to BTPS.

Arm Crank Ergometer

The arm crank ergometer was an adaptation of a cycle ergometer (Monark). The crank unit could be moved so that the shoulder and handle axis were in the same horizontal plane. The wheelchair and seat were placed in such a position that the arm of the subject was in complete extension when the pedal was at its greatest distance. It was possible to adjust the handle crank height and seated position for each subject.

Expired gases were analyzed using an open circuit system (Aerobics Processor 391, San-ei). The analyzer was calibrated before and during test with room air reference gases of known concentration. Heart rate was monitored continuously with a cardiotachometer.

The time course of a test was as follows: After familiarization with arm cranking, the subjects sat quietly for 30 min, and testing physiological data were recorded during the last 5 min. Then the subjects exercised on the arm crank ergometer, and a continuous and progressively increasing work load was applied. It was initiated with the subjects cranking against 20 W resistance at 40 rpm for 4 min, after which, with the same frequency, workload was increased by 20 W every 4 min until 12 min. Then workload was increased by 10 W every 1 min until exhaustion. Since all subjects were strongly motivated, tests were considered maximal when the subjects manifested their inability to work any more.

Results

Results are expressed as mean ($\pm$ SD), and differences between the group were assessed by the t test. Statistical significance of differences was accepted when $p < .05$. Group means for the following pulmonary parameters are presented in Table 3. No significant differences were found between the two groups for any variables measured. The variables in WCBP were not found to be directly related to the level of spinal injury.

Mean values ($\pm$ SD) for maximal oxygen uptake ($\dot{V}O_2$max), maximal heart rate (HR), respiration rate (RR), maximal ventilation ($\dot{V}E$), and exhaustion time are given in Table 4. At maximal exercise, mean $\dot{V}O_2$max reached 28.8 ml/min/kg in AB ($p < .05$). And $\dot{V}O_2$max in WCBP was not found to directly relate to the level of spinal injury. Maximal heart rate, respiration rate, and pulmonary ventilation in WCBP were higher than those in AB. But no significance was found between the two groups. In comparison with AB, the adaptation to submaximal exercise of WCBP was different: For given HR, $\dot{V}O_2$ of WCBP was higher than that of WB (see Figure 1).

Discussion

Previous research has indicated that wheelchair-dependent individuals have below-normal pulmonary function (1) and aerobic fitness. But in the present study, pulmonary function

Table 3   Static Volumes and Dynamic Lung Function

Variables	WCBP ($N = 7$)		AB ($N = 7$)	
	$\overline{X}$	SD	$\overline{X}$	SD
VC (L)	4.3	0.5	4.5	0.9
IRV (L)	1.8	0.5	2.1	0.3
ERV (L)	1.6	0.8	1.7	0.5
FEV 1.0 (L)	3.8	0.4	4.0	0.9
MVV (L)	142	18.6	120	31.8
MMF (L)	5.7	1.2	5.4	1.1
PEFR (L)	9.0	2.5	9.9	2.6

Nonsignificant.

Table 4 Physiological Data from Maximal Arm-Cranking Test

Variables	WCBP ($N = 7$)		AB ($N = 7$)	
	$\bar{X}$	SD	$\bar{X}$	SD
$\dot{V}O_2$ L/min	1.5	0.2	1.4	0.2
ml/min/kg	28.7	5.8	21.2	3.4**
HR beats/min	172.1	12.1	159.9	14.3
RR freq/min	47.9	17.0	40.4	9.1
$\dot{V}E$ L/min	63.9	14.7	55.4	12.8
Exhaustion time/min	15.9	0.7	15.0	1.0

** $p < .05$.

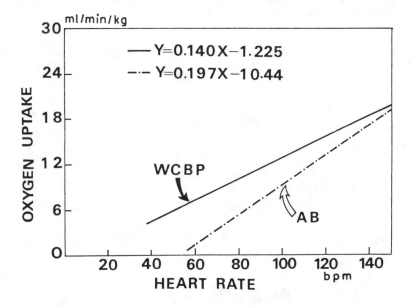

Figure 1. Relationship between HR and $\dot{V}O_2$ during arm ergometry by wheelchair basketball players and able-bodied subjects.

was comparable in wheelchair basketball players and able-bodied subjects. And the $\dot{V}O_2$max (ml/min/kg) in wheelchair basketball players was a higher value than in able-bodied subjects. In comparison with able-bodied subjects, the adaptation to submaximal exercise of wheelchair basketball players was different: For given HR, the $\dot{V}O_2$ values of wheelchair basketball players were higher, suggesting a better efficiency.

The difference between the present and other studies may be related to two factors. First, the majority of the subjects in the present study had low spinal lesions with adaptational innervation to the diaphragm and intercostal muscle. Second, the cardiorespiratory results may reflect the trained condition of the subjects. Kofsky et al. (3) observed that a general association between levels of habitual physical activity and cardiorespiratory propelling did not provide sufficient circulatory stimulus to develop or maintain such a condition among the mobile, sedentary, and incapacitated wheelchair users.

The small sample size in the study prohibits drawing general conclusions about the characteristics of wheelchair basketball players in comparison with able-bodied subjects. This study suggests that sports and recreation are probably more important to physically disabled individuals than to able-bodied persons.

References

1. Bar-Or, O., Zwiren, L.D. Maximal oxygen consumption test during arm exercise-reliability and validity. J. Appl. Physiol. 38:424-426, 1975.

2. Hildebrandt, G., Voigt, E.D., Bahn, D., Berendes, N., Kroger, J. Energy costs of propelling a wheelchair at various speeds: cardiac response and steering accuracy. Arch. Phys. Med. Rehab. 51:131-136, 1970.

3. Kofsky, P.R., Davis, G.M., Shephard, R.J., et al. Cardiorespiratory fitness in the lower limb disabled. J. Appl. Sports Sci. 5, 1980.

Quantitative Analysis of Skeletal Muscles in Dystrophic Mice as a Model of Nonexercise Muscular Atrophy

K. Imaizumi, K. Tachiyashiki, and M. Sekiya

Department of Living and Health Sciences, Joetsu University of Education, Joetsu, Niigata, and Section of Pathology, Niigata Prefectural Central Hospital, Joetsu, Niigata, Japan

Disuse atrophy of skeletal muscle, the loss of muscle mass, has been investigated using human and experimental animal models including limb cast fixation, bed rest, tenotomy, joint pinning, denervation, space flight, cage restraint, and tail-cast suspension (3, 7, 16). The loss of muscle mass in disuse is due at least in part to the loss of muscle proteins (7). The decrease of muscle proteins results from slower protein synthesis, faster protein degradation, or concurrent changes of both processes (4). Atrophy of muscles in immobilized rat hindlimb showed significant changes of both processes to be responsible (5). Little data, however, are available for the intracellular changes of atrophic muscles irrespective of a variety of techniques. It is essential for the complete elucidation of the molecular mechanism of the muscle atrophy to quantitatively study the intracellular changes of atrophic muscle tissues. To clarify this problem, it is very useful to use the homo-type (dy/dy; dystrophic) and hetero-type (dy/?; as control) of the dystrophic model (C57BL/6J-dy) mice as the model animal of nonexercise muscular atrophy (6).

In the present study, as the first step in clarifying the cellular mechanism of nonexercise muscular atrophy, we measured (a) amounts of nucleic acids (deoxyribonucleic acid, DNA and ribonucleic acid, RNA) in hindlimb muscles, (b) amounts of proteins in three fractions of muscles, (c) the frequency distribution of a cross-sectional area of muscle fibers per unit area of muscle tissue, and (d) numbers of nuclei and muscle fibers per unit area of muscle tissue, using the dystrophic (C57BL/6J-dy) mice. Various measured values in hindlimb muscles of dystrophic mice were compared with those of control mice.

Methods and Materials

Male homozygous dystrophic (dy/dy) and phenotypically normal littermate (=control) mice of the C57BL/6J-dy strain (4-9 weeks of age) were used in this study. Dystrophic mice were identified by complete dragging of the hind legs in walking (20). These mice were obtained from CLEA Japan, Inc., Tokyo. The body weight, tail length, and age of each mouse was recorded. The animal was then sacrificed by cervical dislocation. Preparations were made simultaneously from control and dystrophic mice. All muscles of the hindlimb in the right side were removed from the body, skinned, and dissected away from the surrounding connective tissue. The whole muscle tissue was used for the biochemical analysis. In contrast, medial gastrocnemius muscle and soleus muscle from the left side of hindlimb muscles were isolated to use as the sample for histological studies.

Biochemical Analysis

Whole hind-limb muscles were weighed and minced finely with scissors. The muscles were homogenized at 0 °C in a Potter-Elvehjem-type homogenizer with 10 volume of 25 mM phosphate buffer (pH 7.4). Each homogenate was divided into two sample groups. One sample was used as a sample for analyzing nucleic acid (DNA and RNA) contents in muscle tissue. The other sample was employed for fractionating muscle proteins.

RNA and DNA fractions in the muscle homogenate were separated according to the method of Schmidt and Thannhauser (14) with a slight modification. RNA content was determined by the orcinol reaction (15), in which yeast RNA was used as the standard. DNA content was quantified by the diphenylamine reaction according to the procedure of Burton (2). Total value of DNA or RNA in muscle tissue was determined on the basis of total muscle weight.

Muscle homogenate was fractionated into 25 mM phosphate buffer (pH 7.4) soluble fraction (F-1), 1.2M KCl-soluble fraction (F-2), and 1.2M KCl-insoluble fraction (F-3) (6). The protein content was determined by the method of Lowry et al. (10) with bovine serum albumin used as a standard.

Histological Analysis

All muscles isolated were fixed by 4% formaldehyde solution (formalin) at resting length. Histological observations were performed on serial cross sections (3 μm thick) of paraffin-embedded medial gastrocnemius muscle and soleus muscle routinely stained with hematoxylin and eosin. Photomicrographs of the cross sections were enlarged to a final enlargement magnification ($\times$ 400). Each photomicrograph was traced on section paper on which the standard area of the specimen calibrated with a stage micrometer was depicted (19). The cross-sectional area of each muscle fiber was determined by comparing its size with the standard area. The numbers of the nuclei and muscle-fibers per 1 mm^2 of the cross-sectional area of muscle tissue were counted on papers that were enlarged by Xerox copy. Differences between control and dystrophic mice were evaluated by the Student's t test or Welch's t test.

Results

Developmental Changes

The body weight of the control mice increased with age; the rate of increase was 0.35 g • day^{-1} at age from 29 to 47 days (see Figure 1A). In contrast, the body weight of the dystrophic mice increased at a lower rate (0.11 g • day^{-1}) for the same age range. The body weight of the dystrophic mice was 56% and 63% lower at 6 and 9 weeks old, respectively, than those of the control mice, and the growth of body weight was virtually arrested after about 2 months of age.

Biochemical Analysis

The DNA and RNA contents in the whole hind-limb muscles of the control and dystrophic mice are shown in Figure 2. As shown in Figure 2A, DNA content in the muscles of the dystrophic mice was 2.8 ($p < .001$) and 2.5 times ($p < .001$) higher in 6- and 9-week-old mice, respectively, than those of the control. This result is qualitatively in accordance with the other observations (8, 19). DNA content in the muscles decreased with age from 6 to 9 weeks old, being 11% and 20% lower in the control and dystrophic mice, respec-

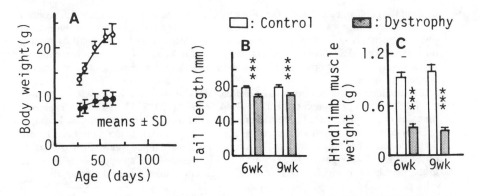

Figure 1. Growth of body weight in control (O) and dystrophic (●) mice (A), and comparison between control and dystrophic mice in tail length (B) and hindlimb muscle weight (C). For further details, see Table I. Values in B and C are shown as means ± *SE*. *** Difference between control and dystrophic mice means significant with $p < .001$.

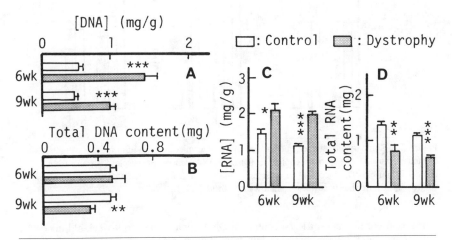

Figure 2. Comparison between control and dystrophic mice in nucleic acid contents in hindlimb muscles of mice. A, DNA contents in muscles; B, total DNA contents in muscles; C, RNA contents in muscles; D, total RNA contents in muscles. Values are expressed as means ± *SE*. Difference between control and dystrophic mice means significant with *$p < .05$, **$p < .01$, ***$p < .001$.

tively. Total DNA content in the muscles showed no significant difference between the control and dystrophic mice in 6-week-old mice (see Figure 2B). However, total DNA content in the muscles of 9-week-old dystrophic mice was 29% ($p < .001$) lower than the control value.

In total DNA content in the muscles of control mice, there was no significant difference between 6- and 9-week-old mice. However, the total DNA content of 9-week-old dystrophic mice was 33% ($p < .001$) lower than that of 6-week-old dystrophic mice. In accordance with results of the DNA content (see Figure 2A), the RNA content in muscles of 6- and 9-week-old dystrophic mice was 1.45 ($p < .02$) and 1.79 times ($p < .001$) higher than

172 Imaizumi, Tachiyashiki, and Sekiya

those of the control, respectively (see Figure 2C). RNA content in muscles of the control and dystrophic mice was 1.32 and 1.07 times higher in 6-week-old mice than 9-week-old mice, respectively. Total RNA contents in the muscles of 6- and 9-week-old dystrophic mice were about 55% of control values (see Figure 2D). Total RNA contents in the muscle of the control and dystrophic mice were about 19% higher in 6-week-old mice than in 9-week-old mice.

It is assumed that indicators of apparent cell volume are given by muscle wet weight per DNA content or protein content per DNA content (6, 19). Therefore, we evaluated the value of each indicator. The results are shown in Figure 3. The ratio of muscle weight to DNA content in the dystrophic mice was about 12% ($p < .001$) of the control (see Figure 3A). The ratio of protein content to DNA content in muscle tissue was 30-34% ($p < .001$) of the control (see Figure 3B). Figure 3A and B indicates that an apparent cell volume in the muscle of dystrophic mice is significantly lower than that of the control.

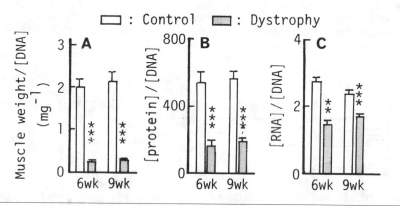

Figure 3. Comparison between control and dystrophic mice in hind-limb muscle weight/DNA content in muscles (A), protein content in muscles/DNA content in muscles (B), and RNA content in muscles/DNA content in muscles. Values are means ± *SE*. *** Difference between control and dystrophic mice means significant with $p < .001$.

The value of the ratio of RNA content to DNA content in 6- to 9-week-old mice was 2.4-2.7 and 1.4-1.7 in the control and dystrophic mice, respectively (see Figure 3C). The value of the ratio of RNA content to DNA content in muscle of dystrophic mice was 53% ($p < .001$) and 72% ($p < .001$) in 6- and 9-week-old mice, respectively, of the control values.

Protein content in hind-limb muscles (see Table 1) of the dystrophic mice was 81% ($p < .01$) and 83% ($p < .001$) in 6- and 9-week-old mice, respectively, of the control. Muscle protein content in both groups showed no significant difference in age from 6- to 9-week-old mice. The total protein content in muscles of the dystrophic mice was 30% ($p < .001$) and 26% ($p < .001$) in 6- and 9-week-old mice, respectively, of the control values. The marked decrease is mainly due to the decrease of the mass (=wet weight) of the hind-limb muscles (see Figure 1C).

Total protein content in the control muscle was almost the same in 6- to 9-week-old mice. The value of total protein content in the muscle of 9-week-old dystrophic mice, however, was about 88% of that of 6-week-old mice.

Muscle protein content of F-1 in the dystrophic mice was about 9% ($p < .01$) lower than the control in 9-week-old mice. Muscle protein content of F-2 in the dystrophic mice was 24% ($p < .05$) and 34% ($p < .001$) lower in 6- and 9-week-old mice, respectively,

Table 1 Comparison Between Control and Dystrophic Mice in Body Weight, Hind-Limb Muscle Weight, and Muscle Protein Content in Each Muscle Fraction

	6-week-old		9-week-old	
	Control ($n = 6$)	Dystrophy ($n = 7$)	Control ($n = 10$)	Dystrophy ($n = 6$)
Body weight (g)	21.6 ± 0.8	10.2 ± 0.5 ***	23.1 ± 0.8	9.2 ± 0.6 ***
Muscle weight[a] (g)	0.93 ± 0.04	0.34 ± 0.03***	0.99 ± 0.04	0.31 ± 0.03***
[Protein][b] (mg/g)	278 ± 9.0	225 ± 10.6 **	264 ± 6.3	220 ± 4.9 ***
Total protein (mg)	259 ± 17.6	77 ± 7.2 ***	261 ± 11.1	68 ± 3.8 ***
F-1 [protein] (mg/g)	54.3 ± 1.0	53.1 ± 1.5	53.9 ± 1.2	49.2 ± 0.6
F-2 [protein] (mg/g)	49.1 ± 2.5	37.1 ± 3.1 *	54.7 ± 11.5	36.4 ± 1.8 ***
F-3 [protein] (mg/g)	174.7 ± 7.3	135.0 ± 7.5 **	155.5 ± 6.7	133.9 ± 2.8 *
F-1 total protein (mg)	50.5 ± 7.4	18.1 ± 1.6 ***	53.4 ± 3.0	15.3 ± 1.3 ***
F-2 total protein (mg)	45.7 ± 5.1	12.6 ± 1.3 ***	54.2 ± 3.5	11.3 ± 1.1 ***
F-3 total protein (mg)	162.5 ± 18.7	45.9 ± 4.8 ***	154.0 ± 6.4	41.5 ± 2.6 ***

Note. Values are means ± *SE*. Difference between control and dystrophic mice means significant with $*p < .05$, $**p < .01$, $***p < .001$. [a]total weight of hind-limb muscles, [b]protein content in the hind-limb muscle. Numbers in parentheses indicate number of mice used.

than those of the control. Muscular protein content of F-3 in the dystrophic mice was 23% ($p < .01$) and 14% ($p < .05$) lower in 6- and 9-week-old mice, respectively, than that of the control. The order of the magnitude of decrease in muscle protein content was F-2 > F-3 > F-1 in 6- and 9-week-old mice, indicating that the degree of protein content is not identical with each muscle fraction.

The ratio of dystrophic mice to the control mice in the total protein content in muscles was 0.29-0.30, 0.21-0.28, and 0.27-0.28 in F-1, F-2, and F-3, respectively. From these results, the order of the magnitude of decrease of total protein content in muscles agrees qualitatively with that for muscle protein content.

Histological Analysis

In the skeletal muscle of adult dystrophic mice, variation of muscle-fiber diameter, atrophic fiber, connective tissue, fiber necrosis and central nucleation and increase in fiber splitting were documented by many investigations (11, 12, 19). These morphological abnormalities in 6- and 9-week-old dystrophic mice were also observed in the present work.

Figure 4 shows numbers of nuclei and muscle fibers in the hind-limb muscles of 9-week-old mice. Figure 4A shows that number of nuclei per 1 mm² of muscle tissue area in the dystrophic mice was 1.56 times ($p < .001$) higher than that of the control. This result may be closely related to the increase of DNA content in the muscle tissues of the dystrophic mice (see Figure 2A). Figure 4B presents numbers of muscle fibers per 1mm² of muscle tissue area. This value in the dystrophic mice was 49% ($p < .001$) of the control value. This phenomenon agrees well with the result obtained by Totsuka (17). Figure 4C depicts numbers of muscle fibers per numbers of nuclei in muscle tissue. This value in the dystrophic mice was 35% ($p < .001$) of the control. A percentage of the presence of the centronucleated muscle fibers per total muscle fibers in a cross section was compared between dystrophic and control mice. The results are indicated in Figure 4D. The percentage of centronucleated muscle fibers in the dystrophic mice was 9.5 times ($p < .001$) higher than in the control.

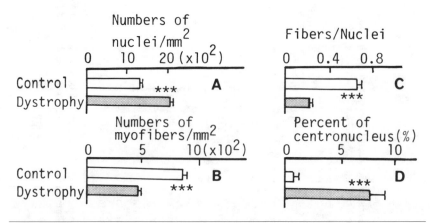

Figure 4. Comparison between control and dystrophic mice in numbers of nuclei/1mm² of muscle tissue area (A), numbers of muscle fibers/1mm² of muscle tissue area (B), numbers of muscle fibers/numbers of nucleus (C), and percentage of centronucleated fibers (D). Each value represents means ± *SE*. *** Difference between control and dystrophic mice means significant with $p < .001$.

Figure 5 shows a cross-sectional area frequency distribution of medial gastrocnemius muscle in 9-week-old mice (A: control, B: dystrophic). The frequency distribution of a cross-sectional area in muscle of the control mice was approximated by the Gaussian distribution curve. The value of a cross-sectional area at peak (=maximal) point was about $7.2 \times 10^2 \mu m^2$. In contrast, the maximal peak of the histogram of a cross-sectional area in the dystrophic muscle was evaluated as about $4.0 \times 10^2 \mu m^2$. However, the histogram showed the cross-sectional area variation. The larger muscle fibers were observed frequently in dystrophic mice (see Figure 5B).

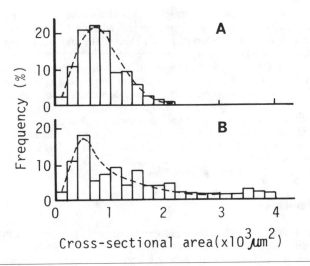

Figure 5. Comparison between control and dystrophic mice in cross-sectional area frequency distribution of medial gastrocnemius muscle in 9-week-old mice. A, control mice ($n = 447$); B, dystrophic mice ($n = 540$).

Discussion

The determination of the intracellular changes in hind-limb muscles of the dystrophic mice provides a quantitative scale, which is related to nonexercise muscular atrophy. For instance, DNA content in the hind-limb muscles was significantly higher in the dystrophic mice than in the control, and the nucleic acid content decreased with age from 6 to 9 weeks (see Figure 2), thus confirming an earlier observation (20).

We now report a significant, positive relation between biochemical changes and histological changes in the hind-limb muscles of dystrophic mice. Such biochemical changes related to histological changes may be one of the most useful ways to clarify the cellular mechanism of muscular atrophy (6). The increase of DNA content in muscles of the dystrophic mice (see Figure 2A) may be related to the increase of numbers of nuclei per unit area of muscle tissue (see Figure 4A).

It is generally accepted that nondividing cells contain very constant amounts of DNA and that the DNA content per whole hind-limb muscles in the control mice is almost constant irrespective of age (see Figure 2B), suggesting little proliferative activity of muscle cell

(20). Moreover, the total DNA content is proportional to the number of cells as described by Vandrely (21). A significant decrease of total DNA content in hind-limb muscles of 9-week-old dystrophic mice (see Figure 2B) may result in (a) the decrease of numbers of muscle fibers per unit area of muscle tissue (see Figure 4B), (b) the decrease of the ratio of muscle fibers to numbers of nuclei (see Figure 4C), (c) the decrease of an apparent cell volume (see Figure 3A and B), and (d) decrease of hind-limb muscle weight (see Figure 1C). These results suggest that the number of fibers per muscle is much smaller in dystrophic muscles than in the control at 9 weeks old (17). The decreased number of muscle fibers in the dystrophic mice may be caused by a defective maturation of dystrophic myofibers, as postulated by Totsuka (18).

The decrease of protein content in muscle tissues of the dystrophic mice (see Table I) may be influenced by the following factors, although additional data are needed to verify this: (a) the decrease of total RNA content (see Figure 2D), (b) the lowering of maximal peak of histogram of the cross-sectional area (see Figure 5B), (c) the decrease of the ratio of RNA content to DNA content (see Figure 3C), (d) the decrease of an apparent cell volume (see Figure 3A and B), and (e) the decrease of protein content in F-2 (see Table I). Recently, Obinata et al. (13) reported that a marked decrease in actin content occurs with the progression of muscular dystrophy. The decrease in actin content may be due to the elevation of the activities of several proteolytic enzymes in dystrophic muscle (1, 9), and seems to be related to the morphological degradation of myofibrillar structure (13).

In conclusion, these results show that biochemical and histological analyses used in the present study provide a basis with which to pursue future investigations of nonexercise muscular atrophy. Further detailed experiments are now going on.

Acknowledgments

We thank Dr. Tsuyoshi Totsuka (Department of Physiology, Institute for Developmental Research, Aichi Prefectural Colony) for useful suggestions. This study was supported in part by a Grant-in-Aid for Scientific Research from the Ministry of Education, Science and Culture of Japan.

References

1. Aoyagi, T., Wada, T., Umezawa, H. Analysis of abnormalities in enzymatic activities in various organs of dystrophic mice. In: Ebashi, S., Ozawa, E., eds. Muscular dystrophy: biomedical aspects. Tokyo: Japan Scientific Society Press, 1983:257-265.

2. Burton, K. A study of the conditions and mechanism of the diphenylamine reaction for the colorimetric estimation of deoxyribonucleic acid. Biochem. J. 62:315-323, 1956.

3. Dasse, K.A., Chase, D., Burke, D., Ullrick, W.C. Mechanical properties of tenotomized and denervated-tenotomized muscles. Am. J. Physiol. 241 (Cell Physiol. 10): C150-C153, 1981.

4. Goldberg, A.L., Goodman, H.M. Relationship between cortisone and muscle work in determining muscle size. J. Physiol. London 200:667-675, 1969.

5. Goldspink, D.F. The influence of immobilization and stretch on protein turnover of rat skeletal muscle. J. Physiol. London 264:267-282, 1977.

6. Imaizumi, K., Tachiyashiki, K., Sekiya, M. Analysis of hindlimb skeletal muscles in the dystrophic mice (C57BL/6J-dy) as the model of non-exercise muscular hypotrophy. J. Physiol. Soc. Jpn. 50(8-9): 536, 1988.

7. Jaspers, S.R., Tischler, M.E. Atrophy and growth failure of rat hindlimb muscles in tail-cast suspension. J. Appl. Physiol.: Respir. Environ. Exer. Physiol. 57:1472-1479, 1984.

8. King, D.W., King, C.R., Jacaruso, R.B. Avian muscular dystrophy: thyroidal influence on pectoralis muscle growth and glucose-6-phosphate dehydrogenase activity. Life Sci. 28:577-585, 1981.

9. Komatsu, K., Tsukada, K., Hosoya, J., Sato, S. Elevations of cathepsin B and cathepsin L activities in forelimb and hind limb muscles of genetically dystrophic mice. Exp. Neurol. 93:642-646, 1986.

10. Lowry, O.H., Rosebrough, N.J., Farr, A.L., Randall, R.J. Protein measurement with the Folin phenol reagent. J. Biol. Chem. 193:265-275, 1951.

11. Maier, H., Southard, J.L. Muscular dystrophy in the mouse caused by an allele at the dylocus. Life Sci. 9:137-144, 1970.

12. Michelson, A.M., Russell, E.S., Harman, P.J. Dystrophia muscularis: a hereditary primary myopathy in the house mouse. Proc. Natl. Acad. Sci. USA 41:1079-1084, 1955.

13. Obinata, T., Shimizu, N., Okamoto, K. Quantitative changes in monomer and polymer actins during development of normal and dystrophic chicken skeletal muscle. In: Ebashi, S., Ozawa, E., eds. Muscular dystrophy: biomedical aspects. Tokyo: Japan Scientific Society Press, 1983:79-88.

14. Schmidt, G., Thannhauser, S.T. A method for the determination of deoxyribonucleic acid, ribonucleic acid and phosphoproteins in animal tissue. J. Biol. Chem. 161:83-89, 1945.

15. Schneider, W.C. Determination of nucleic acids in tissues by pentose analysis. In: Colowick, S.P., Kaplan, N.O., eds. Methods in enzymology, Vol. 3. New York and London: Academic Press, 1957:680-684.

16. Templeton, G.H., Padalino, M., Manton, J., Glasberg, M., Silver, C.J., Silver, P., DeMartino, G., Leconey, T., Klug, G., Hagler, H., Sutko, J.L. Influence of suspension hypokinesia on rat soleus muscle. J. Appl. Physiol.: Respir. Environ. Exer. Physiol. 56:278-286, 1984.

17. Totsuka, T. A paradoxical growth of large myofibers in growth-arrested rectus femoris muscles of muscular dystrophic mice. Cong. Anom. 26:157-167, 1986.

18. Totsuka, T. Centronucleated myofibers having also peripheral nuclei in rectus femoris muscles of muscular dystrophic mice. Cong. Anom. 27:51-60, 1987.

19. Totsuka, T., Watanabe, K. Some evidence for concurrent involvement of the fore- and hindleg muscles in murine muscular dystrophy. Exp. Anim. 30:465-470, 1981.

20. Totsuka, T., Watanabe, K., Kiyono, S. Maturational defects of muscle fibers in the muscular dystrophic mouse. Cong. Anom. 21:253-259, 1981.

21. Vandrely, R. The deoxyribonucleic acid content of the nucleus. In: Chargaff, E., Davidson, J.N., eds. The nucleic acid, Vol. 2. New York and London: Academic Press, 1955:155-180.

Stretch Gymnastic Training in Asthmatic Children

A. Kanamaru, M. Sibuya, T. Nagai, K. Inoue, and I. Homma

Department of Physiology, Showa University School of Medicine, Tokyo, and Department of Pediatrics, Tokyo Metropolitan Hiroo General Hospital, Tokyo, Japan

Dyspneic sensation is the major subjective symptom of an asthma attack. This restricts the patient's activity and impedes self-management. Regarding the mechanism of dyspnea, Homma et al. (2) have proposed a central-peripheral mismatch theory. This theory suggests that when the phase of the intercostal muscle spindle afferent is mismatched with the phase of the central respiratory demand, dyspnea is induced.

Muller et al. (3) have reported activity in the inspiratory intercostal muscle and diaphragm at the end of the expiratory phase in asthmatic patients during attacks. It has not been shown though that the inspiratory muscle spindle afferents are also active throughout the expiratory phase. However, due to γ dependency of muscle spindle sensitivity and α-γ linkage, central-peripheral mismatch may be assumed as a cause of dyspnea during asthma attacks.

The stretch gymnastics reported here were designed to stretch the intercostal muscle spindles and to condition sensitivity. Due to the α-γ linkage, mere stretching of a resting muscle does not stretch the receptor portion of the muscle spindles very powerfully. The muscle has to be contracted and stretched simultaneously for efficient muscle spindle stretching. Thus the right combination of respiration and movement must be found in order to increase muscle afferents in phase with contraction. These stretch gymnastics were clinically instructed to asthmatic children in an outpatient clinic, and the effectiveness on dyspnea and pulmonary function test was studied.

Methods

The effects of stretch gymnastics on the intercostal muscles were studied in 5 normal subjects using EMG. The surface electrodes were attached on the midaxillary line between the 7th and the 10th intercostal spaces and on the midclavicular line in the 2nd or 3rd intercostal space to record the expiratory and inspiratory muscle activity, respectively (4). The movements were evaluated and made into a stretch gymnastics program.

Fifteen asthmatic children (7-12 years old, 5 males and 10 females, 6 severe, 9 moderate, all of them were positive EIA test) participated in the stretch gymnastics program once a week. All patients were required to perform the stretch gymnastics each week, except during a severe attack. Pulmonary function tests were carried out before and after each class. EMG was some of the basic stretch gymnastics recording during to determine each patient's skill.

Results

Comparisons of the EMG activity with and without stretch gymnastics in a healthy trained subject during deep breathing are shown in Figures 1 and 2. The increase in EMG activity

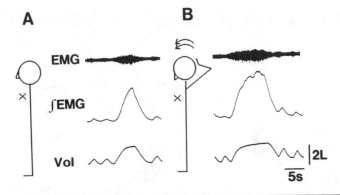

Figure 1. Illustrations representing movement: Upper (EMG in right upper intercostal muscle), middle (EMG integration), lower (respiratory volume). Cross (x) point at which surface electrode was attached was second intercostal space at the parasternal region. A = deep inspiration only. B = tilting the head forward with help of arm. Enhancement was seen in B compared to A.

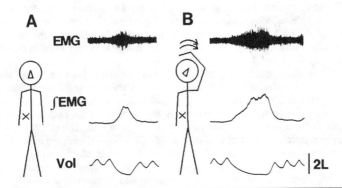

Figure 2. Illustrations representing movement: Upper (EMG in right upper intercostal muscle), middle (EMG integration), lower (respiratory volume). Cross (x) point at which surface electrode was attached was eighth intercostal space to the anterior axillary line. A = deep expiration only. B = tilting the head to the left with help of arm and pushing the right arm down. Enhancement was seen in B compared to A.

in Figures 1B and 2B compared to 1A and 2A could be due to either the load-compensation reflex, mediated by the muscle spindles, or the increase in demand from the cerebral cortex in order to achieve the movement. However, mere movement with no deep respiration did not increase the EMG activities. Thus, it was considered that the intercostal muscles and their muscle spindles were stretched by that particular movement. The combinations of respiratory phase and movements which enhanced EMG activity are shown in Figure 3. The movements A, C, D, E, and F augmented the activity of the upper intercostal muscle during deep inspiration. The movements B, C, D, E, and F augmented the activity of the lower intercostal muscle during deep expiration.

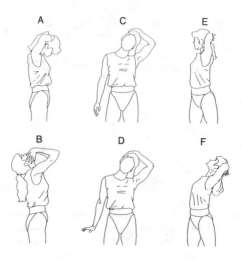

Figure 3. Stretch gymnastic program: A, C, D, E, and F for inspiration and B, C, D, E, and F for expiration.

Table 1 summarizes all the pulmonary function test results from 14 children who underwent the test before and after six gymnastic training periods. The results are divided according to the initial FEV1.0% value. There was no significant change in the average of the before and after values. Moreover, no significant change was seen even in the child with low pulmonary function.

The EMG was examined in 12 of the 15 asthmatic children who have undergone weekly stretch gymnastics instruction for at least 2 years. They performed the following types of stretch gymnastics: (a) tilting the head to both sides, (b) tilting the head forward and backward, and (c) twisting the body while holding the hands at the back of the head. Each movement was performed during both inspiration and expiration. The effects of each movement were evaluated and were scored on a scale of 7. The total average was 3.6; no child was able to perform the exercise perfectly. However, five children who had claimed that the dyspneic sensation decreased and whose pulmonary function test improved by stretch gymnastics with no other treatment or medication had higher scores.

Table 1 Pulmonary Function Test

FEV1.0% (before)	n	%FVC	FEV1.0%	%V$_{50}$
> 85%	21	0.4 ± 9.8	−3.0 ± 4.4	−6.5 ± 15.9
75-85%	41	2.7 ± 10.9	−0.9 ± 6.7	0.4 ± 27.3
< 75%	22	4.2 ± 16.7	0.2 ± 12.3	7.7 ± 31.4
Total	84	2.5 ± 12.3	−1.2 ± 8.1	0.6 ± 26.4

Note. Mean (%) ± *SD*.

Discussion

The mechanism of dyspnea during asthma attacks is still unclear. The involvement of the chest wall afferents has been suggested by Campbell and Howell (1) and by Homma et al. (2). The central-peripheral mismatch theory suggests that when afferent activity from the inspiratory or expiratory intercostal muscle spindles reaches the central nervous system during the expiratory or inspiratory phases, respectively, the mismatched (or out-of-phase) afferent activity reaching the higher center is recognized as a dyspneic sensation. We based stretch gymnastics on this theory.

There are a few reports suggesting that the inspiratory muscles are tonically active in the expiratory phase during asthma attacks in humans (3). This would indicate that the inspiratory muscle spindles are continuously activated and send abnormal afferent information to the central nervous system. It has also been reported that in some cases the functional residual capacity during the attack is larger than the total lung capacity between attacks (5). If this is due at least in part to the tonic inspiratory activity, powerful afferents from the inspiratory muscle spindles would be expected in the expiratory phase. Homma et al. (2) have suggested that such out-of-phase afferents would cause central-peripheral mismatch and may be the mechanism of dyspneic sensation during the asthma attack. In this study, some patients were able to relieve their dyspneic sensation solely by stretch gymnastics. The gymnastics were programmed to stretch intercostal muscles and muscle spindles during the contraction phase. This supports the hypothesis that chest wall afferents are essential in the formation of dyspnea. The stretch gymnastics may improve passive viscosity and elasticity of the muscle spindle and help release the stiffness. This also contributes to the activation of the muscle spindle afferents during the contraction phase.

We have also applied the EMG evaluation method for muscle spindle stretching to intercostal muscles. This method appears quite suitable for the evaluation of the effectiveness of particular muscle stretching movements. There are a few maneuvers known to be effective for asthmatics, such as yoga or taijiquan. It is possible that intercostal muscle spindles are stretched in these maneuvers. It would be of interest to apply the EMG evaluation method to these maneuvers. Clinically, stretch gymnastics have never worsened pulmonary functions, even at severe positive EIA and at low respiratory function. Therefore, stretching can be done in any asthmatic condition.

Acknowledgments

The authors thank Dr. Albert Simpson and Mary Beth Sibuya for reviewing the manuscript. This study was supported by the Environment Agency of Japan.

References

1. Campbell, E.J.M., Howell, J.B.L. The sensation of breathlessness. Br. Med. Bull. 19:36-40, 1963.

2. Homma, I., Obata, T., Sibuya, M., Uchida, M. Gate mechanisms in breathlessness caused by chest wall vibration in humans. J. Appl. Physiol. 56:8-11, 1984.

3. Muller, N., Bryan, A.C., Zamel, N. Tonic inspiratory muscle activity as a cause of hyperinflation in asthma. J. Appl. Physiol. 50:279-282, 1981.

4. Taylor, A. The contribution of the intercostal muscles to the effort of respiration in man. J. Physiol. 151:390-402, 1960.

5. Woolcock, A.J., Read, J. Improvement in bronchial asthma not reflected in forced expiratory volume. Lancet 2:1323-1325, 1965.

Cardiovascular Response of Severely Multihandicapped Individuals to Body Position at Rest

K. Mita, K. Akataki, T. Miyagawa, K. Koyama, and N. Ishida
Institute for Developmental Research, Aichi Prefectural Colony, Kasugai; Rehabilitation Engineering Center for Employment Injuries, Nagoya; and Jiyuu Gakuin Junior College, Nishikasugai, Japan

According to the Child Welfare Law in Japan, severely multihandicapped children are defined as persons below 18 years of age with the double handicaps of severe mental retardation and severe physical disability (3). This term is not used in medical diagnosis but is an exclusive administrative concept in Japan's child welfare services. Similar handicapped persons above 18 years of age are not defined administratively as severely multihandicapped adults. Although the strict definition focuses on only the severely multihandicapped children, the same welfare services are provided even for the handicapped adults in the practical enforcement of the law. We refer generically to the handicapped children and adults as severely multihandicapped individuals in the present report.

Intelligence quotients of severely multihandicapped individuals who are defined under the law remains lower than 35. Posture in daily living is limited to sitting as a result of profound disabilities in limbs. A considerable number of the handicapped individuals are lying down on beds during the entire day. It is extremely difficult for them to perform active and vigorous physical activity. Not only does the physical inactivity lead to a serious risk of decrease in the circulatory function, but it causes consequential diseases such as decubitus, edema, and infectious disease. In order to improve wellness and physical fitness, it is necessary to involve them in physical training, even by passively simulated physical work. Frequent postural changes may be one of several possible methods for stimulating the cardiovascular function.

In the present study, the influence of body position producing hydrostatic pressure shift to cardiovascular function was investigated and the possibility of using passive methods of physical training was discussed.

Methods

The subjects were 19 individuals from a medicare-provided residential institution for the severely multihandicapped. The ages ranged from 5 to 32 years. The diagnoses included cerebral palsy (13), meningitis (3), hydrocephaly (2), and epilepsy (1). Eight of the subjects had been able to take sitting or standing posture in the past. All the subjects had no active motor ability and ambulatory ability and lay on beds during the entire day. However, 14 of them had opportunities to experience a supported sitting position several times a day. We classified the subjects into four groups according to posture in the past and opportunity of sitting position in daily living. The first group (referred to as LDLD) had lain on beds in the past and had not had the opportunity of sitting in daily living. The second group

(STLD) could sit or stand independently in the past but had the same lack of opportunity as the LDLD group in sitting. The third group (LDST) and fourth group (STST) had the opportunity for sitting in daily living. In addition, the LDST group was unable to sit and stand in the past but the STST group was able. Eleven nonhandicapped people aged 19-24 years participated for the control group.

A sitting position with knees extended and hips flexed at 60° was selected to investigate cardiovascular response to hydrostatic pressure stress. This position was fixed with a reclining bed. Supine position was used as the control posture. The measurement was performed in the supine position at rest during a period of 10 min and in subsequent sitting position during the same period.

Electrocardiogram and photoplethysmogram were measured consecutively through a period of the posture-change process. The electrocardiogram was detected by precordial unipolar electrodes and was recorded using a radio system. The heart rate was calculated using the electrocardiogram. The photoplethysmogram was derived from the left big toe. The signal was sampled at a rate of 250 samples per second by means of an A/D converter and power spectral density was computed every minute. The power spectral density was accumulated to determine the power of the photoplethysmogram. The accumulation was performed on the spectral density at the frequencies of more than 0.5 Hz to eliminate artifacts such as body motion. The blood pressure of the right upper arm was measured noninvasively by means of a sphygmomanometer based on the oscillometric method. In order to obtain stationary values of the above parameters, the processing was performed on the signals for a period of 7 min from the 3rd min to the end in each posture.

Results

The heart rate in the sitting position showed a tendency for a higher response than that in supine position. Interindividual mean of the difference was 2.93 ± 3.12 b/min (mean $\pm$ SD) for the handicapped individuals and was 2.47 ± 3.20 b/min for the nonhandicapped. A somewhat greater difference was found for the handicapped individuals than for their control. There was no significant difference in heart rates between the two groups. However, there were significant differences between some of the classified groups, that is, between the LDLD group and the LDST group ($p < .01$) as well as between the LDLD group and the nonhandicapped group ($p < .05$).

The photoplethysmogram reduced to $62.1 \pm 27.4\%$ in sitting position for the handicapped individuals and to $68.8 \pm 25.1\%$ for the nonhandicapped individuals. Significant differences in the photoplethysmogram were detected neither between the two groups nor among the classified groups.

As seen in Figure 1, there was a linear relationship between depression of the photoplethysmogram and difference of the heart rate for the nonhandicapped individuals. The solid line presents regression line for the nonhandicapped individuals ($y = -0.12x + 10.87$, $r = -.97$, $p < .001$) and the broken line indicates double width of the root mean square error (RMS error). A similar correlation between the two parameters as for the nonhandicapped was not found for the handicapped individuals. However, obvious characteristics were detected for the classified handicapped groups according to previous posture and opportunities for sitting in daily living. The points for the LDLD (open squares) and STLD (solid squares) groups except 1 subject located downward on the broken line indicating the -2RMS error. Those for most subjects of the STLD group (open circles) positioned inside the ± 2RMS error lines or upward. The results for the STST group (solid circles) except 1 subject kept inside or around the ± 2RMS error lines.

The systolic pressure in the sitting position was lower by 3.38 ± 5.55 mmHg than that in the supine position for handicapped individuals. It increased slightly by 1.50 ± 3.69 mmHg for the nonhandicapped. The variation of the systolic pressure was significantly

184   Mita, Akataki, Miyagawa, Koyama, and Ishida

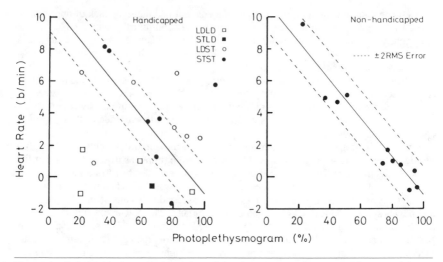

Figure 1. Relationship between depression of the photoplethysmogram and difference of the heart rate.

different between the two groups (p <.05). The variation of the diastolic pressure was -2.25 ± 4.81 mmHg for the handicapped individuals and 1.47 ± 4.14 mmHg for the nonhandicapped individuals. This was also a significant difference ($p < .05$) between the two groups.

Table 1 presents differences of the blood pressure between sitting and supine positions for the classified handicapped group. The systolic pressure lowered sharply for the LDLD, STLD, and LDST groups. There were significant differences among the LDLD and LDST groups and the STST and nonhandicapped groups, interactively. No significant difference between the STST group and the nonhandicapped individuals was found. The diastolic pressure for the LDLD group lowered by -5.58 ± 4.52 mmHg, and it was the greatest variation among the four groups. There was significant differences only between the LDLD

Table 1   Difference of Systolic Pressure and Diastolic Pressure Between Supine and Sitting Positions for the Classified Handicapped Groups

Subject	Systolic pressure (mmHg)	Diastolic pressure (mmHg)
Handicapped		
LDLD	-5.31 ± 3.85 (4)	-5.58 ± 4.52 (4)
STLD	-5.90 (1)	-1.25 (1)
LDST	-6.36 ± 4.09 (7)	-2.07 ± 5.28 (7)
STST	1.21 ± 5.82 (6)	-1.73 ± 4.17 (6)
Nonhandicapped	1.50 ± 3.69 (11)	1.47 ± 4.14 (11)

$*p < .05$, $**p < .01$.

groups and the nonhandicapped. The other three handicapped groups might be placed between the LDLD group and the nonhandicapped individuals.

Discussion

Postural changes resulting in hydrostatic pressure stress bring about noticeable alterations in the cardiovascular system. As reported previously for nonhandicapped people (1, 2, 4), with postural change from supine position to sitting position the blood is pooled in the part of the body below the heart level. The hydrostatic pressure shift dilates the vessels in the lower limbs and reduces the peripheral resistance. Decrease of the venous return and the stroke volume accompanying reduced peripheral resistance causes a fall in arterial blood pressure. However, since the baroreceptor-mediated reflex activates rapid peripheral vasoconstriction, peripheral blood flow is lowered. Consequently, the systolic pressure recovers to the control value and the diastolic pressure increases. The heart rate increases to compensate for decreasing cardiac output.

In order to investigate the above cardiovascular adjustment for the handicapped individuals, we used the heart rate and the systolic pressure as measures of central circulation and the diastolic pressure and the photoplethysmogram as measures of peripheral blood flow. Particularly, the blood flow is determined frequently by venous occlusion plethysmography using a Whitney mercury-in-silastic strain gauge. It was difficult to apply this method to the severely multihandicapped individuals in the present study. We estimated indirectly the peripheral blood flow using the photoplethysmography, which could measure easily the cutaneous volume pulse.

The experimental results showed a negative correlation between the heart rate and the photoplethysmogram for the nonhandicapped individuals. The systolic pressure remained at almost the same level. These results confirmed that cardiovascular control systems at both the central and peripheral levels were adjustable. No distinct change of the diastolic pressure suggested that the sitting position with hip flexed at 60° in this study did not produce a great hydrostatic pressure stress.

The STST group of the severely multihandicapped individuals demonstrated very similar characteristics to the control group. It was believed that the handicapped individuals who had the opportunity to use the sitting position in daily living were able to acquire a cardiovascular function close to nonhandicapped individuals. The LDST group was characterized by a greater increase of the heart rate in association with the reduced peripheral flow and the fall of the systolic pressure. This seemed to indicate lower baroreflex control in the peripheral circulation and greater compensation in heart level. The LDLD group did not show adjustment by heart rate accompanying the peripheral flow change. In addition, both the systolic pressure and the diastolic pressure were reduced. These results suggested serious lower function or dysfunction in both the central and peripheral circulatory systems. Since the STLD group consisted of one subject, it was difficult to estimate a reliable property. The STLD group might have intermediate properties between the LDLD and LDST groups.

In conclusion, cardiovascular control function for severely multihandicapped individuals depends on opportunity for orthostatic posture in daily living in addition to motor ability in the past. We propose that frequent postural change is one of the useful methods for improving cardiovascular function for severely multihandicapped individuals.

Acknowledgments

The authors express their gratitude to Dr. J. Yamakawa, Professor of Japan Women's College of Physical Education, and Dr. H. Nakamura, Director of Ashikaga Hospital, National Sanatoriums for Mentally and Physically Handicapped Children, for their generous support. This work was supported in part by a Grant-in-Aid for Scientific Research (No. 60580119) from Ministry of Education, Science and Culture, in Japan.

References

1. Bevegard, S., Holmgren, A., Jonsson, B. The effect of body position on the circulation at rest and during exercise, with special reference to the influence on the stroke volume. Acta Physiol. Scand. 49:279-298, 1960.

2. Hoshi, T., Kojima, T., Kameyama, S., Matsuda, K. On the influence of postural change upon the cardiac rate in man. Tohoku J. Exp. Med. 62:221-234, 1955.

3. Ministry of Health and Welfare, ed. Graphs and charts on Japan's child welfare services. Tokyo: The Japan Research Institute on Child Welfare, 1987.

4. Reeves, J.T., Grover, R.F., Blount, S.G., Jr., Filley, G.F. Cardiac output response to standing and treadmill walking. J. Appl. Physiol. 16:283-288, 1961.

PART III

HEALTH AND FITNESS OF THE INDUSTRIAL WORKER

The Costs and Benefits of Exercise:
An Industrial Perspective

R.J. Shephard
School of Physical and Health Education and Department of Preventive
Medicine and Biostatistics, Faculty of Medicine, University of Toronto,
Canada

Each of the three major areas explored in this conference lends itself to cost/benefit or
cost/effectiveness scrutiny. A major part of currently spiraling health care costs is due
to prolonged invalidism of the elderly and a resultant need for institutional care for the
elderly. It would thus be very appropriate to examine the costs of fitness programs adapted
to the needs of senior citizens versus a possible reduction in the need for chronic care
after recruitment to such programs. Moreover, prolonged invalidism is almost inevitably
poor quality living, and although it is unlikely that regular endurance exercise will extend
the lifespan of the elderly by more than a few months, it can greatly improve functional
ability and thus the "quality-adjusted" lifespan of the senior (45, 48).

Similar arguments could be advanced with respect to many categories of chronic disability. Those confined to wheelchairs by spinal trauma were at one time dependent members
of society, regarded as doomed to early death from renal infection, respiratory disease,
or ischemic heart disease. However, participation in relatively low cost training programs
or wheelchair sport has now completely changed this gloomy prognosis. Many wheelchair competitors have become confident, productive members of society with a physical
working capacity which has sometimes exceeded that of their able-bodied peers (49).

However, cost/benefit analyses are furthest advanced with respect to industrial fitness
programs. I shall make industry the primary focus of this report. North American industry
currently faces strong and increasing competition from seemingly more productive corporations. Attention has focused on various facets of oriental industrial operations, including not only the organization of the production line but also social features of the work
site, such as the opportunity for mass participation in employee exercise classes. Western
companies have thus viewed the introduction of fitness and lifestyle programs tailored
to the needs of the North American labor force as one possible tactic in the battle to match
oriental production costs. An increasing number of anecdoctal reports from North America
suggest that such initiatives have a favorable impact upon company balance sheets (44, 47).
However, careful, controlled experiments are a rarity. Moreover, a full economic assessment of an employee fitness program is a difficult undertaking (46), and occasional analyses
by experienced health economists still query whether fiscal benefit would result from
enhanced physical activity (43).

The present report thus critically examines the economic gains which supposedly result
from the introduction of corporate fitness and lifestyle programs. It commences with a
brief historical review of key papers leading to the advancement of this hypothesis. The
active individual, and in some instances the government, could both profit from an enhancement of personal activity. However, we shall here consider only advantages to the sponsoring corporation. Possible sources of financial benefit to the employer (44, 47) include

an improved corporate image, facilitation of employee recruitment, an increase in the quality and quantity of production, a decreased rate of absenteeism, a lower turnover of employees, reduced health care costs, and a lower incidence of industrial injuries.

Historical Review

The general idea that worker satisfaction and thus industrial output would be improved by a congenial environment, including the provision of athletic and social facilities, extends back to Quaker philanthropists such as the Cadburys (47). However, the early justification for such initiatives was the shrewd intuition of the entrepreneur rather than any rigidly documented experiment.

Over the past two decades, the emphasis in North American corporations has moved from the organization of industrial sports teams (where there were often more spectators than participants) to the provision of endurance exercise programs open to all employees. One of the first investigators to suggest a linkage between the personal fitness of the worker and the likelihood of absenteeism was Lindén (32). A cross-sectional study related cardio-respiratory fitness data to absenteeism rates for male customs officers and fire fighters, office workers of both sexes, and miscellaneous employees from other nonsedentary jobs. The customs officers were the only group in which a statistically significant correlation between maximum oxygen intake and absenteeism was demonstrated (coefficient of correlation .47). However, further support for the value of endurance fitness as a method of combating absenteeism was adduced from (a) a low maximum oxygen intake in customs officers and firefighters with more than eight absences per year and (b) a high maximum oxygen intake in office workers with no absenteeism over the course of the year. While this study strongly suggested benefit from endurance training, critics have pointed to the perennial problem of self-selection; the active lifestyle and thus the high maximum oxygen intake was determined by the worker and not by the investigator. Employees who were frequently absent generally came from families of low socioeconomic status, and this in turn influenced various aspects of their personal lifestyle, including both smoking habits and their prior participation in active leisure pursuits.

A second important paper was that of Bjurstrom and Alexiou (5). Beginning in 1972, they offered governmental employees in New York State a 15-week program of work site exercise (3 days per week, each session comprising 10 min of warm-up, 25-30 min of walking and jogging, and 5 min of relaxation exercises) with a follow-up personalized lifestyle prescription. Male program participants showed significant gains in physical working capacity and predicted maximum oxygen intake, with a decrease of body fat, but physiological changes were slight in female participants. Sick leave in program participants was reduced by 4.7 h per year relative to their personal experience in the previous year, and the arbitrary cardiovascular risk factor score for the active subjects decreased from 26 to 22 points. The main weakness of the study was the lack of a randomly assigned control group, particularly as those who elected to participate in the program had a below average initial absenteeism rate (46.5 versus 73.5 h per year). A second difficulty was a very low adherence rate, especially among female employees. While 80% of those recruited (about a third of employees) completed the 15-week program, after 1 year adherence to the prescribed exercise had dropped to 61%, and by 5 years the figures were 45% for men but only 11% for women. In 8% of subjects, defections from the program were attributable to a change of job, and in a further 13% there was a physical or a medical reason for noncompliance, but the most common explanation (79%) was loss of interest (including difficulty in meeting the schedule of exercise classes).

In Canada, interest in work site programs was strong enough to warrant a national conference on employee fitness (30). In response to this initiative, available information was drawn together in a short monograph (12), a pilot work site program was introduced into government offices in Ottawa (42), and a controlled trial of an employee fitness program was initiated in Toronto (16, 38). The enthusiasm of health economists for fitness initiatives was further advanced when it was reported to the Ontario government that if a typical worker could be brought to an average level of fitness, there would be large savings in both current health care expenditures and the likelihood of future costs due to ischemic heart disease (40). Again, it should be stressed that the data base for this report was cross-sectional in nature; thus is could not establish whether fitness reduced health care costs or whether the healthy person was also likely to become physically fit. At the Olympic Congress in Quebec City, Pravosudov (39) presented more cross-sectional data, suggesting that Russian worker athletes had a higher productivity and were less vulnerable to a variety of infections than were their sedentary counterparts.

In most of the North American studies cited to date, the participants have tended to be white-collar workers, often with a preponderance of upper management. While such individuals are of considerable value to a company, they are few in number, and they also tend to be quite health conscious. Thus, from the viewpoint of overall corporate health, the hourly (or to use a term now in disfavor, blue-collar) worker presents a much larger reservoir of correctible lifestyle faults, including an inadequate level of habitual activity. The design of exercise programs with ambiance that will attract the hourly worker is currently one of the major challenges facing the industrial fitness community (36).

Employee Fitness and Corporate Image

Lifestyle advertising is currently a popular and apparently a successful technique for marketing a variety of products, at least in North America. Particularly if a company is selling a health-related product such as food, the sponsoring of a corporate fitness program can be linked to such advertising, thereby enhancing corporate image. It has also been argued that employees with a fit appearance are an important asset to organizations such as the armed services, the police, and fire protection agencies. Such concepts make good intuitive sense, but they do not appear to have been tested by empirical research; moreover, it would be hard to assign a convincing dollar value to a specific corporate image.

Fitness Programs and Employee Recruitment

An attractive fitness and lifestyle program may be an inducement to the recruitment of personnel in markets where experienced labor is in short supply. However, the corollary of this argument is that the surplus of labor generated by robotics may soon make recruitment an unimportant problem except in the upper echelons of management.

Bernacki and Baun (4) have argued that companies that adopt a corporate fitness policy enjoy a selective recruitment and retention of high-achieving personnel. Plainly, the economic value of any recruitment incentive varies widely with the market demand for a given type of labor. Selective recruitment may remain very important when seeking key executives, but it is unlikely to be a major fiscal argument favoring the future provision of a fitness/lifestyle program for hourly employees.

Employee Fitness and Productivity

The poor quality and quantity of current production is a major concern of North American industrialists. Low productivity can have many causes, including poor management, a shortage of materials, or restrictive practices by labor unions. Low productivity is often symptomatic of worker dissatisfaction, and in this context estimates of worker satisfaction may be at least as revealing as formal measures of output, which are notoriously difficult to carry out.

The monograph "Work in America" (57) painted a grim descriptive picture of dissatisfied workers. On the contrary, formal evaluations of attitudes, using such tools as the job satisfaction index of Holmes and Rahe (25), have documented relatively high levels of satisfaction among Canadian and U.S. employees (15, 29, 31). Nevertheless, it must be stressed that formal surveys have tended to be conducted in nonunionized, white-collar operations with a history of good industrial relations; if a strike is pending, management is unlikely to want questionnaires circulated on the subject of worker satisfaction! Various anecdotal reports (47) have commented on improved attitudes about work after introduction of an employee fitness program (see Table 1) and support for these comments may be inferred from a reduction of absenteeism and health care costs as workers became more active. However, formal assessments of work satisfaction over the controlled trial of an employee fitness program have demonstrated surprisingly little change (15).

The quantity of production is particularly hard to assess in most white-collar occupations. Howard and Michalachki (26) noted no increase in the productivity of middle managers

Table 1   Influence of Employee Fitness/Lifestyle Programs Upon Industrial Productivity

Author	Benefit
Rohmert (1973)	Less fatigue, faster recovery
Laporte (1966)	Greater strength, hand steadiness, less eye-fatigue
Pravosudov (1978)	Output standard +2-5% to +10-15%
Réville (1970)	31% decrease of errors
Geissler (1960)	Reduced fatigue
Manguroff, Channe, & Georgieff (1960)	Reduced fatigue
Galevskaya (1970)	Reduced fatigue
Pravosudov (1978)	Greater creativity, less fatigue
Heinzelmann (1975)	Greater self-reported productivity
Howard & Michalachki (1979)	No benefit in middle managers
Finney (1979)	No benefit from recreational programs
Stallings, O'Rourke, & Gross (1975)	No effect on teaching or research output
Blair et al. (1980)	No effect on supervisor assessments, merit pay or promotions
Health & Welfare Canada	4% gain in productivity
Mealey (1979)	39% increase in police officer commendations
Briggs (1975, February)	Improved memory, muscle control, work performance
Shephard et al. (1981)	2.7% gain in productivity

Note. See Shephard, 46 for details of references.

after 6 months of participation in an employee fitness program, and there have been other negative reports from Finney (19) and Stallings et al. (55). The only controlled trial seems that of Cox et al. (16); they compared the observed to the standard time for various office tasks, finding in the year after introduction of an employee fitness program a 7% gain in productivity at the experimental company, compared with a 4.3% change at the control company. The inference seems that there was a "Hawthorne effect" at both work sites due to the trial, but that there was also a net benefit of 2.7% attributable to the exercise program. Other earlier studies noted a decrease in errors on the part of both telegraph operators (34) and textile workers (41) in response to relatively brief fitness breaks; here, the explanation seems a relief of boredom.

In certain forms of physical work, there is a more obvious relationship between productivity and physical working capacity. Hughes and Goldman (27), for example, demonstrated that in self-paced work, performance was commonly adjusted to use about 40% of aerobic power. Thus, if the aerobic power of the worker is increased by a program of endurance training, an improvement of production might be anticipated in self-paced work, with a lessening of fatigue and its associated adverse consequences in machine-paced tasks. Apparently on the basis of such reasoning, Pravosudov (39) argued that Russian worker-athletes had a 4-10% advantage over their sedentary peers in terms of their capacity for the performance of physical work. In Ontario, Danielson and Danielson (17) examined the productivity of forest fire fighters as kilometers of firebreak cut per day. In general, endurance training did not increase the performance of this group of employees, but it did prove an advantage when work was performed under very hot and arduous conditions.

Fitness and Absenteeism

Absenteeism, much of it unrelated to health, causes losses of 10 or more of 220 working days per year in many Canadian companies. Taking account also of the high cost of hiring temporary replacements (a typical allowance is 1.75 times the hours lost), absenteeism can boost production costs by as much as 7-8%.

One major difficulty in addressing the absenteeism problem through the introduction of a corporation-wide fitness program is that a minority of employees (15-20%) account for most of the absenteeism, and the characteristics of the absentees are such that they are unlikely to participate in a fitness initiative (4, 13). A number of studies (see Table 2) have suggested that there is some reduction in absenteeism (company-wide gains of 0.5-1.5 days per year, with effects of up to 2.8 days per year in exercisers) following introduction of a corporate fitness or comprehensive health promotion program (3, 5, 6, 7, 16, 20, 24). Unfortunately, questions of self-selection remain; those who elect an exercise program have a low inherent rate of absenteeism, and in cross-sectional comparisons this factor accounts for a large part of the apparent benefit from exercise. However, recent multiple regression analyses have shown an association between increases of aerobic fitness and decreases of absenteeism even after allowance for worker satisfaction (15) and initial absenteeism (7), strongly suggesting that physical activity makes a causal contribution to the improved attendance record.

Fitness and Employee Turnover

The economic cost of employee turnover depends in part on the length and complexity of training that is required for a given job. However, even in a task such as bus driving (in which formal training lasts only a few weeks), there is a substantial economic advantage to ensuring a stable labor force, since there is a progressive decrease in the number of

Table 2   Influence of Fitness Upon Industrial Absenteeism

Author	Benefit
Lindén (1969)	Correlation of low absenteeism, high $\dot{V}O_2$max
Condon (1978)	23% decrease in absenteeism
Barhad (1979)	Decrease in absenteeism
Pafnote et al. (1979)	Decrease in absenteeism
Keelor (1970)	50% decrease in absenteeism
Pravosudov (1978)	Decrease 4.0 days per worker-year
Mealey (1979)	Decrease of 34% (1.4 days per worker-year)
Wilbur (1983)	Decrease of 22%
Bjurstrom & Alexiou (1978)	Decrease of 0.59 days per worker-year
Blair et al. (1980)	No effect
Richardson (1974, May/June)	Decrease of 0.82 days per worker-year
Garson (1977)	Decrease of 47% (2.8 days per worker-year)
Cox et al. (1981)	Decrease of 23% (1.3 days per worker-year)

Mean of percentage changes: 33%

Mean decrease of absences: 1.8 days per worker-year

Note. See note to Table 1.

chargeable vehicular accidents over several years of employment, irrespective of the age at recruitment to a bus company (37).

In the Canada Life Assurance Study (16), the cost of training office staff was estimated at $13,600 for executives and $6,400 for clerical personnel (both figures being measured in 1983 Canadian dollars). Prior to introduction of the employee fitness program, employee turnover amounted to 18% per annum. In the year immediately following introduction of the program, the turnover among regular program adherents dropped to 1.8%. One possible explanation could be that the fitness program recruited an unusually conscientious and stable segment of the labor force (56). The preexperimental period of service with the Canada Life Assurance Company of the regular program participants was much the same as those who did not join the exercise classes (see Table 3), but on the other hand there was selective recruitment of program participants from the upper ranks of the company hierarchy. It is thus possible that the fact of promotion had increased the stability of the active employees within the company.

Tsai et al. (56) distinguished upper echelon from less skilled workers in the Tenneco Corporation. In both categories of employment, there was some advantage of retention rates for exercisers (at one year, 97% versus 88% in upper echelon staff and 92% versus 77% in other categories of worker; at 4 years a lesser benefit of 70% versus 64% in upper echelon staff and 60% versus 48% in others). Unfortunately, this study did not examine the longevity of employment prior to introduction of the exercise program.

A decrease of employee turnover could make a valuable contribution to the profitability of many corporations. However, actual savings would depend on the relative proportions of executive and lower echelon workers in the company, their relative participation in the fitness/lifestyle program, and their relative susceptibility to a change of turnover rate

Table 3   Turnover Rate for Various Categories of Employees Prior to Introduction of an Employee Fitness Program

Subject group	Average duration of service (yr)	Estimated[a] < 1 yr of service (%)	Actual < 1 yr of service (%)	Estimated[b] turnover rate (%)
Controls	8.3	6.02	—	12.0
Nonparticipants	11.3	4.42	6.00	8.9
Dropouts	9.8	5.10	8.06	10.2
Low adherents	8.1	6.17	2.86	12.3
High adherents	9.7	5.15	5.84	10.3

Note. Calculated from reported duration of service. From "Influence of an Employee Fitness Programme Upon Fitness, Productivity and Absenteeism" by M. Cox, R.J. Shephard, and P. Corey, 1981, *Ergonomics*, 24, pp. 795-806. [a]Calculated as (2/average duration of service)100. [b]Calculated as (1/average duration of service)100.

as a result of the exercise classes. Moreover, any benefit would likely be fairly long-term in nature; it is doubtful whether a person considering an early change of employment would invest either time or money in a corporate fitness program.

Fitness and Health Care Costs

In Canada, all health care costs are met by a prepaid governmental insurance scheme, and the impact of spiraling health care costs upon industrial corporations comes only indirectly—through provincial and federal taxation. In the United States, most companies provide health coverage as part of their package of fringe benefits, and steeply rising insurance premiums are a serious concern (2, 18, 43). Given the ability of regular exercise to reduce the risk of developing a number of major chronic diseases such as myocardial infarction, it has been argued that an employee fitness program (particularly if coupled with more general health promotion measures) could generate substantial savings. Not only would companies reduce the direct insured costs of illness (premiums for hospital admission and immediate medical care), but they would see indirect benefits through a reduction in absence from work and premature death of key employees (see Table 4).

In a long-term perspective, such savings may indeed accrue, although it would be exceedingly difficult to obtain empirical proof of the benefits hypothesized from changes in the risk factors for chronic disease (5, 6, 50, 52). However, the savings demonstrated immediately after health promotion or exercise program introduction ($100-$400/year; see Table 5) have appeared far too rapidly to reflect any change in the incidence of chronic disease (2, 3, 8, 9, 16, 18, 21). Moreover, while the exercisers typically make fewer demands for health care than their sedentary counterparts (an average cost of $600 versus $1,269 per year in the study of Baun et al. [3]), the fiscal benefit from the introduction of a health promotion program seems in some instances (51)—but not all (21)—to extend to the entire company. Shephard et al. (52) found only a very modest relationship between individual gains of fitness and reductions in health care costs. Among male participants in an employee

Table 4   Direct and Indirect Costs Attributable to Chronic Cardiovascular Disease

Cost[a]	M = Million
Direct costs	
Hospital services	$ 497M
Physicians' services	116M
Pharmaceuticals	116M
Medical education and research	Excluded
Total	$ 729M
Indirect costs	
Total	$ 744M
Grand total (direct and indirect costs)	$1,473M
($538 per worker-year)	

Note. From *The Relationships Between Physical Fitness and the Cost of Health Care* (p. 11) by Quasar, 1976, Toronto: Quasar Systems, Ltd. These costs might be reduced up to 50% by an effective employee fitness program.
[a]Expressed in 1983 Canadian collars.

Table 5   Immediate Effects of Employee Fitness Program Upon Prepaid Costs of Medical Care

| | Company A | | Company B | | Net |
Claims	1977	1978	1977	1978	saving
Hospital bed-days ($ per employee-year)	43.20	14.39	27.18	81.55	83.18
Medical costs ($ per employee-year)	134.63	135.92	135.12	181.81	45.40
Total					$128.58

Note. Company B served as control throughout. Hospital beds cost $160/day (1983 dollars). (See Shephard, 1986b).

fitness program, hospital days were significantly correlated with exercise heart rate, while other medical costs showed a similar but statistically nonsignificant trend. In female employees, on the other hand, there were no statistically significant trends.

The main explanation of the reduced demand for medical services on the part of active workers is probably that perceived health (23) has improved. Many of the patients who are seen in a doctor's consulting room, and even in a hospital, are not affected by any clear-cut pathology. Rather, dissatisfaction with their current situation at work or at home has displaced their perceptions to the right on a continuum linking good and ill health. In a similar manner, any improvement in the work situation can cause a leftward displacement of health perceptions in the direction of good health.

The demonstration of management interest manifested by the introduction of a fitness program could thus have an indirect effect upon health care utilization by boosting the morale of employees. The likelihood that exercise participation has a more specific effect is suggested not only by the weak statistical associations noted above but also by comments that participation in an activity class makes an individual "feel better." Exercise may provide an arousing stimulus, relief of boredom, or an outlet for frustration and hostility. A chemical elevation of mood through an enhanced secretion of endorphins is also a theoretical possibility, although such a response is unlikely to be realized with the intensities of exercise that are encountered in the usual employee fitness class. A trimmer figure may improve self-image, and if aerobic power is increased, less fatigue will be sensed in physically demanding work.

Fitness and Industrial Injuries

In a typical white-collar operation there are few industrial injuries, and there is thus little scope for improving this item on the company balance sheet by improving the fitness of employees. However, in some resource industries such as lumbering, a high injury rate is currently a major component of labor costs. In 1974, 1,400 Canadian hospital beds were occupied by patients with work-related injuries, and there were 1,465 work-related deaths (1 per 6,000 worker-years). Average medical claims amounted to $128 per worker-year, and indirect costs (loss of productivity, material damage, and industrial retraining) were estimated at a further $451 per worker-year (11).

In theory, regular exercise could reduce the incidence of injury in several ways. A better self-image and job satisfaction might encourage safe working habits. Greater personal arousal might also be helpful when watching for the mistakes of others. Stronger muscles would reduce the likelihood of internal injuries while carrying and lifting. Finally, greater work satisfaction would encourage a speedy return to employment after recovery from injury.

Russian reports (39) have suggested less industrial traumatism in cross-sectional comparisons between worker athletes and their sedentary peers, while other reports have suggested back injuries were more likely in supervisors (22) or recent immigrants (33) who were unaccustomed to heavy lifting. Cady et al. (10) made a prospective comparison of 320 initially healthy fire fighters. Comparing the 20 most flexible with the 20 least flexible employees, the average cumulative injury cost was $231 versus $448, and respective back injury costs were $44 versus $250. Comparing the strongest 20 with the weakest 20 employees, analogous figures were $295 versus $431 and $55 versus $154. Injury costs were also lower in the 20 individuals who had the highest PWC_{170} and in the 20 employees who were the thinnest. In another prospective study, Mealey (35) noted a substantial decrease of back injuries among police officers after introduction of a work site fitness program. Most recently, in a remarkable initiative at a Safeway bakery, a combination of shop floor calisthenics and peer pressure reduced a high compensable injury rate to zero (28).

It is less clear that such benefits would be achieved by the involvement of workers in a typical light aerobics class. The dominant problem in many industries is a high incidence of back injuries, and the individuals concerned would benefit more from general muscle strengthening and specific back exercises than from standard jogging or light calisthenic classes.

Costs of Employee Fitness Programs

Against the various benefits of a work site fitness program must be set the costs of facilities, equipment, leadership, lost opportunities, and possibly an increased demand for certain types of medical services. The method of program financing varies from one company to another, but in most instances workers are expected to meet at least a part of the expense for facilities, equipment, and professional leadership. In Canada, about one third of corporations meet all costs; in one third, the expenses are shared; in the remaining third they are met by the employees. A small monthly payroll deduction ($5-$10) does not seem to have any substantial deterrent effect on program participation (53), and indeed partial payment may encourage utilization of the exercise facilities.

Costs of Fitness Facilities

The perceived cost of facilities varies with their scale, their location, and the completeness of accounting. Some companies have been content to install showers for employees who cycle to work, while others have developed lavish facilities including large gymnasia, indoor tracks, and Olympic-size swimming pools. For those offering on-site facilities, a minimum standard of 25 m² floor area for administration and testing, 25-50 m² for personalized activities, and 0.25 m² per employee for group activities has been suggested (12). In some cases, companies have merely assessed the costs of refurbishing a basement or storage area, which might incur a capital expense of no more than $2-$3 per participant. Other reports have cited total program costs of $100-$150 per participant, which stand in sharp contrast with the usual fees of equivalent commercial establishments. However, if an economic rental is assessed for fully serviced facilities in a prime location, the operating cost of the facility alone could easily mount to $500-$1,500 per participant per year.

Costs for Equipment

There is an equally wide variation in the scale of exercise equipment provided for work site fitness programs. Seemingly, if a basic minimum of apparatus is available, recruitment and adherence to a program are not improved by a more lavish investment in equipment such as Nautilus weight training machines (38). Indeed, if the majority of employees are women, such equipment may have little utilization. On the other hand, if a major goal of the program is to provide a status-giving fringe benefit to upper echelon employees, then provision of an impressive range of equipment may be useful in satisfying this objective.

Costs of Trained Leadership

Adequate and well-trained professional leadership is essential to a safe and successful employee fitness program. While there are at present no mandatory standards for fitness staff, some Canadian provinces are strongly recommending the qualification of class leaders through the Canadian Association of Sport Sciences certification program.

At the same time, over-stringent requirements for preliminary medical clearance and class supervision can rapidly make a fitness program uneconomic. Exercise scientists do a serious disservice to the potential exerciser if they follow the common U.S. practice (1, 14) of insisting upon a costly and rather ineffective medical clearance as a preliminary to program participation. Small companies may also incur unnecessary expense through hiring a full-time exercise class leader when program needs could be met adequately through a combination of part-time professional leadership and lay assistance.

Opportunity Costs of an Exercise Program

Any effective exercise program demands a substantial investment of time in order to induce physiological changes and realize the potential benefits discussed above. Particularly in unionized companies, there is much discussion as to whether this time should be supplied by the corporation or the individual participants; the unions argue that since productivity is likely to improve as a result of the exercise classes, the company should provide what could easily amount to 3 hr out of a 37-hr working week, potentially an 8% increase in payroll costs.

In practice, most companies have finally persuaded employees to exercise in their own time. The one concession from management has typically been some flexibility in scheduling, so that class members can take an extended lunch break or exercise before starting work. In discussions with employees, it can be stressed that because traveling is eliminated, the opportunity cost of exercise is much lower when pursued in a company exercise facility than when community resources are used. Moreover, a complete analysis should be set against the opportunity cost of "lost personal time," certain personal "opportunity dividends"—an increased alertness, a greater ability to undertake physical tasks, a trimmer figure, an improved self-image, and other benefits summarized under the rubric "feeling better."

Medical Costs of Exercise

Participation in an employee fitness program could conceivably increase the demand for specific medical services such as preliminary screening and the treatment of exercise-induced injuries. However, in practice, overall medical costs per worker have decreased in response to program initiation. In the Canada Life Assurance study, there was no evidence of an increased demand for either electrocardiographic or orthopedic services in the year following introduction of an employee fitness program. In Sweden, an employee sports and fitness program which included various team sports generated negligible orthopedic costs (55). Nevertheless, insistence upon an unnecessary initial medical clearance or subsequent medical supervision of classes could drastically modify these figures. Taking account only of the corporate expenses involved in operation of an employee fitness program, estimated costs vary widely from $100-$400 per employee, or (with a 20% active participation in the program) $500-$2,000 per participant per year.

Cost/Benefit Analyses

A cost/benefit analysis would translate all known costs and benefits of a fitness program into their dollar equivalents, attempting to develop a rigid balance sheet covering both sides of the ledger (see Table 6). In contrast, a cost-effectiveness analysis sets a specific corporate goal (for example, a 20% decrease in absenteeism) and then compares the relative costs of achieving this goal through various types of fitness and health promotion programs.

There are currently several major objections to adopting a rigid cost/benefit approach. Inevitably, it imposes a hierarchical system upon a corporation. There is much greater apparent benefit in servicing the fitness needs of the company president than in meeting the needs of those who are working on the shop floor. A second difficulty is that many

Table 6   Industrial Benefits to be Weighed Against Costs of an Employee Fitness Program

Benefit	Fiscal saving
Employment in fitness services	Labor-intensive
Worker satisfaction	Higher quality production-less warranty work
Productivity	$116 per worker-year
Absenteeism	$ 30 per worker-year
Turnover	$324 per worker-year
Industrial injury	$ 43 per worker-year
Health insurance premiums	Reduced (?32%)
Company image	Enhanced by in-house program
Total	$513 per worker-year

Note. See Shephard, 1986b.

of the benefits of exercise such as a reduction of ischemic heart disease and an extension of working years are long-term in nature; thus the magnitude of the supposed economic gains cannot easily be tested by direct experiment. Moreover, the estimates are highly susceptible to assumptions regarding the discount rate (the willingness of a company to sacrifice current profits or incur indebtedness in order to improve future employee performance). Finally, there are as yet no precise figures for many items which should be included on either the cost or the benefit side of the ledger. While the net balance sheet currently looks quite favorable to an amateur economist, the individual figures remain too uncertain to convince a sceptical business manager.

Marginal costs and benefits are a further source of uncertainty for an expanding program. While one can calculate relatively accurate program costs for current exercise participants, a much greater investment in both promotion and facilities might be necessary in order to interest those employees who are presently nonparticipants. Furthermore, even if the latter group could be persuaded to start exercising, it is less certain that they would contribute equivalent cost savings to the company as a consequence of their enhanced activity.

Cost/effectiveness analysis avoids many of the difficulties associated with cost/benefit analysis. It is fairly easy to check whether the investment of a $100,000 basement renovation and an annual salary of $25,000-$30,000 for a professional fitness class leader can achieve such objectives as a 20% reduction in absenteeism or a 25% decrease in medical claims. However, there remains the important problem that the main impact of the exercise classes is upon the healthy rather than the needy segment of a corporation. In a company of 1,000 employees, a typical experience is that some 300 employees enroll in a fitness program, 200 attend classes intermittently, and about 100 become committed exercise enthusiasts (47). Moreover, detailed activity histories suggest that many of the 100 enthusiasts were physically active prior to introduction of the employee fitness program. Thus, in terms of physiological objectives such as an increase of maximum oxygen intake or a reduction of body fat, the impact of a corporate fitness program may be relatively weak (6, 16).

Many companies have now recognized that there are economies of scale associated with multiphasic health promotion programs rather than exercise classes per se, making future evaluation of exercise alone even more difficult. An effective work site program merges exercise prescription with specific classes for dieting, stress reduction, smoking withdrawal, and alcohol and substance abuse. Development of an accurate balance sheet for such a complex operation is a tremendous challenge to health economists. At the present time, a specific health commitment on the part of the company president and an appeal to good corporate citizenship are thus likely to be the most effective weapons in gaining support for a fitness and health program. Most sports scientists have the training and the expertise to win the exercise commitment of key company officials. In contrast, they lack both the data and the educational background to prove the fiscal viability of employee fitness programs to the comptroller of a corporation. Although the economic balance sheet of the work site exercise class looks favorable, the fitness director is thus advised to put a major emphasis upon seeking the personal physical commitment of corporate decision makers.

Acknowledgment

The research support of Fitness Canada and the Canadian Fitness and Lifestyle Institute and the cooperation of Canada Life, North American Life, and General Foods Corporation are acknowledged with thanks.

References

1. American College of Sports Medicine. Guidelines for graded exercise testing and exercise prescription and behavioral objectives for physicians, program directors, exercise leaders and exercise technicians. Philadelphia: Lea & Febiger, 1975.

2. Barker, F. Worksite health promotion—today and tomorrow. In J. Hurley Meyer, ed., Decreasing barriers—a blueprint for workplace health in the 90s. Dallas: American Heart Foundation, 1987.

3. Baun, W.B., Bernacki, E.J., Tsai, S.P. A preliminary investigation: effect of a corporate fitness program on absenteeism and health care costs. J. Occup. Med. 28:19-22, 1986.

4. Bernacki, E.J., Baun, W.B. The relationship of job performance to exercise adherence in a corporate fitness program. J. Occup. Med. 26:529-531, 1984.

5. Bjurstrom, L.A., Alexiou, N.G. A program of heart disease prevention for public employees. J. Occup. Med. 20:521-531, 1978.

6. Blair, S.N., Piserchia, P.V., Wilbur, C.S., Crowder, J.H. A public health intervention model for worksite health promotion: impact on exercise and physical fitness in a health promotion plan after 24 months. J. Am. Med. Assoc. 255:921-926, 1986.

7. Blair, S.N., Smith, M., Collingwood, T.R., Reynolds, R., Prentice, M.C., Sterling, C.L. Health promotion for educators: impact on absenteeism. Prev. Med. 15:166-175, 1986.

8. Bly, J.L., Jones, R.C., Richardson, J.E. Impact of worksite health promotion on health care costs and utilization: evaluation of Johnson & Johnson's Live for Life Program. J. Am. Med. Assoc. 256:3235-3240, 1986.

9. Bowne, D.W., Russell, M.L., Morgan, J.L., Optenberg, S.A., Clarke, A.E. Reduced disability and health care costs in an industrial fitness program. J. Occup. Med. 26:809-816, 1984.

10. Cady, L.D., Thomas, P.C., Karwasky, R.J. Program for increasing health and physical fitness of firefighters. J. Occup. Med. 27:110-114, 1985.

11. Chisholm, D.M. Occupational health—a priority and a challenge. Can. J. Pub. Health 68:189-191, 1977.

12. Collis, M. (Minister of State for Fitness and Amateur Sport Health and Welfare, Canada). Employee fitness. Ottawa: Queen's Printer, 1977.

13. Conrad, P. Who comes to worksite wellness programs? A preliminary review. J. Occup. Med. 29:317-320, 1987.

14. Cooper, K.H. Guidelines in the management of the exercising patient. J. Am. Med. Assoc. 211:1663-1667, 1970.

15. Cox, M.H., Shephard, R.J., Corey, P. Physical activity and alienation in the work place. J. Sports Med. Phys. Fit. 27:429-436, 1987.

16. Cox, M.H., Shephard, R.J., Corey, P. Influence of an employee fitness programme upon fitness, productivity and absenteeism. Ergonomics 24:795-806, 1981.

17. Danielson, R., Danielson, K. Exercise program effects on productivity of firefighters. Toronto: Ontario Ministry of Culture and Recreation, 1982.

18. Dedmon, R. Barriers and opportunities in providing wellness for hourly and salaried employees. In: Meyer, J.H., ed. Decreasing barriers—a blueprint for workplace health in the 90's. Dallas: American Heart Foundation, 1987.

19. Finney, C. Recreation: its effects on productivity. A recent study and its unexpected results. Rec. Manag. 21:10, 1979.

20. Gettman, L.R. Cost/benefit analysis of a corporate fitness program. Fitness in Bus. 1:11-17, 1986.

21. Gibbs, J.O., Mulvaney, D., Henes, C., Reed, R.W. Work site health promotion: five year trend in employee health costs. J. Occup. Med. 27:826-830, 1985.

22. Guthrie, D.I. A new approach to handling in industry. A rational approach to the prevention of low back pain. S. Afr. Med. J. 3:651-656, 1963.

23. Herzlich, C. Health and illness. London: Academic Press, 1973.

24. Hoffman, J.J., Hobson, C.J. Physical fitness and employee effectiveness. Personnel Admin. 4:101-126, 1984.

25. Holmes, T.H., Rahe, R.H. The social readjustment rating scale. J. Psychomatic Research 11:213-218, 1967.

26. Howard, J., Michalachki, A. Fitness and employee productivity. Can. J. App. Sport Sci. 4:191-198, 1979.

27. Hughes, A.L., Goldman, R.F. Energy cost of hard work. J. Appl. Physiol. 29:570-572, 1970.

28. Humphreys, S., Jacobson, R. The equation for employee involvement (employee authorship and professional expertise) × fun = participation "Buns on the Run". In J. Hurley Meyer, ed., Decreasing barriers—a blueprint for workplace health in the 90s. Dallas: American Heart Foundation, 1987.

29. Kaplan, R.H. How do workers view their work in America? Monthly Labor Review June:46-48, 1973.

30. Keir, S. Employee physical fitness in Canada. Ottawa: Fitness and Amateur Sport, 1975.

31. King, M., Murray, M., Atkinson, T. Background, personality, job characteristics and satisfaction with work in a national sample. Can. J. Behav. Sci. 13:44-52, 1981.

32. Lindén, V. Absence from work and physical fitness. Br. J. Industr. Med. 26:47-53, 1969.

33. Magora, A., Taustein, I. An investigation of the problem of sick leave in the patient suffering from low back pain. Industr. Med. 38:80-90, 1969.

34. Manguroff, J., Channe, N., Georgieff, N. Tempo, Dosieurung, Anzahl und Charakter der Übungen für Berufsgymnastik. Vuprosi na Fiz. Kuly. (Sofia) 5:161, 1960.

35. Mealey, M. New fitness for police and firefighters. Physic. and Sportsmed. 7:96-100, 1979.

36. Meyers, J.H. Decreasing barriers—a blueprint for workplace health in the 90s. Dallas: American Heart Association, 1987.

37. Norman, L.G. Medical aspects of road safety. Lancet 1:989-994, 1039-1045, 1960.

38. Peepre, M. Employee fitness and lifestyle project. Ottawa: Fitness and Amateur Sport, 1978.

39. Pravosudov, V.P. Effects of physical exercises on health and economic efficiency. In: Landry, F., Orban, W.A.R., eds. Physical activity and human well-being. Miami: Symposia Specialists. 1978:261-271.

40. Quasar Corporation. The relationships between physical fitness and the cost of health care. Toronto: Quasar Systems, 1976.

41. Réville, P.H. Sport for all. Physical activity and the prevention of disease. Strasbourg: Council of Europe, 1970.

42. Richardson, B. Don't just sit there—exercise something. Fitness Living 49(May/June), 1974.

43. Russell, L.B. Is prevention better than cure? Washington, DC: Brookings Institute, 1986.

44. Shephard, R.J. The impact of exercise upon medical costs. Sports Med. 2:133-143, 1985.

45. Shephard, R.J. Physical activity and the quality of life. Quality of Life and Cardiovascular Care 1:40-44, 1985.

46. Shephard, R.J. The economic benefits of enhanced physical fitness. Champaign, IL: Human Kinetics, 1986a.

47. Shephard, R.J. Fitness and health in industry. Basel, Switzerland: Karger, 1986b.

48. Shephard, R.J. Physical activity and aging. 2nd ed. London: Croom Helm, 1987.

49. Shephard, R.J. Physical activity in special populations. Current fitness status and response to training. Champaign, IL: Human Kinetics, 1988.

50. Shephard, R.J., Corey, P., Cox, M. Health hazard appraisal—the influence of an employee fitness program. Can. J. Pub. Health 73:183-187, 1982.

51. Shephard, R.J., Corey, P., Renzland, P., Cox, M.H. The influence of an industrial fitness programme upon medical care costs. Can. J. Pub. Health 73:259-263, 1982.

52. Shephard, R.J., Corey, P., Renzland, P., Cox, M. The impact of changes of fitness and lifestyle upon health care utilization. Can. J. Pub. Health 74:51-54, 1983.

53. Shephard, R.J., Morgan, P., Finucane, R., Schimmelfing, L. Factors influencing recruitment to an occupational fitness program. J. Occup. Med. 22:389-398, 1980.

54. Sorensen, C.H., Sonne-Holm, S. Social costs of sports injuries. Br. J. Sports Med. 14:24-25, 1981.

55. Stallings, W.M., O'Rourke, T.W., Gross, D. Professorial correlates of physical exercise. J. Sports Med. Phys. Fit. 15:333-336, 1975.

56. Tsai, S.P., Baun, W.B., Bernacki, E.J. The relationship of employee turnover to exercise adherence in a corporate fitness program. J. Occup. Med. 29:572-575, 1987.

57. Work in America: report of a special task force to the Secretary of Health, Education and Welfare. Cambridge: MIT Press, 1973.

The Psychobiological Effects
of Industrial Respirator Wear

P.B. Raven and J.R. Wilson

Department of Physiology, Texas College of Osteopathic Medicine, Fort
Worth, Texas, U.S.A.

With the enactment of the Occupational Safety and Health Act in 1970, the need to develop
measures by which individuals can be assessed for respirator wear has become an issue
of medical, legal, and practical importance. For example, the U.S. Nuclear Regulations
Commissions Guide states:

> Workers must be evaluated by competent medical personnel to ensure that they are
> physically and mentally able to wear respirators under simulated and actual working
> conditions. These evaluations should be an important part of the employee's periodic
> examinations routinely given in most industrial medical facilities. Adequate medical
> supervision of respirator users is indispensable in determining the extent of individual
> tolerance and in preventing potential physiological derangements (NUREG 0041. sec.
> 7.4., Medical Limitations). (pp. 7-11)

Unfortunately, this statement of responsibility does not provide the physician with the
objective criteria for assessing a worker's ability to use a respirator. In an effort to provide
some guidance, the American National Standards Institute asked a group of concerned
physicians and researchers to provide a practical guideline for the "Physical Qualification for Respirator Use," euphemistically termed Z88.6. The following information will
highlight background information on the biological and psychological aspects used for
development of the standards as well as provide specific recommendations, based on our
own investigations, for the evaluation of worker capability for respirator wear.

In an initial review of the literature, Raven et al. (13) identified that the primary effect
of all types of respirators was discernible decrements in pulmonary function (11, 14, 15).
In addition, Myhre et al. (10) and Raven et al. (12) have documented in healthy normal
workers that wearing a self-contained breathing apparatus (SCBA) or rebreather type
apparatus results in an additional work requirement because of the weight of the apparatus.
This increased weight (approximately 35 lb or 16 kg) is seen as a 20% average increase
in energy requirements for a given submaximal work load, and consequently results in
a 20% decrease in maximal work performance (12, 19). The effect of the additional weight
appears to be the definitive factor and overrides the effects of different breathing modes
and the increased resistance to breathing of specific respirators. We suggest that the effects
of additional weight are linear and hence predict that for each 1 lb of apparatus weight
that the increased energy requirements or decrease in maximal work capacities will be
0.6%. However, the important concept to note is that for any respirator that involves significant weight, a measurable increase in work load requirements will occur. Therefore, it
is essential that the physician be informed of the type of respirator and the maximal level
of work the job will place on the worker. As a consequence of the above, workers required

to use an SCBA or rebreather type respirator for emergency work should be evaluated using a maximal exercise stress test.

If maximal work effort is limited because of cardiopulmonary disease (ischemia, arrhythmia, asthma, ventilation/perfusion, and diffusion/perfusion inequality), the ANSI Z88.6 recommendations preclude a worker from respirator wear. It is our contention that the interaction between specific stable cardiopulmonary diseases (e.g., bronchitis, asthma, and history of myocardial infarction and hypertension) is unaffected by respirator wear. The problem for the physician is discerning the degree of lung impairment that is a contraindication to respirator wear, regardless of the specific etiology of the disease, whether it be restrictive, obstructive, or diffusion limiting. This decision is multifactorial and is related to the normal work load usage and the duration of the work. While the physician has available those tests needed to determine pulmonary function capacity, it is unlikely that the examining physician is aware of the work load or the duration for which the respirator is to be used. Consequently, it is important that the job description in terms of time and metabolic demands be provided by the company to the examining physician. In return, the physician must be aware of the maximal exercise capacity and maximal ventilatory capacity of the worker as well as the expected decrement in both exercise and ventilatory capacity that will occur while wearing an industrial respirator.

A complete pulmonary function screening of workers can be done, yet in the interest of time and the need for mass screenings of industrial workers a single item pulmonary function test for suitability for respirator wear should be the practical test of choice. Support for a single item screening test lies in the fact that several of the standard pulmonary function measures are highly correlated with each other (19). The physiologically discernable changes in normal pulmonary function are directly related to the increased resistance of the respirator on inspired and expired flow (15). Consequently, with flow as a component part of these measures of pulmonary function, maximum voluntary ventilation in 15 s MVV_{25}, forced vital capacity (FVC), forced expiratory volume in 1 s (FEV_1), MVV_{25}, and peak inspired flow (PF_I) were proposed as reasonable candidates for selection as a single item screening test.

Because of the complexities of respiratory control imposed by a respirator, a single item screening test of clinical pulmonary function should be able to account for all possible conditions. Previously, Raven et al. (15) had suggested that MVV_{25} should be the test of choice. The basis for this recommendation was three-fold. First, it was a test of lung function that has been shown to be related to lung and chest wall mechanics as well as respiratory muscle fatigue (6, 16, 18). Second, it was a simple and inexpensive screening test that could be conducted in the doctor's office. Third, sufficient data existed relating the MVV_{25} score to (a) the 4-min MVV assessment of respiratory muscle fatigue (3, 6), (b) the sustained maximal exercise ventilation (3, 4, 6, 18), and (c) the effect of respiratory resistance on the MVV_{25} score (15). In order to validate the use of the MVV_{25} score as a single item screening test, this study determined the pulmonary function responses of a large, heterogeneous population to respirator wear at rest and during work, and subsequently used these responses to predict worker capability for respirator wear during work (20).

An air-line supplied, full face piece, pressure demand respirator was used in this study; thus, the added weight of an SCBA was not a factor and the focus was directed toward pulmonary and metabolic changes due to the added resistances of the respirator to inspired and expired flows. Table 1 presents the demographic data of the 38 subjects completing the study while Table 2 lists the results of pulmonary function tests with (W) and without (W/O) the respirator. Linear regression analyses were used to predict work performance in both maximal exercise tests and submaximal exercise tests to exhaustion. Table 3 indicates that while the relationship was not strong, the scores on the MVV_{25} did significantly predict maximal exercise performance both with and without the respirator. Table 4 indicates the average decrease in MVV_{25} that may be expected due to respirator wear in the present

Table 1 Descriptive Demographic Data and Pulmonary Function Measures Compared to Age and Height Normative Data

Variable	Mean	Range	Predicted[a]
Age (yr)	31.8 (8.1)	24 to 51	
Height (cm)	178.7 (9.6)	152.5 to 198.0	
Weight (kg)	80.7 (15.4)	53.8 to 121.3	
Forced vital capacity (L)	4.95 (1.0)	3.11 to 8.56	5.20 (95%)
Forced expiratory volume in 1 s (L)	4.17 (0.08)	2.40 to 6.12	4.09 (102%)
FEV$_1$/FVC (%)	81.5 (6.2)	66 to 91	80.7 (101%)
Total lung capacity (L)	7.23 (1.21)	4.66 to 9.98	7.18 (101%)
Residual volume (L)	2.09 (0.60)	1.39 to 4.84	1.98 (105%)

Note. Mean ($\pm$ SD). Adapted from "Clinical Pulmonary Function Tests as Predictors of Work Performance During Respirator Wear" by J.R. Wilson and P.B. Raven, 1989, American Industrial Hygiene Association Journal, 50, p. 52.

[a]Predictions based upon data of Bates et al., 1955.

Table 2 Mean Values for Pulmonary Function Measures With and Without a Full Face Piece, Pressure-Demand Respirator

Pulmonary measure	With	Without
Forced vital capacity[a]	4.95 $\pm$ 1.0	5.60 $\pm$ 1.0
Range	1.0 to 8.56	3.11 to 8.56
Forced expiratory volume in 1 s (L)	4.17 $\pm$ 0.9	4.50 $\pm$ 0.8
Range	2.27 to 5.88	2.40 to 6.12
FEV$_1$/FVC (%)[a]	85.4 $\pm$ 6.1	81.6 $\pm$ 6.2
Range	62 to 95	66 to 99
Peak flow, expired[a] (L/s)	7.1 $\pm$ 1.7	8.4 $\pm$ 1.4
Range	3.0 to 10.3	5.2 to 10.9
Flow at 50% vital capacity (L/s)	4.9 $\pm$ 1.5	4.9 $\pm$ 1.4
Range	1.90 to 9.51	2.40 to 8.38
Flow at 50% vital[a] capacity (L/s)	2.4 $\pm$ 0.9	2.0 $\pm$ 0.7
Range	1.12 to 4.08	0.76 to 4.00
Maximum voluntary[a] ventilation (L/min)	156.2 $\pm$ 37.5	186.6 $\pm$ 39.2
Range	62.5 to 237.7	83.1 to 256.7

Note. Mean ($\pm$ SD). Adapted from "Clinical Pulmonary Function Tests as Predictors of Work Performance During Respirator Wear" by J.R. Wilson and P.R. Raven, 1989, American Industrial Hygiene Association Journal, 50, p. 52.

[a]Differences statistically significant at the .05 level.

Table 3   Prediction of Work Performance from Clinical Pulmonary Function Tests

Work performance time to exhaustion	Variable	r-squared[a]
Maximal exercise test (W)[b]	MVV_{25} (W)	0.31
Maximal exercise test (W/O)[c]	MVV_{25} (W)	0.26
Endurance exercise test (W)	PF_I	0.36

[a]The value for r-squared provides an indication of how much variability can be accounted for by that variable in the prediction of work performance. The closer the R-squared value is to 1.0, the stronger the variable is in actually determining the value in question. [b]with respirator. [c]without respirator.

Table 4   Changes in Maximal Ventilatory Volumes Due to Respirator Wear Based on Present (20) and Our Earlier Study (11)

	Average decrease due to respirator wear		
MVV_{25} (L/min)	(L/min)	(%)	(%, ref. #11)
250	24.4	9.8	N/A
200	17.4	8.7	N/A
150	10.4	6.9	35
100	3.4	3.4	30
50	N/A	N/A	20

Note. Adapted from "Clinical Pulmonary Function Tests as Predictors of Work Performance During Respirator Wear" by J.R. Wilson and P.R. Raven, 1989, *American Industrial Hygiene Association Journal*, 50, p. 55.

study and in an earlier study (11). These data provide a range of decrements that may occur in pulmonary function and suggests that any type of respiratory protection that presents the wearer with resistance to breathing must be evaluated in light of work intensity and the worker's capacity. It is evident from these data as well that individuals with smaller or impaired lung capacities may be less affected by respirator wear. However, these individuals may not have enough reserve capacity for the increased ventilatory demands of work and respirator wear, especially if the work is prolonged (14). Even at the 50% MVV_{25} levels that Freedman (6) concluded could be sustained "ad infinitum," the progressive increase in work ventilation along with decrements of 7%-33% in MVV_{25} will impose limitations on the intensity and duration of work performance with a respirator.

As mentioned, the problem for the physician is in matching worker capability, decrement in worker capacity due to the added resistances of a respirator, and the intensity of the work task. Since the manual work tasks of industry have been generalized to a semiquantitative and qualitative description, the industrial hygienist should be able to provide information on work tasks to the physician. An example of classification is shown in Table

5. This information, coupled with the results of the MVV_{25} test, will provide the physician with the data needed to assess worker capability for respirator wear. For example, a physician might screen a worker for potential respirator wear and find that the worker has an MVV_{25} of 130 L/min, BTPS (see Table 6). With respirator wear, this MVV_{25} of 130 L/min could be reduced by 7.6% (122.4 L/min) to as much as 28% (92.6 L/min) (15). Assuming a maximal tolerance steady state exercise ventilation of 64% MVV_{25} (3), ventilatory requirements for the tasks could not exceed 78.3 L/min to 59.3 L/min during respirator

Table 5   Work Load Ventilations in Metabolic Equivalents (METS)^a

Job description	Energy cost (O_2 uptake)	Required ventilation
Light work	up to 0.5 L/min (1-2 METS)	6-15 L/min
Moderate work	0.5 - 1.0 L/min (2-4 METS)	15-25 L/min
Heavy work	1.0 - 1.5 L/min (4-6 METS)	25-40 L/min
Very heavy work	1.5 - 2.0 L/min (6-8 METS)	40-60 L/min
Extremely heavy work	2.0 - 3.0 L/min (8-12 METS)	60-90 L/min
Exhaustive work	> 3.0 L/min (12-15 METS)	90-120 L/min

Note. Adapted from *Textbook of Work Physiology*, 2nd ed. (p. 681) by Åstrand and Rodahl, 1977, New York: McGraw Hill.
^{a}One MET = 3.5 ml/kg/min $\dot{V}O_2$.

Table 6   Example of Screening a Worker for Respirator Wear

Worker's MVV_{25}	130 L/min	
With respirator	7.6% (present study)	28% (ref #11)
Maximum steady state exercise ventilation = 64% MVV_{25} (industrial hygienist)	122.4 L/min	92.6 L/min
Example of work intensity from Table 5	$\dot{V}_E \leqslant$ 78.3 L/min	$\dot{V}_E \leqslant$ 59.3 L/min
a) $\dot{V}O_2$ = 1.0 - 1.5 L/min		
b) $\dot{V}_E$ = 25 - 40 L/min		
c) Ventilatory creep (up to 30 L/min)	$\dot{V}_E$ = 55 to 70 L/min	$\dot{V}_E$ = 55 to 70 L/min
d) 25 L/min + 30 = 55 L/min 40 L/min + 30 = 70 L/min	maximal steady state ($\dot{V}_E$ approached)	maximal steady state ($\dot{V}_E$ exceeded)

Note. Adapted from "Clinical Pulmonary Function Tests as Predictors of Work Performance During Respirator Wear" by J.R. Wilson and P.R. Raven, 1989, *American Industrial Hygiene Association Journal*, 50, p. 56.

wear. With information provided by the industrial hygienist regarding energy cost of the work task, the required ventilatory costs can be estimated from Table 5. A work intensity of 1.0-1.5 L/min would require a ventilation of 25-40 L/min. If this intensity is greater than 60% of the worker's maximum capacity, a progressive increase of up to 30 L/min (4) could occur over time, placing the worker at 55 L/min to 70 L/min, which approaches or exceeds this worker's ability to continue for more than 30 min (Table 6). Thus, the physician must know the worker's functional lung capacity, as well as the demands of the work task that must be performed, to appropriately evaluate worker capability for respirator wear.

Another important consideration with respect to worker capacity and respirator wear is the effect of the resistances imposed by the respirator upon the maximal exercise capacity of that worker. Workers of varying body sizes and physical and ventilatory capacities will not all be affected to the same degree by the respirator. The purpose of the second stage of our study was to describe the biological and perceptual changes of a large subject population, heterogeneous in regard to body size, age, and fitness level, up through and including maximal exercise (21). The average work performance time to maximal levels decreased -24.1 s when wearing the respirator ($p < .01$) and ranged from a maximum decrease of -125 s to an actual increase of $+77$ s. Table 7 presents the physiological data at termination of the maximal exercise test, which used a ramping protocol to assess maximal capacity. Maximal oxygen uptake ($\dot{V}O_2$max), tidal volume (V_T), expired pressure (PP_e), and dyspnea index (DI) were all significantly greater while wearing the respirator, while breathing frequency (f_B) and expired flow (PF_E) were significantly lower with the respirator. The greater scores on the breathing scale (BrSc) while wearing the respirator approached significance.

The results of this portion of the study indicate that some biological and perceptual parameters are altered by respirator wear during exercise to maximum levels and that these parameters are altered in such a way as to significantly reduce performance time ($p < .05$). The biological and perceptual data with and without the respirator at maximal exercise (see Table 7) indicated no significant differences in ventilation volume ($\dot{V}_E$), heart rate (HR_{max}), perceived exertion (RPE), and PF_I. The lack of significant difference in PF_I, with and without the respirator, is probably due to the positive-pressure mode of breathing, which tends to aid peak inspired flow despite an increased inspired resistance. While equivalent $\dot{V}_E$s were measured at maximal exercise, other indicators of ventilatory load were significantly higher during respirator wear. These indicators of increased ventilatory load include biological (PF_E, PP_e, and DI) as well as a perceptual parameter (BrSc) and are reflected in a significantly greater $\dot{V}O_2$max with the respirator. The significantly greater PF_E with the respirator resulting in a significantly lower flow indicated an increased work of breathing, which may have contributed not only to the increased $\dot{V}O_2$max but to the decreased performance time as well.

The third portion of this investigation focused on the effects of an air-line supplied, full face piece, pressure demand respirator on exhaustive endurance work. The majority of studies investigating physiological responses to respirator wear or an increased resistance to breathing during exercise have examined responses during progressive exercise to maximal levels or submaximal exercise for periods of 5-30 min (1, 7, 11, 14, 20, 21). Many of these investigations have examined the physiological effects of various types of protective respirator masks, that is, air purifying, air supplied, or self-contained breathing apparatus (1, 7, 11, 14, 20, 21) and increased resistances to inspiration and exhalation (1, 5). With the exception of the study by Deno et al. (5), the maximum length of exercise has been 30 min (1). There are, however, instances of industrial usage where respirator wear exceeds this time frame. Therefore, it becomes imperative to examine the effects of respirator wear on the biological and perceptual responses during prolonged work (>30 min).

Table 7   Physiological Data at Termination of the Ramp Test Without (w/o) and With (w) Full-Face Respirator

Variable	Without respirator	With respirator	p value
$\dot{V}O_2$max (ml/kg/min)	42.18 ± 1.4	44.11 ± 1.3	0.0001
$\dot{V}_E$ (L/min)	119.6 ± 5	118.7 ± 4	0.774
f_B (breaths/min)	42 ± 3.1	38 ± 1.3	0.001
V_T (L)	2.6 ± .1	3.1 ± 0.1	0.001
PF_I (L/min)	281.0 ± 9	268 ± 7	0.063
PF_E (L/min)	324.0 ± 13	289 ± 12	0.0001
PP_I (cmH$_2$O)	−6.43 ± 0.3	−7.65 ± 0.8	0.071
PP_e (cmH$_2$O)	10.69 ± 0.5	13.05 ± 0.7	0.001
HR_{max} (bpm)	185.0 ± 2	184 ± 2	0.447
DI (%)	70.9 ± 2.3	76.0 ± 2.3	0.033
RPE	17.5 ± 0.5	17.6 ± 0.5	0.606
BrSc	4.6 ± 0.16	5.1 ± 0.16	0.057

Note. Means (± *SE*). Adapted from "Effects of Pressure-Demand Respirator Wear on Physiological and Perceptual Variables During Progressive Exercise to Maximal Levels" by J.R. Wilson, P.B. Raven, W.P. Morgan, S.A. Zinkgraf, R.G. Garmon, and A.W. Jackson, 1989, American Industrial Hygiene Association Journal, 50, p. 88.

Data collected at the conclusion of each endurance walk to exhaustion are presented in Table 8. A final 5-min collection of data was obtained on each subject regardless of performance time. As a result, the final value represents the data point at which their own estimation of exhaustion compelled each subject to terminate the exercise. A significant decrease in the average work performance time of −13.5 min (p < .02) also occurred when wearing the respirator and ranged from a maximum decrease of −72 min (with to without) to an actual increase of +16 min. A comparison of final values for oxygen uptake indicated that the $\dot{V}O_2$ and percent oxygen uptake (% $\dot{V}O_2$max) at the conclusion of the endurance walk were greater with the respirator than without the respirator (p < .05). The data in Table 9 illustrate the time course of changes in selected ventilatory measures with and without the respirator. These data are the means at 30, 60, 90, and 120 min. The significantly greater $\dot{V}_E$ was due to an increased V_T, as the f_B values were not significantly different with or without the respirator during the first 60 min of exercise. The change in the combination of f_B and V_T with the respirator represents an attempt by the subjects to attain the most efficient means of ensuring adequate oxygen uptake. With the exception of the average measures at 30 min of exercise, V_T with the respirator was always greater than without.

The breathing scale was used to quantify respiratory distress by asking subjects to rate their breathing (BrSc) on a seven point scale (9). The ratings at 5 and 30 min of exercise (see Table 9), when subject number was equal, were significantly greater with the respirator

Table 8   Physiological and Perceptual Data at Termination of the Exhaustive Walk (Last Time Values)

Variable	With respirator	Without respirator	p value
Performance time (min)	55.6 (3.8)	69.1 (4.4)	0.015
*$\dot{V}O_2$ (ml/kg/min)	34.4 (1.1)	31.9 (1.1)	0.001
%$\dot{V}O_2$max	84.0 (2.0)	76.0 (1.0)	0.001
HR (beats/min)	177 (3)	178 (3)	0.535
$\dot{V}_E$ (L/min BTPS)	89.2 (3.4)	73.4 (3.7)	0.001
V_T (L)	2.06 (0.7)	1.75 (0.08)	0.003
f_B (number/min)	39 (1)	37 (1)	0.177
Inspired flow (L/min)	211.4 (7.5)	190.9 (7.8)	0.001
Expired flow (L/min)	202.2 (9.6)	212.9 (9.3)	0.195
Inspired pressure (cmH_2O)	−3.04 (0.35)	−3.99 (0.18)	0.001
Expired pressure (cmH_2O)	+10.38 (0.45)	+5.26 (0.31)	0.001
D.I. ($\dot{V}_E$ max/MVV_{25})	58.6 (2.1)	44.6 (2.0)	0.001
Breathing distress	4.4 (0.2)	4.0 (0.2)	0.085
Perceived exertion	17.2 (0.4)	17.2 (0.4)	0.998

Note. Means ($\pm$ *SE*). Adapted from "Alterations in Physiological and Perceptual Variables During Exhaustive Endurance Work While Wearing a Pressure-Demand Respirator" by J.R. Wilson, P.B. Raven, S.A. Zinkgraf, W.P. Morgan, and A.W. Jackson, 1989, American Industrial Hygiene Association Journal, 50, p. 143.

than without. In addition, perceived exertion with the respirator was significantly greater than without the respirator at 30 min of exercise. From 30 to 60 min of exercise, more than 20 subjects had terminated their exercise test with the respirator, while only 12 subjects ended their exercise test without the respirator. With an equal number of subjects continuing the endurance walk through 30 min, one half hour of exercise appears to be representative of the time in which to expect a heterogeneous population to continue work with a respirator. However, despite the two tests being carried out at equivalent work loads, the subjects perceived the work as greater with the respirator than without ($p < .05$).

Respirator wear during endurance exercise to exhaustion results in a significant increase in the physiologic effort of breathing to overcome the added resistances. The increased effort of breathing increases the perception of exercise intensity and results in an earlier termination of exercise by an average of 13.5 min. The continued increase in PP_e over the first 30 min appears indicative of an excessive ventilation response. At 30 min of exercise those individuals who continued for a significantly shorter period of work time with the respirator were experiencing respirator and psychological distress, as evidenced by the sharp increase in RPE and BrSc. Thus, we agree with Louhevaara et al. (7) that, given the current respirator designs, continuous use of these devices should be limited to a maximum of 30 min.

Table 9 Time Course of Changes in Ventilatory Measures With and Without the Respirator

Time (minutes)	5		30		60		90		120	
	With	Without	With	Without	With	Without	With	Without	With	Without
Subjects	38	38	32	32	10	20	3	5	1	1
Tidal volume	2.47* (0.8)	2.11 (.07)	2.17 (.08)	2.10 (.09)	2.30 (.15)	1.98 (.09)	2.48 (.04)	2.00 (.12)	2.53	1.56
Breathing frequency (breaths/min)	28 (1)	26 (1)	33 (1)	31 (1)	32 (2)	30 (2)	29 (2)	38 (3)	26	44
Heart rate	154 (3)	150 (3)	168 (3)	169 (3)	173 (4)	171 (3)	158 (10)	171 (6)	150	180
Breathing scale	2.8* (.2)	2.2 (.1)	3.6* (.2)	2.7 (.2)	3.4 (.3)	3.1 (.3)	3.3 (.3)	3.5 (.7)	3	4
Ratings of perceived exertion	12.3 (.2)	12.0 (.3)	14.9* (.3)	13.6 (.4)	15.5 (.8)	14.8 (.6)	14.3 (.7)	14.8 (1.4)	16	15

Note. Means ($\pm$ *SE*). Adapted from "Alterations in Physiological and Perceptual Variables During Exhaustive Endurance Work While Wearing a Pressure-Demand Respirator" by J.R. Wilson, P.B. Raven, S.A. Zinkgraf, W.P. Morgan, and A.W. Jackson, 1989, American Industrial Hygiene Association Journal, 50, p. 144.

$p < .05$. Mean ($\pm$ *SE*).

Psychological Aspects

From a practical standpoint, a respirator designed for a large population should consider subjective assessment. It is equally as important to ensure that these individuals who need respiratory protection can and will use the respirators. Respirator wear and the consequent increase in breathing resistance is accurately detected by approximately 90% of any given sample of test subjects during both resting and exercise conditions (8). Ventilatory cues provide the basis for the perception of effort during hard physical work; consequently, claustrophobic or high anxiety workers who perceive that the effort is greater due to the increased resistance to breathing should not be given jobs requiring respirator wear. The major problem in selecting workers for tasks in which industrial respirators must be worn is the isolation of the 10% in any given sample who experience anxiety attacks when exposed to a hostile environment and respirator wear. A portion of the individuals in this 10% are classified as hyperventilators or individuals known to ventilate at levels in excess of the ventilatory demand of a given work load. Those individuals who experience the hyperventilation syndrome with the resulting symptoms are considered at greater risk when performing tasks during vigorous exercise while breathing in a respirator mask. It is possible to administer standardized psychological inventories designed to measure trait anxiety. Thus far, research in the area of physiological and psychological responses to respirator wear have observed the level at which stress responses occur. In one experiment, Morgan and Raven (9) considered the predictability of determining those individuals who would experience difficulty while wearing a respirator mask during an exercise stress. Forty-five volunteer subjects were required to exercise on a motor driven treadmill while wearing an SCBA. Five of these subjects had elevated scores (above the group mean) on a standard measure of trait anxiety (17). It was predicted a priori that 5 of the subjects would experience difficulty on the treadmill tests. Six of the 45 subjects experienced dizziness, claustrophobia, or anxiety attacks during heavy exercise while wearing an SCBA. The 5 subjects with elevated scores were among the 6 who actually experienced anxiety attacks (see Table 10). These results support Morgan's theory that certain "types" of individuals were more likely to experience anxiety attacks while wearing an SCBA and performing hard physical work. Furthermore, these individuals can be identified in advance with an acceptable degree of accuracy (83% or 5 out of 6). A similar ratio of prediction was observed in the more recent studies of progressive maximal work and exhaustive maximal work carried out by

Table 10 Absolute Frequencies of Observed and Predicted Respiratory Distress in the "Demand" and "Pressure-Demand" Experiments Combined

| | | Predicted distress | | | Predicted rate |
		Yes	No	Sum	
Actual distress	Yes	5	1	6	83% (5 of 6)
	No	1	38	39	97% (38 of 39)
Total		6	39	45	

Note. From "Prediction of Distress for Individuals Wearing Industrial Respirators" by W.P. Morgan and P.B. Raven, 1985, *American Industrial Hygiene Association Journal,* 46, p. 364.

Raven and Wilson and described above. These data indicate that both biological and psychological information can be effective in predicting distress, however, we suggest that a psychobiological screening approach is more powerful than either approach alone.

References

1. Arborelius, M., Dahlback, G.L., Dakar, P.-G. Cardiac output and gas exchange during heavy exercise with a positive pressure respiratory protective apparatus. Scand. J. Work Environ. Health 9:471-480, 1983.

2. Bates, D.V., Boucot, N.G., Cormes, A.E. The pulmonary diffusing capacity in normal subjects. J. Physiol. 129:237-250, 1955.

3. Clarke, T.J.H., Freedman, J., Campbell, E.J., Winn, R.R. The ventilatory capacity of patients with chronic airway obstruction. Clin. Sci. 36:307-316, 1969.

4. Dempsey, J.A., Vidruk, E.J., Mastenbrook, S.M. Pulmonary control systems in exercise. Fed. Proc. 39:1498-1505, 1980.

5. Deno, N.S., Kamon, E., Kiser, D.M. Physiological responses to resistance breathing during short and prolonged exercise. Am. Ind. Hyg. Assoc. J. 42:616-620, 1981.

6. Freedman, S. Sustained maximum voluntary ventilation. Respir. Physiol. 8:230-244, 1970.

7. Louhevaara, V.A. Physiological effects associated with the use of respirator protection devices. Scand. J. Work Environ. Health 10:275-281, 1984.

8. Morgan, W.P. Psychological factors influencing perceived exertion. Med. Sci. Sports 5:97-103, 1979.

9. Morgan, W.P., Raven, P.B. Prediction of distress for individuals wearing industrial respirators. Am. Industr. Hyg. Assoc. J. 46:353-369, 1985.

10. Myrhe, L.G., Holden, R.D., Baumgardner, F.W., Tucker, D. Physiological limits of firefighters: unclassified Technical Report No. ESL-RT-79-06, 1979. Available from: Tyndell AFB, Pensacola, Florida.

11. Raven, P.B., Bradley, O., Rohm-Young, D., McClure, F.L., Skaggs, B. Physiological response to "pressure-demand" respirator wear. Am. Industr. Hyg. Assoc. J. 43:773-781, 1982.

12. Raven, P.B., Davis, T.O., Shafer, C.L., Linnebur, A.C. Maximal stress test performance while wearing self-contained breathing apparatus. J. Occup. Med. 19:802-806, 1977.

13. Raven, P.B., Dodson, A.T., David, T.O. The physiological consequences of wearing industrial respirators: a review. Am. Industr. Hyg. Assoc. J. 40:517-534, 1979.

14. Raven, P.B., Jackson, A.W., Page, K., Moss, R., Skaggs, B., Bradley, O. The physiological responses of mild pulmonary impaired subjects while using a "demand" respirator during rest and work. Am. Industr. Hyg. Assoc. J. 42:247-257, 1981.

15. Raven, P.B., Moss, R.F., Page, K., Garmon, R.G., Skaggs, B. Clinical pulmonary function and industrial respirator wear. Am. Industr. Hyg. Assoc. J. 42:897-903, 1981.

16. Roussos, C.S., Macklem, P.T. Diaphragmatic fatigue in man. J. Appl. Physiol.: Respir. Environ. and Ex. Physiol. 43:189-197, 1977.

17. Spielberger, C.D., Gorsuch, R.L., Lushene, R.E. The state-trait anxiety inventory manual. Palo Alto: Consulting Psychologists Press, 1969.

18. Tenney, S.M., Reese, R.E. The ability to sustain great breathing efforts. Respir. Physiol. 5:187-201, 1968.

19. Weil, H. Pulmonary function testing in industry. J. Occup. Med 15:693-699, 1973.

20. Wilson, J.R., Raven, P.B., Zinkgraf, S.A., Morgan, W.P., Jackson, A.W. Clinical pulmonary function tests as predictors of work performance during respirator wear. Am. Industr. Hyg. Assoc. J., 50:51-57, 1989.

21. Wilson, J.R., Raven, P.B., Zinkgraf, S.A., Morgan, W.P., Jackson, A.W. Effects of pressure-demand respirator wear on physiological and perceptual variables during progressive exercise to maximal levels. Am. Industr. Hyg. Assoc. J., in press.

Work Load and Demanded Physical Performance Capacity Under Different Industrial Working Conditions

J. Rutenfranz, J. Ilmarinen, F. Klimmer, and H. Kylian
Institute of Occupational Health at the University of Dortmund, FRG, and
Institute of Occupational Health, Helsinki/Vantaa, Finland

At the beginning of this century, heavy physical work was normal for about 75% of the working population; this is still true for many of the developing and industrializing countries but no longer true for most of the industrialized countries. Therefore, the public in most industrialized countries more or less accepts the following statements:

- There exists today a high mechanization of all work places combined with a low energy expenditure for all workers. Robots are typical signs of our state of industrialization.
- Workplaces requiring hard physical work no longer exist. The problems of this type of work have been solved during the last century by using scientific knowledge of work physiology and new technologies like mechanization, automation, and microprocessors.

From my experience with physiological studies of about 1,000 work places during the last 30 years, the above mentioned statements are too simplistic. Therefore, I would like to describe the actual situation in industrial work places in a more realistic manner.

To describe the general industrial developments of the last 150 years, consider the industrial changes in iron and steel production. The developments in this area can be summarized as follows:

- The dramatic changes in industrial work places reach even traditionally hard muscular work industries like iron and steel production.
- The speed of development has increased, especially during the last 20 years.
- The direction of development can be described as moving from work places characterized by physical labor to work places characterized by "converting information into action."
- The question remains whether all work places could participate in these developments or if we are only impressed by the outstanding technical developments of some processes and therefore neglect the remaining traditional working conditions.

Systems for Formal Classification of the Work Place

To generalize the experiences from the cited example, we need systems that allow us to classify the working conditions of several work places in several industries under restricted categories. Such systems have been developed in the last 20 years as "Position Analysis

Questionnaire'' (PAQ) by McCormick et al. (33, 34, 35) and as ''Arbeitswissenschaftliches Erhebungsverfahren zur Tätigkeitsanalyse'' (AET) by Rohmert and Landau (38), for which English and Finnish versions are now available (41, 42). Both systems are based on the evidence that professions no longer determine the specific load of work places but rather ''positions'' during work. Positions may be similar in different professions. Therefore, any analysis of working conditions must be based on positions instead of professions. According to Rohmert and Rutenfranz (42) these positions may be generally described by the following five categories:

1. producing forces,
2. coordinating motor and sensory functions,
3. converting information into action,
4. converting input into output, and
5. producing information.

These formal categories are based mainly on the theory of the man-machine system.

The classification of positions follows a standardized system of a combination of observation and interview, which includes 216 items. These items have to be answered by using scales of different levels (nominal scales to ordinate scales). The generalization is possible by using statistical methods, including cluster analysis, to identify groups belonging to the same categories. This position analysis system is also based on the stress-strain concept. This means that there are objective and subjective aspects of any real working condition that have to be identified if you want to classify them.

The above mentioned systems classify only the objective stress of a given working condition. Therefore, their advantage consists of observing only one or a few work places and interviewing only one or a few position holders in order to characterize the stress on identical or similar work places. We must remember, however, that identical stress in these work places may be combined with very different strain according to the individual differences among the different workers.

Examples of the Different Categories

Producing Forces

This category includes dynamic and static work with different levels of energy expenditure or muscular force. Characteristic examples of this type of work are jobs in the concrete or construction industry, which may reach high levels of energy expenditure (see Figure 1), jobs in the iron and steel industry (see Figure 2), jobs in the chemical industry (see Figure 3), jobs in the service sector (24), as well as jobs loading aircraft (see Figure 4) (21, 29, 45, 46). This work is still characterized by frequent bending, lifting, and carrying, which often have to be done under a very low ceiling in awkward positions and which need high levels of energy expenditure, even if the levels are related to the maximal aerobic power of the individual workers (see Figure 5).

Coordinating Motor and Sensory Functions

This category includes a broad spectrum of positions from assembly line work to different types of modern manipulatory jobs like forestry work (Figure 6); container handling between trains and merchant vessels with Van-Carriers (see Figure 7); or steering different modern

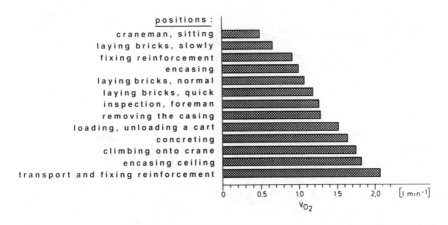

Figure 1.   Energy expenditure for different tasks in the construction industry (from Klimmer et al., 1983).

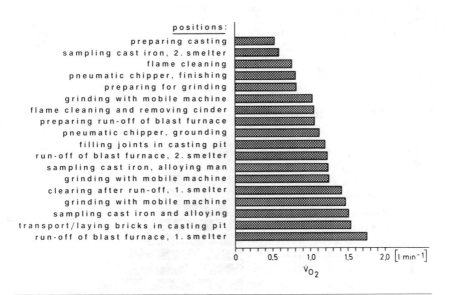

Figure 2.   Energy expenditure for different tasks in the iron and steel industry (from Klimmer et al., 1984).

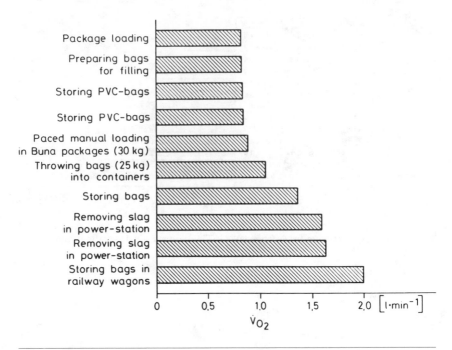

Figure 3. Energy expenditure for different tasks in the chemical industry (from Rutenfranz and Bolt, 1988).

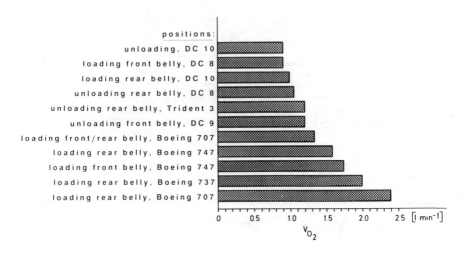

Figure 4. Energy expenditure for loading and unloading aircraft.

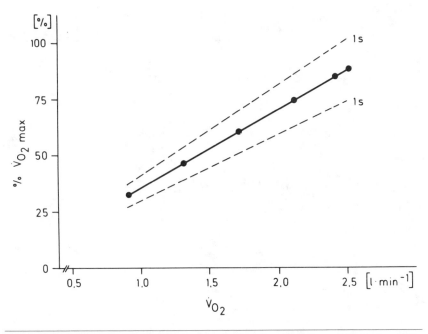

Figure 5. Energy expenditure for loading and unloading aircraft relative to individual aerobic power.

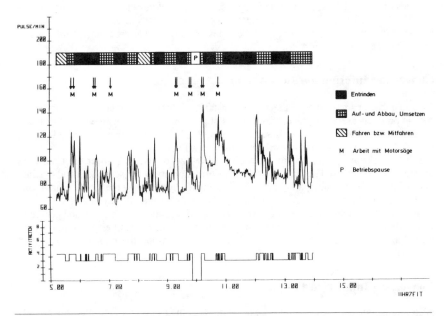

Figure 6. Heart rate and physical activities during steering and driving of machines for unbarking trees in forestry (from Klimmer and Rutenfranz, 1983).

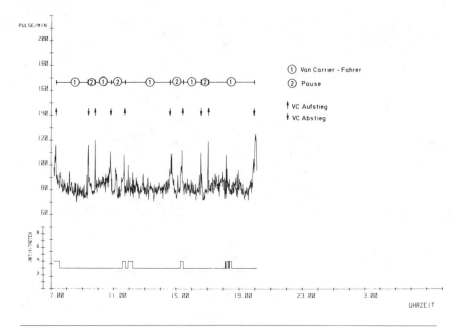

Figure 7. Heart rate and physical activities of a Van-Carrier driver at a container terminal (from Klimmer et al., 1981b).

vehicles like cars, trains, aircraft, helicopters, or merchant vessels used in inland navigation (3, 17, 22, 23, 26). These jobs must be performed mostly in a sitting position with low levels of energy expenditure, but they may include special problems of mental and emotional stress (see Figure 8).

Converting Information Into Action

Typical jobs for this category are inspection tasks. Information about the suitability of special products as well as the different types of possible failures must be stored in short-term memory. Coin production is such an example (36). The woman in Figure 9 had to inspect 1,100,000 coins daily, or 150 coins/s (see Figure 10).

Similar tasks are performed by train dispatchers, who have to inspect the train flow through specific areas. They have to follow information about the sequences and destinations of the different trains, and in this semiautomated system they must only react if one of the systems fails, which is detectable by changes on some displays (19).

Normally these jobs have to be performed sitting with continuous attention and generally with only a few breaks. The responsibility for materials or human beings as well as the mental and emotional load is high, and the type of work is mostly monotonous and even boring (25).

Converting Input Into Output

Positions in this category include many of the so-called modern jobs. Typical for this category are radar controllers, who are characterized by high levels of catecholamine excre-

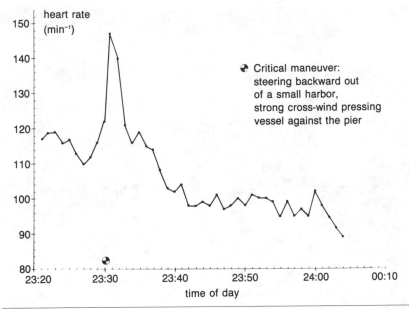

Figure 8.   Heart rate of a captain on an inland waterway boat during a critical incidence (from Klimmer, 1978).

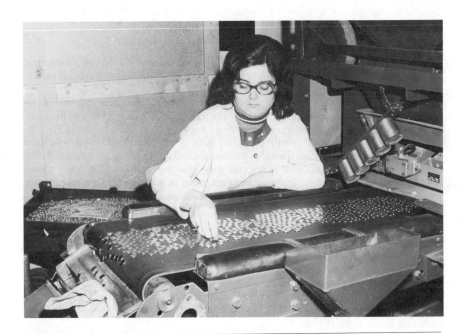

Figure 9.   Quality control of coins (from Rohmert and Rutenfranz, 1975).

224 Rutenfranz, Ilmarinen, Klimmer, and Kylian

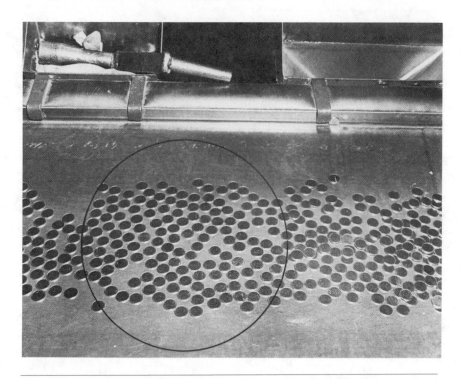

Figure 10. Sector of the conveyor belt with the coins to be controlled per second.

tion and who have to convert analog and digital input information into output information for pilots. This conversion often involves the development of special strategies for starting or landing aircraft (7, 18, 38).

To the same category belong the Japanese train controllers, who guide and control the Shinkansen trains. This job includes not only the traditional dispatcher but also the tasks of the engine driver. The Shinkansen has only an engine driver, and other tasks are performed by people in a central control room in Tokyo (see Figure 11). These people have to monitor all information concerning environmental influences like typhoons and earthquakes in addition to normal time tables, and they have to convert this into information needed for speed. These jobs are normally performed in a sitting position and include low levels of energy expenditure but require high attention and responsibility.

Producing Information

This category involves positions like journalists, clerks, scientists, poets, and several other creative jobs (28). Their special work is mostly done in sitting positions but may include walking and standing. Because they are mostly "free artists," the time pressure may be very different at different times. They often have no fixed working hours and no fixed breaks but a greater variation in work, which at times can lead to high rates of adrenaline excretion in the urine (Figure 12).

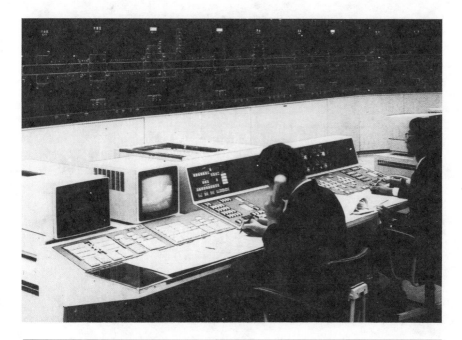

Figure 11. Supervision task in the central railway control room (Tokyo).

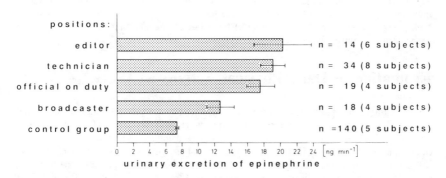

Figure 12. Urinary excretion of adrenaline for different positions in broadcasting (from Kylian et al., in press).

Characteristic for Categories 4 and 5 is the increasing use of visual display units (6, 27). This may reduce many professions to the same type of work or to very similar positions (see Figure 13).

Another yet unmentioned development may be the "dehumanization of work," or displacing human beings from work and giving the positions to robots, which began with

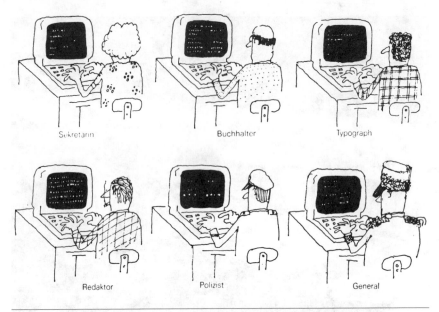

Figure 13.   Unification of positions for different professions using Visual Display Units.

car production. This development clearly diminishes the possibility for physical activities at work, because robots have taken those jobs that mainly include hard physical work. The workers who are handling robots are not mainly involved in programming but in maintaining and repairing the robots. These jobs may include physical activities with a high energy expenditure for several short tasks but are mostly characterized by waiting for actions and observing processes.

Evaluation of Daily Physical Activity at Work

The meaning of the optimal level of daily physical activity at work is ambiguous, extremely hard work seems to be as dangerous to health as work with low levels of energy expenditure. The idea that extremely heavy work should be dangerous to health is an old axiom of occupational medicine. This axiom, however, is based mainly on experiences from the last century, where morbidity among workers under those working conditions was very high. Those working conditions were, however, not only characterized by the high level of energy expenditure but at the same time included prolonged working hours, work by children, a high percentage of work with dangerous toxic agents, unsanitary conditions at work and at home, and malnutrition, as well as other factors (45).

To the best of my knowledge there have been up to now no sound epidemiological studies made as to whether extremely heavy work for long periods damages health and longevity, assuming nutrition and basic hygienic standards are sufficient. This must not exclude the indirect negative health effects of very hard muscular work. Such effects may consist of extremely high fatigue and diminishing protective functions of the muscles on the backbone and may in some cases lead to acute or chronic lower back pain syndrome.

On the other hand, the decrease in daily physical activity brought about by the changes in working conditions in the industrialized countries is regarded as a risk factor for cardiovascular disease. Many classical epidemiological studies in industrialized countries have concluded that a lack of daily physical activity represents a behavior parameter that in itself is a minor risk factor or quite obviously may aggravate other risk factors (32, 48, 50). Apart from this, the lack of physical activity can diminish physical fitness whereby possibilities for leisure activities are reduced.

Because of these great differences in the amount of work with high or low energy expenditure in industrialized countries, I would like to explain the problems on the basis of the stress-strain concept. This concept describes different energy expenditures by means of three physiological facts (see Figure 14): (a) Because the energy expenditure in a particular activity is the same for everyone (if the same load is reached), the stress in such work can be objectively described by measuring the oxygen consumption during work. (b) The strain that occurs in work involving high or low energy expenditure can be best registered by a continuous measurement of the heart rate (47). This does not, however, result directly from the level of energy expenditure but is dependent on (c) the cardiopulmonary fitness of the individual. This can be defined operationally as the individual oxygen consumption at maximal ergometrical load (e.g., the maximal aerobic power).

In Figure 14, it can be seen that the same stress caused by an oxygen consumption of 0.9 L • min^{-1} means a very different percentage of $\dot{V}O_2max$ for young children, male or female young adults, older people, and young athletes. The strain, measured by heart

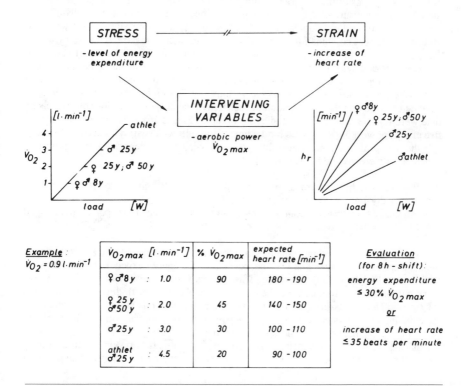

Figure 14. Stress-strain concept of dynamic work.

rate, may differ for such individuals between heart rates of 90 and 190 min^{-1}, whereas the stress is the same.

This may raise the question of what is the optimal level of daily physical activity either in leisure time or during working hours. According to experience gained in exercise physiology, one can assume that optimal daily physical activity occurs when the larger muscle groups are worked dynamically, corresponding to a level of 50% of the individual maximal oxygen intake for at least 60 min, or to a level of 85% of the individual maximal oxygen intake, for at least 15 min/day and at least three to five times a week (1).

In contrast to those prescribed minimum levels of daily physical activity, occupational medicine and work physiology tries to prescribe the upper limits for daily energy expenditure during the working hours. In accordance with the discussions of Legg and Myles (31), we propose the upper limit of energy expenditure as follows: 30% $\dot{V}O_2$max for dynamic work without special rest pauses or 50% $\dot{V}O_2$max for mixed dynamic/static work, or for dynamic work with rest pauses. If we evaluate the working conditions for the individuals, mentioned in Figure 14, only the young male adult and the young athlete could do this work unstrained without rest pauses according to the assumptions of Bonjer (2) (see Figure 15).

As we have mentioned before (Figures 1 to 4), these upper levels were exceeded at several work places even in industrialized countries. The number of such work places in unknown due to the lack of appropriate statistics in most of the countries. The percentage for our nation is about 15-20%. Häublein et al. (8) counted the incidence of such places for the other parts of our nation as 25%.

Since it is not always possible to realize either the demands of occupational medicine or the prescriptions of the American College of Sports Medicine (1), one has to consider the working and leisure time conditions together if one wants to evaluate the daily physical activities of the working population (30). Such studies therefore always deal with four groups of different combinations of activity levels. In such a cross-sectional study of 120 men, 23-60 years old, belonging to the five different work place (position) categories described previously, Ilmarinen et al. (11, 13, 15, 16) performed intense time and position studies including energy expenditure measurements and continuous heart rate recordings during the entire shift. Additionally, the various risk factors for cardiovascular diseases were determined and the participation of each individual at sports activities during leisure time were registered (9). These studies showed (see Figure 16) a distinct ranking for the five groups of working categories for the time of the shift with heart rates above 120 min^{-1}.

If the group of 120 men were split to the following four categories some interesting conclusions were reached (11, 13, 16).

- Physically light work (mean heart rate/shift below 110 min^{-1}), no sports activities;
- Physically light work, active in sports;
- Physically heavy work (mean heart rate/shift above 110 min^{-1}), no sports activities; and
- Physically heavy work, active in sports.

For example, excess weight could only be prevented if the workers included sports among their leisure time activities that was independent of the energy expenditure level at work (see Figure 17). Especially interesting was the fact that workers with physically heavy work but no sports activities were the most overweight. Similar findings were presented for systolic blood pressure (see Figure 18). The best conditions were again attributed to the combination "physically heavy work, active in sports", and the worst to the combination "physically heavy work, no sports activities."

Ilmarinen et al. (11, 13) concluded from these studies that the preventive effect of daily physical activity even of heavy physical work was not sufficient for most cardiovascular

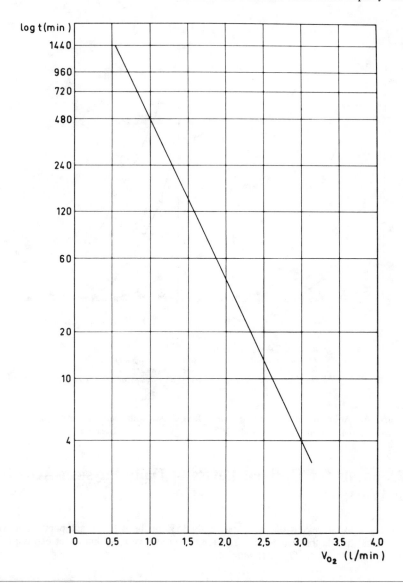

Figure 15. Allowable oxygen intake for work as a function of working time (from Bonjer, 1971).

risk factors. This may be explained by the fact that even heavy physical work in today's working conditions includes a high percentage of static work, the preventive effects of which are rather small (16).

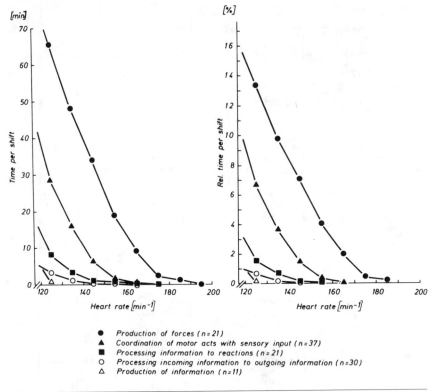

● Production of forces (n = 21)
▲ Coordination of motor acts with sensory input (n = 37)
■ Processing information to reactions (n = 21)
○ Processing incoming information to outgoing information (n = 30)
△ Production of information (n = 11)

Figure 16. Absolute and relative times per shift in classes with heart rates over 120 min^{-1} in five AET-groups (from Ilmarinen et al., 1978).

Proposals for Optimal Levels of Daily Physical Activity at Work

According to the review of Vuori (50), only 15% of the working age population even in Finland fulfills the stringent criteria for preventive exercise and about one third the less strict criteria. As Oja (37) showed,

> Jogging-running is, by its nature—provided, that the minimum requirements for exercise frequency and duration are met—an efficient form of preventive exercise. Walking is equally effective for previous untrained individuals. Cross-country skiing has high energy demands and is suitable for aerobic conditioning. Cycling is an excellent form of cardiorespiratory conditioning although its effect may be more task specific than jogging-running. Swimming is a suitable form of activity for good swimmers but presents problems for less-skilled individuals. Conventional calisthenics and weight training have little value as aerobic exercise. In the circuit training form they improve muscular strength, endurance and flexibility but have negligible aerobic effects even though the cardiocirculatory stress may be considerable. Non-running ball games such as volleyball and tennis are inefficient aerobic exercises at a low skill level, and their effects may be marginal even among more skilled players.

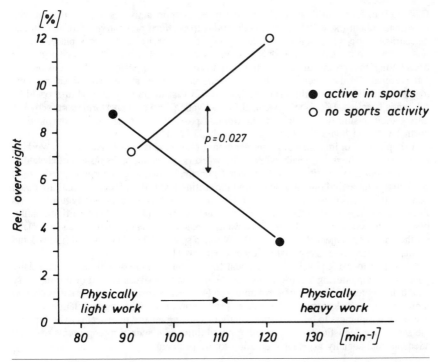

Figure 17.   Relationship between weight, heart rate at work, and sports activity during leisure time in 120 middle-aged men (from Ilmarinen et al., 1980b).

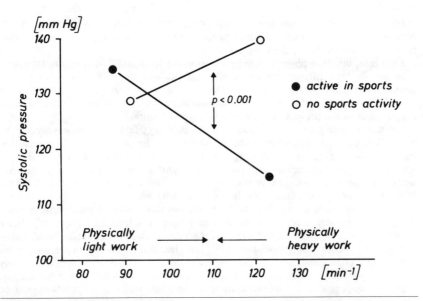

Figure 18.   Relationship between systolic pressure and daily physical activity during work and leisure time (from Ilmarinen, 1978).

Oja's (37) excellent evaluation of different types of sport activities in combination with experience about the willingness of populations to perform preventive exercise (50) can discourage those who want to introduce preventive exercise in the work place.

According to my experience, only a limited percentage of work places have organized breaks long enough in time and of appropriate frequency to perform substantial on-the-job exercise. On the other hand, it seems to be impossible, at least for ethical reasons, to rearrange working conditions in such a manner that the energy expenditure could be substantially raised. Because the potential for motivating workers to perform sports activities during their leisure time is limited, the training possibilities of the workers during their normal working hours should be encouraged (5, 12, 15).

A simple form of implementing considerations of this kind is to motivate workers working in high-rise buildings, especially white collar workers, to use the stairs instead of elevators. Since the working conditions of these groups normally lead to an energy expenditure at work that is increased only a little beyond the resting level, the energy expenditure could quite clearly be increased by using the stairs instead of the elevators (see Figure 19). As Ilmarinen et al. (12) have demonstrated, it is necessary to climb at least 25 floors daily, best done in sections of five floors, if one wants to reach sufficient training effects, especially for the untrained subjects (see Figure 20). Within a span of 10 weeks physical fitness could be distinctly increased, especially in weak persons (15).

According to work physiology, physical fitness can be increased either by hard daily physical training during leisure time when the occupational work is light or through very hard daily professional work of a dynamic type (4). Because professional work is becoming more and more sedentary for the greater proportion of the working population and because the willingness to perform sports activities during leisure time seems to be limited, the search for realistic on-work training possibilities like stair climbing seems to be an adequate and socially acceptable solution to the problem.

Conclusions

Public opinion does not adequately reflect physical activity at work. This is understandable, because we are often more impressed by the 1,000 robots working at a company than by the 99,000 workers at the same company.

Therefore, the daily physical activity situation—at work and during leisure time—has to be described in a different manner. In industrialized countries, about 20% of work places involve more heavy physical work but include substantial sedentary work. At those work places the energy expenditure is high but the sedentary work components of these positions negate some of the preventive effects of this type of work.

For each of these professions or positions, minimal physical performance is needed and can be defined. Such values have to be calculated from the energy expenditure measurements for the limiting peak loads (14), referring to 30% (no rest pauses) or 50% (with rest pauses) of the individual aerobic power as criteria for the upper limits of energy expenditure during work. The maximal aerobic power should therefore be two or three times the level of the energy expenditure for their critical work phases.

Using the 30% criteria we came to the conclusion that male or female workers in the construction industry need a maximal aerobic power of at least 2.75 l/min (45). If we compare this criterion with the histograms of maximal aerobic power for unselected middle European female and male populations (49), it is clear that depending on age and gender only selected populations meet this criteria (see Figure 21). This demonstrates additionally the need for training, especially for older workers even in such highly selected groups.

In other work places, energy expenditure for the whole shift is still too low to produce preventive effects. The work must be done sitting or standing and does not always allow for organized breaks, because the work has to be done more or less continuously.

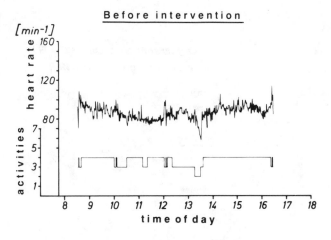

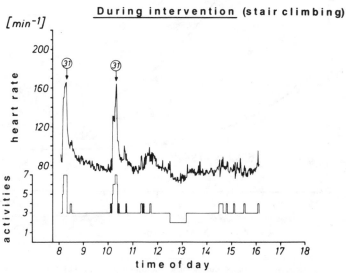

Figure 19. Heart rate and physical activities before and during an intervention study with stair climbing (from Ilmarinen, 1978).

Organized sports during working hours in the work sites could be a desired solution, and this is realized in some countries. But one has to be faced with the difficulties not only of convincing the employers but also of motivating the workers themselves. This is already possible for only a small percentage of countries, companies, and workers. Using the normal possibilities for increasing the daily physical activity on the work sites, like stair climbing instead of using elevators, seems to have a potential not always used.

The possibilities of motivating workers for sports activities after work are limited. But as the development in the United States shows, there may be a greater potential than realized for Europe.

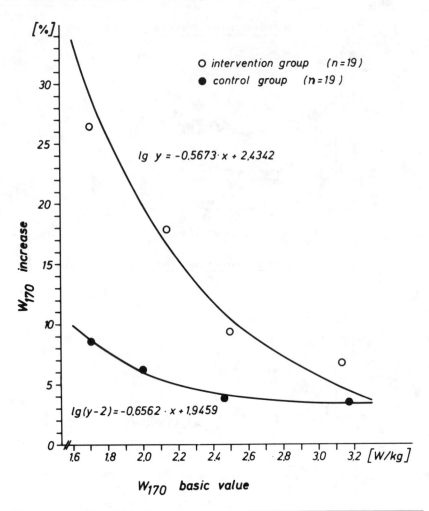

Figure 20.   Effects of stair climbing during office hours on physical performance capacity (W_{170}) (from Ilmarinen et al., 1978).

References

1. American College of Sports Medicine. Position statement on the recommended quantity and quality of exercise for developing and maintaining fitness in healthy adults. Med. Sci. Sports 10:7-10, 1978.

2. Bonjer, F.H. Temporal factors and physiological load. In: Singleton, W.T., Fox, J.G., Whitfield, D., eds. Measurement of man at work. London: Taylor and Francis, 1971:41-44.

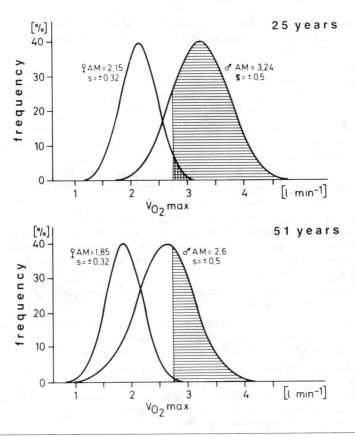

Figure 21. Histogram of maximal aerobic power for males and females at the age of 25 and 51 years (critical levels for the construction industry are marked) (from Rutenfranz et al., 1982).

3. Böttger, M., Klimmer, F., Knauth, P., Nachreiner, F., Rutenfranz, J. Analyse der Tätigkeitsanforderungen für Binnen-schiffahrtssteuerstände. Arbeitsmed. Sozialmed. Präventivmed. 11:254-258, 1973.

4. de Boorder, T. Energiebesteding en lichamelijk prestatievermogen. Amsterdam, 1971. Dissertation.

5. Fardy, P.S., Ilmarinen, J. Evaluating the effects and feasibility of an at work stair-climbing intervention program for men. Med. Sci. Sports 7:91-93, 1975.

6. Grandjean, E., Vigliani, E., eds. Ergonomic aspects of visual display terminals. Proceedings of the International Workshop, 1980 March, Milan. London: Taylor and Francis, 1980.

7. Grandjean, E.P., Wotzka, G., Schaad, R., Gilgen, A. Fatigue and stress in air traffic controller. Ergonomics 14:159-165, 1971.

8. Häublein, H.-G., Heuchert, G., Schulz, G., Blau, E., u.a. Methodische Anleitung zur arbeitshygienischen Professiografie. Forschungsverband Arbeitsmedizin der DDR. Berlin, 1979 December.

9. Ilmarinen, J. Beziehungen zwischen beruflicher und sportlicher körperlicher Aktivität und kardiopulmonaler Leistungsfähigkeit. Untersuchungen bei Männern mittleren Alters unter besonderer Berücksichtingung prophylaktischer Aspekte der koronaren Durchblutungsstörungen. Koln, 1978. Dissertation.

11. Ilmarinen, J., Ilmarinen, R., Korhonen, O., Nurminen, M. Circadian variation of physiological functions related to physical work capacity. Scand. J. Work Environ. Health 6:112-122, 1980.

12. Ilmarinen, J., Ilmarinen, R., Koskela, A., Korhonen, O., Fardy, P., Partanen, T., Rutenfranz, J. Training effects of stair-climbing during office hours on female employees. Ergonomics 22:507-516, 1979.

13. Ilmarinen, J., Knauth, P., Rutenfranz, J., Karvonen, M.J. Untersuchungen über unterschiedliche präventive Effekte von habituellen körperlichen Aktivitäten in Beruf bzw. Freizeit: I. Prävalenz von Risikofaktoren für Herz- und Kreislaufkrankheiten in Gruppen mit unterschiedlicher habitueller körperlicher Aktivität. Int. Arch. Occup. Environ. Health 45:15-33, 1980b.

14. Ilmarinen, J., Rutenfranz, J. Occupationally induced stress, strain and peak loads as related to age. Scand. J. Work Environ. Health 6:274-282, 1980.

15. Ilmarinen, J., Rutenfranz, J., Knauth, P., Ahrens, M., Kylian, H., Siuda, A., Korallus, U. Uber den Einfluß einer berufsnahen Trainingsmöglichkeit auf die körperliche Leistungfähigkeit von Angestellten. Europ. J. Appl. Physiol. 38:25-40, 1978.

16. Ilmarinen, J., Rutenfranz, J., Kylian, H., Klimmer, F., Ahrens, M., Ilmarinen, R. Untersuchungen über unterschiedliche präventive Effekte von habituellen körperlichen Aktivitäten in Beruf bzw. Freizeit: II. Die Wirkung von körperlichen Aktivitäten im Beruf bzw. in der Freizeit auf die kardiopulmonale Leistungsfähigkeit. Int. Arch. Occup. Environ. Health 49:1-12, 1981.

17. Klimmer, F. Analyse mentaler und emotionaler Beanspruchung des arbeitenden Menschen. Darmstadt, 1978. Dissertation.

18. Klimmer, F., Aulmann, H.M., Rutenfranz, J. Katecholaminausscheidung im Urin bei emotional und mental belastenden Tätigkeiten im Flugverkehrskontrolldienst. Int. Arch. Arbeitsmed. 30:65-80, 1972.

19. Klimmer, F., Aulmann, H.M., Wittgens, H., Rutenfranz, J. Arbeitsmedizinische Untersuchungen an Personen im Stellwerksdienst det Deutschen Bundesbahn. Der Ärztliche Dienst 35:97-101, 1974.

20. Klimmer, F., Kylian, H., Ilmarinen, J., Ilmarinen, R., Meyer, R., Piekarski, C., Rutenfranz, J. Belastung und Beanspruchung bei Tätigkeiten in der Eisen- und Stahlindustrie. Arbeitsmed. Sozialmed. Präventivmed. 19:49-54, 1984.

21. Klimmer, F., Kylian, H., Ilmarinen, J., Rutenfranz, J. Arbeitsmedizinische und arbeitsphysiologische Untersuchungen bei verschiedenen Tätigkeiten im Bauhauptgewerbe. Arbeitsmed. Sozialmed. Präventivmed. 18:143-147, 1983.

22. Klimmer, F., Kylian, H., Rutenfranz, J. Einfluß det Arbeitszeit, Schicht- und Pausengestaltung auf die Beanspruchung bei der Containerverladung im Hafen. In: Landau, K., Rohmert, W., eds. Fallbespiele zur Arbeitsanalyse. Ergebnisse zum AET-Einsatz. Bern: Huber, 1981a:189-200.

23. Klimmer, F., Kylian, H., Rutenfranz, J. Untersuchungen über Belastung und Beanspruchung bei der Containerverladung im Hafen. In: Schäcke, G., Stollenz, E., eds. Epidemiologische Ansätze im Bereich der Arbeitsmedizin. Bericht uber die 21. Jahrestagung der Deutschen Gesellschaft für Arbeitsmedizin e.V., Berlin, 13.-16.5.1981. Stuttgart: Gentner:1981b:421-426.

24. Klimmer, F., Kylian, H., Rutenfranz, J., Grund-Eckardt, R. Belastungs- und Beanspruchungsanalyse verschiedener Tätigkeiten bei der Müllabfuhr. Z. Arb. Wiss. 36(8NF):90-94, 1982.

25. Klimmer, F., Löwenthal, I., Rutenfranz, J., Analyse einer rechner- und bildschirmgestützten Personalplanung auf einem Großflughafen. In: Landau, K., Rohmert, W., eds. Fallbespiele zur Arbeitsanalyse. Ergebnisse zum AET-Einsatz. Bern: Huber, 1981a:105-113.

26. Klimmer, F., Rutenfranz, J., Zur Belastung und Beanspruchung durch Tätigkeiten auf Entrindungsmaschinen bei der mechanisierten Holzernte. Arbeitsmed. Sozialmed. Präventivmed. 18:2-5, 1983.

27. Krueger, H., Müller-Limmroth, W. Arbeiten mit dem Bildschirm—aber richtig! München: Bayerisches Staatsministerium für Arbeit und Sozialordnung, 1980.

28. Kylian, H., Klimmer, F., Neidhart, B., Ernst, S., Rutenfranz, J. Belastung und Beanspruchung bei Tätigkeiten in Nachrichtenredaktionen von Rundfunkanstalten, in press.

29. Kylian, H., Rutenfranz, J., Lowenthal, I., Klimmer, F., Knauth, P. Arbeitsanforderungen und zeitliche Organisation bei Ladetätigkeiten auf einem Grossflughafen. In: Landau, K., Rohmert, W., eds. Fallbespiele zur Arbeitsanalyse. Ergebnisse zum AET-Einsatz. Bern: Huber, 1981:177-188.

30. Lange Andersen, K., Masironi, R., Rutenfranz, J., Seliger, V. Habitual physical activity and health. Copenhagen: WHO Regional Publications, European Series No. 6, World Health Organization, 1978.

31. Legg, S.J., Myles, W.S. Maximum acceptable repetitive lifting workloads for an 8-hour work-day using psychophysical and subjective rating methods. Ergonomics 24:907-916, 1981.

32. Leon, A.S. Epidemiological aspects of physical activity and coronary heart disease. Finnish Sports and Exercise Medicine 2:10-27, 1983.

33. McCormick, E.J., Cunningham, J.W., Thornton, G.C. The prediction of job requirements by a structured job analysis procedure. Personnel Psychology 20:431-440, 1967.

34. McCormick, E.J., Jeanneret, P.R., Mecham, R.C. The development and background of the Position Analysis Questionnaire (PAQ). Lafayette, IN: Occupational Research Center, Purdue University, 1969.

35. McCormick, E.J., Jeanneret, P.R., Mecham, R.C. A study of job characteristics and job dimensions as based on the Position Analysis Questionnaire (PAQ). J. Appl. Psychol. 56:347-368, 1972.

36. Nachreiner, F., Klimmer, F., Knauth, P., Lange, W., Rutenfranz, J. Untersuchungen über lesitungsbegrenzende Bedingungen bei einer optischen Kontrollaufgabe. Int. Arch. Arbeitsmed. 34:247-268, 1975.

37. Oja, P. Comparison of the physiological effects of different forms of physical activity. Finnish Sports and Exercise Medicine 2:62-71, 1983.

38. Rohmert, W. Psycho-physische Belastung und Beanspruchung von Fluglotsen. Schriftenreihe ''Arbeitswissenschaft und Praxis'' Band 30, Berlin: Beuth, 1973.

39. Rohmert, W., Landau, K. Das Arbeitswissenschaftliche Erhebungsverfahren zur Tätig-keitsanalyse (AET). Bern: Huber, 1979.

40. Rohmert, W., Landau, K. AET, tyon profiilin kuvausmenetelmä. Vantaa: Työter-veyslaitos, 1981.

41. Rohmert, W., Landau, K. A new technique for job analysis. London: Taylor and Francis, 1983.

42. Rohmert, W., Rutenfranz, J. Arbeitswissenschaftliche Beurteilung der Belastung und Beanspruchung an unterschiedlichen industriellen Arbeitsplätzen. Bonn: Der Bundes-minister für Arbeit und Sozialordnung, 1975.

43. Rutenfranz, J. Recent advances in the field of work physiology: Heavy work, body positions, shiftwork. Conferenza tenuta alla Fondazione Carlo Erba, giugno 1982. Milano: Fondazione Carlo Erba, Sezione di Medicina del Lavoro e Igiene Ambien-tale, 1982.

44. Rutenfranz, J., Bolt, H.M. The impact of physical and mental activity on toxicokinetics and toxicodynamics of workplace chemicals. In: Notten, W.R.F., Herber, R.F.M., Hunter, W.J., Monster, A.C., Zielhuis, R.L., eds. Health surveillance of individual workers exposed to chemical agents. Proceedings of the International Workshop on Health Surveillance of Individual Workers Exposed to Chemical Agents, Amsterdam. October 29-31, 1986. Berlin: Springer, 1988:121-123. (Int. Arch. Occup. Environ. Health, Suppl.)

45. Rutenfranz, J., Klimmer, F., Ilmarinen, J. Arbeitsphyiologische Überlegungen zur Beschäftigung von weiblichen Jugendlichen und Frauen im Bauhauptgewerbe. Schriftenreihe Arbeitsmedizin, Sozialmedizin, Präventivmedizin, Band 70. Stuttgart: Gentner, 1982.

46. Rutenfranz, J., Löwenthal, I., Kylian, H., Klimmer, F., Flöring, R., Gärtner, K.H., Brockmann, W. Arbeitsmedizinische Untersuchungen über Ladearbeiter auf einem Grossflughafen: I. Ergebnisse arbeitsphysiologischer Zeit- und Positionsstudien. Int. Arch. Occup. Environ. Health 47:129-141, 1980.

47. Rutenfranz, J., Seliger, V., Andersen, K.L., Ilmarinen, J., Flöring, R., Rutenfranz, M., Klimmer, F. Erfahrungen mit einem transportablen Gerät zur kontinuierlichen Registrierung der Herzfrequenz für Zeiten bis zu 24 Stunden. Europ. J. Appl. Physiol. 36:171-185, 1977.

48. Salonen, J.T. Physical activity and risk of myocardial infarction, stroke and death. Finnish Sports and Exercise Medicine 2:28-42, 1983.

49. Seliger, V., Bartůněk, Z., eds. Mean values of various indices of physical fitness in the investigation of Czechoslovak population aged 12-55 years. International Bio-logical Programme Results of Investigations 1968-1974. CSTV, Praha (CSSR): Czechoslovak Association of Physical Culture, 1976.

50. Vuori, I. The potential for primary prevention of coronary heart disease by physical activity. Finnish Sports and Exercise Medicine 2:43-53, 1983.

Analysis of the Relationship Between Physical Fitness Level and Risk Factors of Cardiovascular Disease in Workers

K. Aoki, Y. Suzuki, A. Noji, R. Yanagibori, and A. Gunji

Department of Health Administration, Faculty of Medicine, University of Tokyo, Japan

Modernization of industrial work styles has on one hand decreased the physical work load while on the other hand increased the mental load of workers. The changing work load pattern causes inactivity problems for workers, which often lead to an increase in the risk level for cardiovascular diseases. It is important for industrial health administration to take proper means to activate the workers' lives to prevent the incidence of cardiovascular diseases.

Some cross-sectional studies indicate that the risk level for coronary heart disease (CHD) is lower in physically fit persons than in those who are not fit. In some experimental studies, it was shown that physical exercise is effective in reducing the risks of CHD as observed from the changes in total cholesterol, triglycerides, or obesity. Moreover, some recent studies have revealed blood pressure reduction in hypertensives as a result of mild endurance training. Accordingly, physical activity is an important factor in preventing the occurrence of cardiovascular diseases.

In each of these studies, however, only a single relationship between one specific risk factor and a fitness level is referred to. A comprehensive structure of relationships among many risk factors and many kinds of physical fitness levels has not yet been revealed. The purpose of this study is to define such a structure by analyzing relationships between some risk factors of cardiovascular diseases and physical fitness levels.

Methods

Three different data sets were used for analysis. The first data set was obtained from 88 male workers over 35 years of age who engaged mainly in clerical work in an office (Data Set A). The second data set was collected from 107 male workers over 30 years of age who mainly work out of offices to provide services for the maintenance of office machines (Data Set B). The final data set was collected from 182 males over 20 years of age who work at different companies visiting the same medical clinic for health checkups (Data Set C).

Clinical tests included serum total cholesterol, high density lipoprotein cholesterol (HDL-C), triglycerides, blood sugar, uric acid, and blood pressure. Physical fitness tests consisted of vertical jump, side steps, grip strength test, standing trunk flexion, sit-ups, and maximal oxygen uptake ($\dot{V}O_2$max). $\dot{V}O_2$max was estimated from bicycle ergometer using the three steps loading method and Åstrand's nomogram. Body size and composition were measured for height, body weight, and percent fat estimated by skinfolds.

Correlation coefficients between variables obtained from clinical tests and those representing fitness or body dimensions were computed for each data set. Factor analysis was performed using the principal factor method and varimax rotation, plotting each variable on a two-dimensional plane of two axial factors.

Results

Correlation coefficients between the variables obtained from the clinical tests and those of fitness or body dimensions are shown in Tables 1 to 3. Table 1 shows the correlation coefficients for data set A. Of the fitness variables, $\dot{V}O_2$max had negative correlations with total cholesterol ($r = -.19$) and triglycerides ($r = -.25$) while having a positive correlation with HDL-C ($r = .21$). Side step had a negative correlation with uric acid ($r = -.26$). Vertical jump and standing trunk flexion had negative correlations with total cholesterol ($r = -.12$, $-.20$). In the meantime, grip strength had positive correlations with triglycerides ($r = .18$), HDL-C ($r = .14$), and uric acid ($r = .13$). As to the body dimensions, height showed positive relation with HDL-C ($r = .28$) while the percent body fat showed negative correlation with HDL-C ($r = -.24$). Body weight had positive correlation with uric acid ($r = .22$).

Table 1   Correlation Coefficients Between Clinical Test Variables and Fitness Variables (Data Set A)

Physical fitness and body dimension	Clinical tests			
	Total cholesterol	HDL-C	TG	Uric acid
Side step	−0.07	−0.04	−0.00	−0.26
Vertical jump	−0.12	0.07	0.06	−0.13
Grip strength	0.04	0.14	0.18	0.13
Trunk flexion	−0.20	−0.03	−0.01	−0.02
$\dot{V}O_2$max	−0.20	0.22	−0.25	−0.02
Height	−0.02	0.28	−0.05	−0.02
Weight	0.04	−0.02	0.10	0.22
Body fat	0.02	−0.24	0.05	0.00

Table 2 shows the correlation coefficients between the clinical test variables and the fitness variables computed for Data Set B. On the fitness variables, $\dot{V}O_2$max had negative correlations with systolic blood pressure (SBP; $r = -.08$), diastolic blood pressure (DBP; $r = -.23$), total cholesterol ($r = -.26$), triglycerides ($r = -.30$), blood sugar ($r = -.25$), and uric acid ($r = -.26$). On the other hand, grip strength showed positive relationships with these clinical test variables, especially with uric acid ($r = .32$). Grip strength had negative correlation coefficient with HDL-C ($r = -.25$). On the body dimension variables, body weight showed positive correlations with SBP ($r = .23$), DBP ($r = .40$), blood sugar ($r = .30$), and uric acid ($r = .33$). Percent body fat also showed positive correlations with SBP ($r = .19$), DBP ($r = .42$), and total cholesterol ($r = .13$). Body weight and percent body fat both had positive correlation coefficients with HDL-C ($r = -.34$, $-.16$).

Table 2 Correlation Coefficients Between Clinical Test Variables and Fitness Variables (Data Set B)

Physical fitness and body dimension	Clinical tests						
	SBP	DBP	Total cholesterol	HDL-C	TG	Blood sugar	Uric acid
Vertical jump	−.04	0.02	−0.02	−0.22	−0.12	0.05	0.21
Grip strength	0.20	0.22	0.06	−0.25	0.16	0.18	0.32
Trunk flexion	0.06	0.12	0.05	0.12	0.07	−0.11	0.12
Sit-ups	0.01	0.00	−0.07	−0.09	−0.01	−0.08	0.19
$\dot{V}O_2$max	−0.08	−0.23	−0.26	0.10	−0.30	−0.25	−0.26
Height	−0.11	−0.18	−0.12	−0.27	−0.03	0.02	0.13
Weight	0.23	0.40	0.14	−0.34	0.26	0.30	0.33
Body fat	0.19	0.42	0.13	−0.16	0.33	0.06	0.21

Table 3 shows correlation coefficients between the variables for Data Set C. $\dot{V}O_2$max showed positive relation with HDL-C ($r = .20$) and negative relations with triglycerides ($r = -.16$) and uric acid ($r = -.27$). Body weight was positively correlated with SBP ($r = .16$), DBP ($r = .23$), triglycerides ($r = .13$), blood sugar ($r = .14$), and uric acid ($r = .17$) and negatively correlated with HDL-C ($r = -.20$).

Two main factors were chosen by factor analysis for each data set. Percentages of contribution of the specific factors are shown in Table 4. Total percentage of contributions reached 35-40% in each data set.

Variables were plotted on two-dimensional factor planes according to the factor loading scores. Figure 1a shows the relationships among the variables on the factor plane of Data Set A. The horizontal axis represents the loading score of Factor 1 and the vertical axis

Table 3 Correlation Coefficients Between Clinical Test Variables and Fitness Variables (Data Set C)

Physical fitness and body dimension	Clinical tests						
	SBP	DBP	Total cholesterol	HDL-C	TG	Blood sugar	Uric acid
Side step	−0.06	−0.08	−0.07	−0.04	−0.13	−0.07	−0.02
Vertical jump	0.03	0.03	0.01	−0.09	−0.02	−0.05	−0.00
Trunk flexion	−0.00	−0.09	−0.10	0.17	−0.04	−0.11	−0.10
Sit-ups	−0.06	−0.10	0.05	0.23	−0.04	0.04	−0.01
$\dot{V}O_2$max	0.03	−0.02	−0.05	0.20	−0.16	−0.06	−0.27
Height	−0.02	0.02	0.05	0.05	−0.12	−0.13	−0.02
Weight	0.16	0.23	0.17	−0.20	0.13	0.14	0.17

Table 4   Percentage of Contribution of Factors by Factor Analysis

Data set	A	B	C
Factor 1	24.0%	24.6%	18.7%
Factor 2	17.9%	17.2%	15.7%
Total	42.0%	41.8%	34.4%

that of Factor 2. Variables showing high positive relationships with Factor 1 were side step and vertical jump, while that having a high negative relationship was age. Thus, this Factor 1 seemed to show a general fitness level of workers. On Factor 2 axis, high positive relations were observed with relative weight (body weight/height), triglycerides, total cholesterol, and percent body fat. $\dot{V}O_2$max and HDL-C were plotted on negative field of Factor 2. Factor 2 seemed to be a body composition Factor. Under the definitions of the two factors, $\dot{V}O_2$max as an index of cardiovascular fitness level is related with body composition factors and not with the general fitness factor.

Figure 1b shows variables plotted on a factors plane for Data Set B. In this figure, the horizontal axis shows body composition factor as Factor 1, and the vertical axis shows general fitness factor as Factor 2. What is represented by each axis interchanges in Figures 1a and 1b. DBP, SBP, triglycerides, total cholesterol, blood sugar, percent body fat, and relative body weight were positively related with the body composition factor, and $\dot{V}O_2$max was negatively related with this factor. On the axis of general fitness factor (Factor 2), vertical jump, grip strength, and sit-ups were plotted as positive loading scores, while age and HDL-C were plotted as negative loading.

Figure 1c shows variables plotted for Data Set C. Factor 1 seemed to show a general fitness factor, and Factor 2 showed body composition factor as in the case of data set A. Age was negatively related with general fitness factors. Triglycerides, SBP, DBP, blood sugar, total cholesterol, and uric acid had strong positive relations to the body composition factor. HDL-C and $\dot{V}O_2$max were negatively related with this factor.

Discussion

Risk factors for cardiovascular diseases are reported in many studies, but the relationships with the physical fitness level have not been analyzed sufficiently. In this study, correlation coefficients were computed for the observation of relationships between risk factor variables and the fitness variables. The results proved no strong relationships between them. Among the fitness variables, $\dot{V}O_2$max related with almost all of the clinical test variables, seeming to be a negative risk factor for cardiovascular diseases. Inversely, grip strength related with risk factors positively. It is suggested that not all kinds of physical fitness are necessarily beneficial for the prevention of cardiovascular diseases. Indeed, it was reported that isometric training such as hand gripping increased blood pressure levels significantly. Body weight or percent body fat was positively related with risk factors. From these results, it seems that $\dot{V}O_2$max as an index of cardiovascular fitness and weight and percent body fat as indices of obesity are useful in assuming the risk level for cardiovascular diseases.

From the results of factor analysis, two main factors were chosen. One was named the general fitness factor and the other the body composition factor. These two factors were

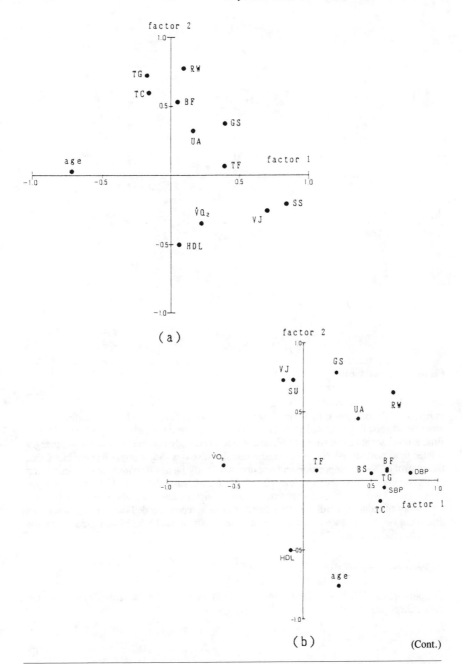

Figure 1. The variables plotted on factor plane: (a) Data Set A, (b) Data Set B, (c) Data Set C. (SS) side step, (VJ) vertical jump, (GS) grip strength, (TF) body trunk flexion, (SU) sit-ups, (VO₂) VO₂max, (RW) relative weight, (BF) percent body fat, (SBP) systolic blood pressure, (DBP) diastolic blood pressure, (TC) total cholesterol, (HDL) HDL-cholesterol, (TG) triglycerides, (BS) blood sugar, (UA) uric acid.

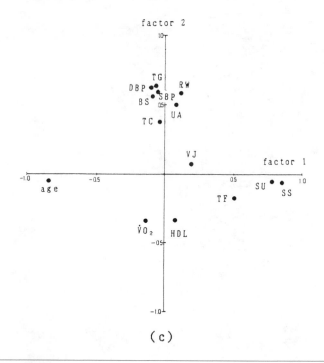

(c)

Figure 1.   (Continued)

independent of each other; therefore, it seems that general fitness level, not including cardio-vascular fitness, is not related to body composition or cardiovascular risk factors. General fitness level seems to be strongly related to age. The body composition factor is strongly related to almost all risk factors of cardiovascular diseases. So, it might be concluded that the control of body composition and obesity, with body fat as one component, is important in decreasing cardiovascular risk levels. Of the fitness variables, only $\dot{V}O_2$max was nega-tively related with the body composition factor, which means that endurance training has a possibility of reducing cardiovascular risk levels. It is recommended that physical exercises that increase cardiovascular fitness should be a part of health administration programs for industrial workers.

Acknowledgment

The authors thank Mr. Shin Doya, Mr. Tetsuo Tomatsu, and Nobuyoshi Shimizu for the data collection.

Exercise Program for Increasing Health and Physical Fitness of Workers

I. Itoh, K. Hanawa, and S. Okuse

Division of Cardiology, NTT Tokyo Central Health Administration Center, Minato-ku, Tokyo, Japan

Even though the incidence of hazardous occupational disease is now generally decreasing, the problem of adult diseases such as diabetes mellitus, obesity, and hypertension must still be addressed. These are particularly prevalent among white-collar workers. One way to tackle the problem is through exercise.

In Japan, a policy of promoting health and fitness in elderly or middle-aged people, called the "Silver Health Plan," has been advocated by the Labor Ministry. A new law came into effect in October 1988 that promotes the health and physical fitness of workers. Under this law the company is recommended to adopt a systemic approach including medical check-ups, data evaluation, prescription of exercise programs, and follow-up.

However, so far only a few companies have adopted such a system, and there has been only limited success among those who have, due to factors such as disinterest on the part of the workers, lack of recreation time to exercise, and the difficulty of implementing regular medical check-ups. As a trial of the above plan, this study has been aimed at improving the health and physical fitness of workers through a prescribed exercise program and at confirming the importance of a medical check-up before or during the exercise program.

Materials and Methods

Subjects were five male sedentary workers with NTT (Nippon Telegraph and Telephone Corporation) who were divided by job category into four office clerks and one researcher (see Table 1). They were all interested in exercise. Two of them ran regularly and two subjects were smokers.

In 1984, when the study began, their ages ranged from 39 to 54 years (the average age being 46.4). One of them had chest pain when exerting himself and mild hypertension (150/96 mmHg). Echocardiography was performed using the Toshiba SSA-90A by sector scanning with parasternal and four-chamber view.

Routine blood tests were carried out including measuring HDL and total cholesterol. Respiratory function was tested at the same time. Supine flexibility and muscular strength performance were also estimated.

The Treadmill test (multistage exercise tolerance test) was performed as follows. The Marquette model CASE II was used to evaluate the estimated maximum oxygen consumption ($\dot{V}O_2$max) by the protocol of Bruce. Consequently this test also included observing electrocardiographic response (ST segments changes and rhythm disturbances), hemodynamic response (heart rate and blood pressure before, during, and after exercise), and functional capacity. The criteria for the end point of the exercise test was mainly that the subject had leg fatigue, that the subject's heart rate reached the target heart rate, or that the subject developed any abnormal ECG findings.

Table 1   Profile of the Subjects in 1983

Case no.	Age	Height (cm)	Weight (kg)	Weight (1988)	$\dot{V}O_2$max (ml/kg/min)	$\dot{V}O_2$max (1988)	Remarks
1	39	168	61	59	53.5	57.0	Ran regularly
2	48	162	58	55	45.5	52.5	Smoking
3	46	158	55	51	52.5	52.5	Ran regularly
4	46	164	62	62	38.5	45.5	Smoking
5	52	166	71	65	42.0	49.0	Mild hypertension, chest pain

Note. Case 4 quit smoking a year later.

The target heart rate was calculated by the Scandinavian method (3). Each subject had a follow-up once a year for more than 3-5 years. The exercise program was prescribed as to mode, intensity, time, frequency, and progression of activity. As a rule, running was selected as the mode of exercise. The intensity of the exercise was determined by the running speed equivalent to the heart rate, which was 50-70% of maximum heart rate. The conversion from the heart rate to the running speed was made using the regression line of the running speed over the heart rate based on the data of 100 workers classified by the age groups. The subjects themselves determined the amount of exercise they took, which ranged from 20 min to 1 hr two or three times a week.

Depending on the results of the exercise test, the subjects' exercise program was modified every year with regard to length of time spent exercising, frequency of exercise, and especially running speed. After completing the prescribed exercise program for one year, the subjects had electrodes attached to their bodies using the CM5 lead. This made it possible to determine whether or not their heart rates at the maximum point of the exercise was within the prescribed range. The results were stored and analyzed using the "memory mac" (VINE Bionics System). Before and after the subjects were prescribed the exercise program, a questionnaire study was done relating to their exercise habits, change of feeling about their condition, and their well-being, including their motivation for work.

Results

After being examined, all the subjects were diagnosed as being fit to do exercise. The result of the test for the maximum oxygen consumption ($\dot{V}O_2$max) at the first check-up showed that the 2 subjects who ran regularly performed well for their age (see Table 1). The running speed stated above was set at 130-180 m/min after determination of heart rate.

The result of the exercise test carried out every year showed an increase of endurance performance on treadmill time in 4 subjects, which meant an increase in maximum oxygen consumption (see Table 1). None of them had ECG abnormalities such as greatly abnormal ST depression or arrythmia. No subject had any abnormality in his biochemical data except a slightly high total cholesterol level in one. Moreover no respiratory disorders were found among the subjects. There was no great difference in vital lung capacity between smokers and nonsmokers.

Supine flexibility and muscle strength were within the standard range for age. Flexibility was generally improved whereas muscle strength did not change. An increase of HDL cholesterol was observed in 3 of the subjects 2 years later. In terms of echocardiography for the subjects, left ventricular hypertrophy (LVH) was observed in one of them; however this seemed to be the same as that observed in most athletes. Hypertrophic cardiomyopathy (HCM) was not found among them.

The exercise program was upgraded for the 4 subjects mentioned above according to the increase in their $\dot{V}O_2$max. One, who had complained of dubious chest pain, lost that symptom a year later in the course of exercise, and his blood pressure was normalized (138/82 mmHg).

One subject developed pain in the knee joints. He was therefore taken off the training for 3 weeks, and his exercise was changed to walking. Two subjects exceeded the prescribed range of heart rate during the exercise, although they did not develop any severe dyspnea. They were ordered to slow down (Figure 1).

The questionnaire revealed that all of them felt better than before (i.e., less stressful and more motivated at work). Weight loss occurred in 4 subjects. That was a strong factor in their feeling of well-being, according to their answers.

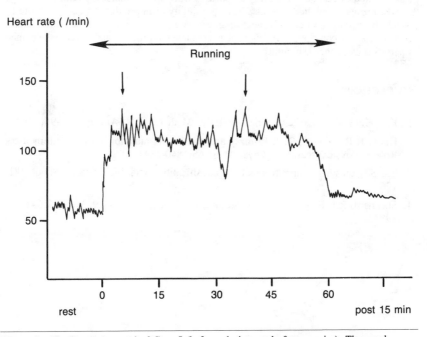

Figure 1. The heart rate trend of Case 5 (before, during, and after exercise). The graph shows that heart rate sometimes exceeded the prescribed upper limit (arrowhead).

Discussion

Within industry many companies are interested in reducing the direct and indirect costs of their health service. It is well known that for those companies one way to decrease their expenses is to shift the emphasis from treating sickness that has already occurred to preventive medicine through programs promoting health and fitness of senior white-collar workers.

These sedentary elder workers suffer from a significant decline in their physical abilities, which can impair their work performance and sense of well-being. Though exercise programs can have an impact on those losses, they can also carry significant risks for the potential participants (1). Thus it is necessary, when determining the goals and conducts of the exercise programs, that a careful assessment of each individual's medical condition and exercise tolerance take place.

We could prescribe a well-designed and safe exercise program with the aid of a work team. Considering the troubles experienced even in our small group of participants, it seems important that each company should employ a medical staff to work as a team, including a health care trainer and a health care leader (2).

In terms of exercise mode, if pursuing safety rather than our method, the possibility of utilizing walking, which is the first form of exercise and now fashionable in the United States, must be entertained. Moreover, in order to check the volume of exercise, using a bicycle for exercise is more suitable.

Concerning the effect on mental status, the efficacy of this program is suggested by the report in the questionnaire of a more positive work attitude and less strain. It is thought that when properly applied, exercise has a possibility of improving the quality of life for the elderly, and the cost effectiveness of an exercise program will soon be widely understood by Japanese companies (4). We hope to continue this program and increase the number of participants in the near future.

References

1. Fitzgerald, P.L. Exercise for the elderly. Med. Clin. N. Am. 69:189-96, 1985.

2. Huhn, R.R., Volski, R.V. Primary prevention programs for business and industry. Role of physical therapist. Phys. Ther. 65:1840-1844, 1985.

3. The Scandinavian Committee on ECG classification. Acta. Med. Scand. (Suppl. 481), 1967.

4. Shephard, R.J. Employee health and fitness: The state of art. Prev. Med. 12:644-653, 1983.

Effects of a Ten-Year Corporate Fitness Program on Employees' Health

K. Okada and T. Iseki

Osaka Gas Health and Fitness Center, Chiyozaki, Nishi-ku Osaka, and Osaka College of Physical Education, Ibaragi-shi Osaka, Japan

In a technologically advanced society, labor-saving measures mean less opportunity for physical activities as part of daily routine. This sedentary lifestyle has led to a decrease in basic physical fitness and deterioration in health with an increased incidence of adult diseases and mortality (4). The extension of retirement age has resulted in an increase in the average age of employees in Japan. Given this situation, helping employees stay well means improving their morale, increasing productivity, and reducing the absentee rate due to sickness (5, 6). To attain these objectives, corporate fitness programs as well as regular medical checkups have very important roles to play. The purpose of this study was to evaluate the effects of a 10-year corporate fitness program on employees' health and physical fitness levels.

Subjects and Methods

The subjects consisted of 1,657 male employees of Osaka Gas Company over 40 years of age who had taken health care exams successively between October 1976 and March 1986. These exams provided data used to evaluate the results of medical checkups and physical fitness tests (see Figure 1).

The corporate fitness program consists of health care exams (medical checkups, physical fitness tests, and a health care seminar) and a physical exercise program on an individual basis. The medical checkups include questionnaires, physical measurement (height, body weight, skinfolds, chest and abdominal circumferences), urine and blood tests, ECG and blood pressure (at rest and after exercise), chest X-rays, and physical examination by a physician. The physical fitness test consists of six items: step test, vertical jump, side step, trunk extension, standing trunk flexion, and sit-ups. According to the results of these tests, physical fitness levels are evaluated as "good," "average," and "poor" (3).

A physical exercise program is prescribed for each individual employee according to his physical condition. Health care trainers conduct exercise classes at the branch offices as well as at the health and fitness center on a regular basis. Regular medical checkups and health education are also provided for the employees with medical abnormalities.

Results and Findings

Though the average age of employees who took health care exams increased by 7.2 years, body weight increased by only 1.3kg during this 10-year period. Skin folds also increased,

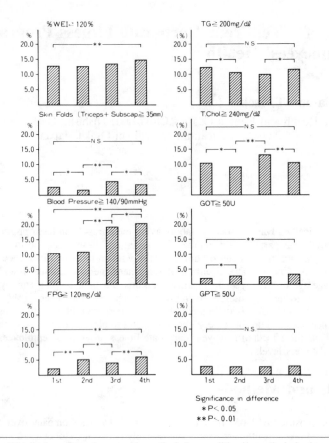

Figure 1. Distribution of employees with medical abnormalities in medical checkup ($N = 1657$).

but only slightly (see Table 1). Resting heart rate decreased while systolic and diastolic blood pressures elevated significantly between the first and fourth exams. Similar results were found in the blood pressures after the Master double two-step test. The indicators of pulmonary function, %VC and FEV 1.0%, improved significantly (see Table 2).

The prevalence of employees who were overweight (%WEI ≥ 120) increased significantly between the first and fourth exams. However, the prevalence of those with obesity (skin folds: triceps + subscapula ≥ 35mm) between the first and fourth exams had no significant change. These results show the preventive effect of a physical exercise program and health education on body fat increase.

The prevalence of abnormal blood pressures and high fasting plasma glucose levels increased significantly. Further medical procedures to cope with these abnormalities should be considered in the near future.

Triglyceride (first exam: 127.1 ± 71.6mg/dl; fourth exam: 124.9 ± 82.6mg/dl, $p <$ .01) and total cholesterol levels (first exam: 197.8 ± 34.4mg/dl; fourth exam 195.4 ± 35.8mg/dl, $p < .01$) decreased significantly. Also, HDL-cholesterol levels which were measured only in the third and fourth exams (third exam: 49.5 ± 13.8mg/dl; fourth exam 51.3 ± 14.7mg/dl, $p < .01$) improved significantly. Our previous data also showed that a physical exercise program improved lipid metabolism among middle-aged employees

Table 1 Change in Age and Physical Characteristics ($N = 1657$)

		1 st Exams	2 nd Exams	3 rd Exams	4 th Exams
Age	(y.o.)	44.5± 2.7	46.9± 3.2*	50.1± 3.5*	51.7± 2.9*†
Body Weight (kg)		60.7± 7.7	61.2± 8.1*	61.6± 8.4	62.0± 7.9*†
%I.B.W.	(%)	105.0±12.4	105.1±12.0	106.4±11.7*	106.9±11.9*†
Chest C.	(cm)	88.0± 4.8	88.7± 4.8*	89.0± 5.8	88.0± 4.8*
Abdom. C.	(cm)	79.5± 7.2	80.2± 6.7*	81.0± 7.3*	81.0± 6.8†
Skin Folds (mm)	Triceps	8.6± 2.6	7.5± 2.3*	10.0± 3.4*	9.4± 3.0*†
	Subscap.	12.6± 4.0	12.3± 4.2*	12.8± 4.2	13.1± 4.3*†
	Abdomen	13.7± 5.7	13.7± 5.5	15.7± 6.3*	16.9± 6.3*†

Values are means± S.D.
Significance in difference from the former exams' value (*$P<0.01$) and between
1st exams' value and 4th exams value (†$P<0.01$)

Table 2 Change in Heart Rate, Blood Pressure, and Pulmonary Function ($N = 1657$)

		1 st Exams	2 nd Exams	3 rd Exams	4 th Exams
Heart Rate	(bpm)	73.2±11.3	72.5±11.1*	72.3±11.2	70.9±10.7*†
B.P. (mmHg) Rest	Systolic	121.2±14.1	120.3±14.4*	125.1±15.2*	127.0±13.8*†
	Diastolic	67.9± 9.8	69.5±10.7*	72.0±12.2*	76.0±10.3*†
B.P. *(mmHg) Imm After	Systolic	143.5±16.0	144.6±18.7*	144.4±19.0	150.9±20.6*†
	Diastolic	69.2±12.1	69.4±11.8	68.1±14.1*	73.2±11.3*†
B.P. *(mmHg) 5mins After	Systolic	122.9±12.9	121.3±13.8*	121.4±15.1	126.4±15.4*†
	Diastolic	70.9±10.4	71.1±10.6	69.9±12.4*	75.5±10.2*†
Pulmonary Function	%V.C.	97.3±16.7	97.0±15.2	109.2±16.3*	110.0±17.0*†
	FEV$_{1.0\%}$	81.7± 7.0	82.9± 8.3*	87.3± 8.6*	82.1± 7.1*†

Values are means± S.D.
Significance in difference from the former exams' value (*$P<0.01$) and between
1st exams' value and 4th exams' value (†$P<0.01$)
* 1st Exams N=1654
  2nd Exams N=1655
  3rd Exams N=1650
  4th Exams N=1645

(2). The improvement of lipid metabolism is expected to prevent possible atherosclerotic diseases such as ischemic heart disease (1). As to the liver function, GOT and GPT were tested. The prevalence of employees with abnormal GOT level (≥ 50) increased significantly. GPT, however, had no marked change between the first and fourth exams. It is necessary to consider how to cope with the alcohol-induced liver disturbances in our corporate health programs, as alcohol is a major cause of liver damage.

The evaluation of the physical fitness tests is shown in Figure 2. The prevalence of the employees with an evaluation of "good" increased markedly between the first and fourth

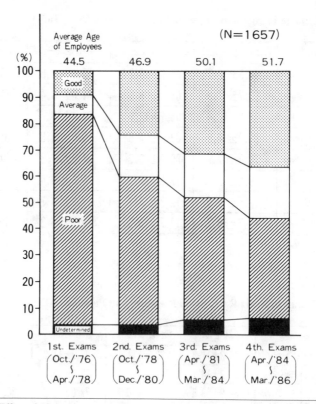

Figure 2. Effect of 10-year corporate fitness program on physical fitness evaluation.

exams (first exam: 9.4%; fourth exam: 37.5%). Further, those with a "poor" rating decreased dramatically from 79.5% to 36.9%. Improved results in the step test in particular during this 10-year period suggest enhanced cardiopulmonary fitness. These results signify the heightened level of overall physical fitness among middle-aged employees through the long-term corporate fitness program.

The benefits of a corporate fitness program are generally thought to be health improvement, decrease of absentee rate, decrease of medical costs, and improvement of employee morale, job performance, and productivity. Our absence rate due to sickness remained low throughout this period despite the increase of the average age of employees (see Figure 3).

Conclusion

This study shows the longitudinal effects of a corporate fitness program on employee's health. These results suggest that a corporate fitness program is effective in improving employees' health and fitness levels and in preventing the progression of adult diseases.

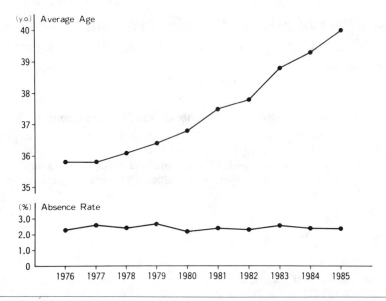

Figure 3. Changes of average age of employees and absence rate due to sickness.

References

1. Gordon, T., Kannel, W.B., Castelli, W.P., Dauber, T.R. Lipoproteins, cardiovascular disease, and death—the Framingham Study. Arch. Intern. Med. 141:1128-1131, 1981.

2. Okada, K., Iseki, T. Physical fitness for middle aged employees with poor health—effect of physical exercise therapy in employees with metabolic disorder. Sumitomo Bull. Industr. Health 20:37-43, 1984.

3. Osaka Gas Health and Fitness Center. Report of 2nd health care exams. Osaka Gas, 1981.

4. Paffenbarger, R.S., Hyde, R.T., Wing, A.L., Hsieh, C.-C. Physical activity, all-cause mortality and longevity of college alumni. N. Eng. J. Med. 314:605-613, 1986.

5. Rudman, W.J. Do onsite health and fitness programs affect worker productivity? Fitness in Bus. 2:2-8, 1987.

6. Shephard, R.J. Practical issues in employee fitness programming. The Physician and Sportsmed. 12:160-166, 1984.

The Effect of a Daily Exercise Program of Industrial Employees on Selected Physical Fitness Components

H. Ruskin, S.T. Halfon, O. Rosenfeld, and G. Tenenbaum

Cosell Center for Physical Education, The Hebrew University of Jerusalem Department of Medical Ecology, School of Public Health, and Community Medicine, Hebrew University—Haddassah Medical School, Jerusalem, Israel, Research Department, Wingate Institute of Physical Education and Sports, Israel

The main purpose of this study, as part of a larger study to determine to what extent a daily program of physical activity in industry will affect psychosocial, functional, and physiological variables of employees, was to estimate the effect of structured physical exercise on selected variables of physical fitness in the work place. The research aim was to estimate these effects while neutralizing the effect of attentiveness to the experimental group and the effect of leisure time physical activity. Also the research aimed to achieve the main purpose of affecting the level of physical fitness through a low-cost system which used workers who functioned as physical training instructors, instead of professional physical education instructors, and a system to reduce dropouts as much as possible.

Methods

During 1984-1985, 540 employees of two pharmaceutical factories of the TEVA Concern participated in a daily structured physical activity program. In order to evaluate the effects of physical activity on the employees' functioning and fitness variables, the participants were randomly divided into two groups of equal size. The experimental group participated in regular physical exercise for 15 min (employer's time) daily, 5 days a week for 7 months, before lunch. The control group was requested to play social games while seated for the same time period. The physical activity program included various stretching and relaxation exercises as well as muscular strength and aerobic exercises. Six exercise charts were prepared, which contained the same basic components but different exercises. The program was carried out by employee-instructors in small units of 15-20 employees. These instructors were trained by the researchers and supervised by a professional teacher of the team. A special program to minimize dropouts was administered. As a result, the adherence rate was 90% throughout the duration of the study. The physical fitness variable changes in the experimental and the control group over the 7-month period were examined by physical fitness examinations before and after the study. Examinations included an ergometric bicycle test to obtain $\dot{V}O_2$max according to the Åstrand protocol (Åstrand, 1960), a grip dynamometer muscular strength test, and a sit-and-reach trunk flexibility test. The results of the pre- and posttests were compared by means of repeated measures MANOVA. The analysis allowed the testing of the group effect, time and reciprocal relation, and group and time over the dependent variables. The other variables, such as occupation (employment category), gender, age, origin, education, and religious status were combined in a multivariable analysis and their specific interactive effect with group and time were also calculated in the multivariate model.

Findings

1. By the end of the study, in comparison to its beginning, there were no significant differences in aerobic capacity between the physical activity–experimental group and the social activity–control group nor between the sexes.

As the age group increased, a significant decline in aerobic fitness was noticed. The young employees (< 39) were at a medium level of aerobic capacity, while the older ones were at a low level in comparison to the aerobic fitness norm of the active population in Israel. In comparison to the "international" (Åstrand) aerobic fitness level, the employees were below average (see Tables 1 and 2).

2. There was a significant improvement in muscular strength as assessed by hand grip among the employees by the end of the study in comparison to its beginning. The most substantial improvement was obtained among the younger males (< 29) and all females in the physical activity group, as opposed to the decline in hand grip among the social activity group employees. Hand grip declined, as expected, with an increase in age. In comparison to national norms, employees in this study were ranked between the 25th and 50th percentiles (see Tables 3 and 4).

3. A relative improvement in flexibility was obtained among the males in all age groups of physical activity. In the social group, the significant improvement was among females over the age of 40. With an increase in age, a decline was recorded in flexibility. However, there were no differences in flexibility as tested by a trunk sit and reach test between the females in the physical and social activity groups where similar results were obtained in all age groups. The flexibility rank of male and female employees in this study was in the 50th percentile in comparison to the national active population (see Tables 5 and 6).

4. In addition to the above mentioned findings, a decrease in weight and skinfolds especially among females and a decrease in the incidence of smoking were found among the physical activity group in comparison to the social activity group.

Table 1 Pre- and Posttests, Aerobic Capacity (Males)

Age group	Social activity		Physical activity	
	Pre	Post	Pre	Post
< 29	33.9 ± 8.0 (7)	31.7 ± 6.0 (7)	39.3 ± 3.2 (4)	40.5 ± 5.1 (4)
30-39	30.0 ± 7.5 (11)	28.8 ± 5.6 (11)	31.3 ± 5.7 (35)	31.8 ± 5.7 (35)
40-49	26.5 ± 7.6 (13)	26.7 ± 7.3 (13)	26.7 ± 7.1 (23)	26.3 ± 4.3 (23)
> 50	23.1 ± 3.4 (9)	23.6 ± 5.8 (9)	24.7 ± 6.2 (20)	25.6 ± 5.2 (20)
Total	28.0 ± 7.6 (40)	27.5 ± 6.6 (40)	28.8 ± 7.0 (82)	29.1 ± 6.4 (82)

Note. Mean and *SD* of $\dot{V}O_2max$ (ml · Kg^{-1} · min^{-1}).

Table 2 Pre- and Posttests, Aerobic Capacity (Females)

Age group	Social activity		Physical activity	
	Pre	Post	Pre	Post
< 29	35.9 ± 6.2 (11)	31.7 ± 6.1 (11)	32.8 ± 7.6 (22)	31.6 ± 7.1 (22)
30-39	29.0 ± 8.2 (6)	27.7 ± 3.6 (6)	28.5 ± 7.2 (26)	27.5 ± 5.8 (26)
40-49	27.1 ± 5.5 (10)	25.4 ± 4.5 (10)	26.1 ± 4.4 (14)	26.1 ± 6.6 (14)
> 50	22.3 ± 7.1 (10)	28.1 ± 10.8 (10)	24.3 ± 5.0 (11)	23.9 ± 4.4 (11)
Total	30.0 ± 7.4 (37)	28.4 ± 7.2 (37)	28.7 ± 7.1 (73)	27.9 ± 6.6 (73)

Note. Mean and *SD* of $\dot{V}O_2$max (ml • Kg^{-1} • min^{-1}).

Table 3 Pre- and Posttest, Hand Grip Muscular Strength (Males)

Age group	Social activity		Physical activity	
	Pre	Post	Pre	Post
< 29	52.4 ± 7.1 (18)	50.5 ± 6.2 (18)	45.4 ± 4.5 (5)	50.4 ± 6.6 (5)
30-39	44.9 ± 6.1 (12)	45.4 ± 10.6 (12)	47.7 ± 6.5 (36)	49.4 ± 6.5 (36)
40-49	44.5 ± 4.4 (15)	47.3 ± 6.5 (15)	43.9 ± 6.9 (25)	44.7 ± 6.5 (25)
> 50	38.9 ± 7.2 (12)	41.9 ± 6.8 (12)	40.8 ± 7.2 (26)	42.2 ± 7.4 (26)
Total	44.4 ± 8.0 (47)	45.9 ± 8.5 (47)	44.6 ± 7.3 (92)	46.1 ± 7.3 (92)

Note. Mean and *SD*, kg.

Table 4 Pre- and Posttest, Hand Grip Muscular Strength (Females)

Age group	Social activity		Physical activity	
	Pre	Post	Pre	Post
< 29	28.5 ± 6.5 (13)	30.1 ± 6.8 (13)	28.6 ± 4.6 (25)	29.4 ± 4.5 (25)
30-39	26.9 ± 4.0 (8)	28.3 ± 5.2 (8)	29.1 ± 4.9 (33)	30.1 ± 5.9 (33)
40-49	22.5 ± 5.6 (15)	23.5 ± 7.0 (15)	25.1 ± 5.7 (18)	27.2 ± 7.2 (18)
> 50	25.5 ± 7.0 (17)	25.7 ± 4.7 (17)	24.5 ± 4.1 (18)	25.6 ± 4.5 (18)
Total	25.6 ± 6.1 (53)	26.6 ± 6.0 (53)	27.3 ± 5.0 (94)	28.5 ± 5.2 (94)

Note. Mean and *SD*, kg.

Table 5 Pre- and Posttests and Trunk Flexibility (Males)

Age group	Social activity		Physical activity	
	Pre	Post	Pre	Post
< 29	56.1 ± 4.6 (8)	56.0 ± 7.4 (8)	49.9 ± 8.7 (5)	53.6 ± 7.0 (5)
30-39	54.1 ± 9.4 (11)	53.5 ± 10.1 (11)	50.9 ± 8.2 (34)	52.8 ± 9.4 (34)
40-49	53.1 ± 8.4 (14)	54.2 ± 8.8 (14)	48.5 ± 2.2 (22)	51.0 ± 7.2 (22)
> 50	46.7 ± 4.3 (10)	51.9 ± 9.0 (10)	45.5 ± 6.9 (21)	49.5 ± 8.3 (21)
Total	52.4 ± 7.7 (43)	51.9 ± 10 (43)	48.8 ± 8.0 (82)	50.5 ± 9.3 (82)

Note. Mean and *SD*, cm.

Table 6   Pre- and Posttests and Trunk Flexibility (Females)

Age group	Social activity		Physical activity	
	Pre	Post	Pre	Post
< 29	53.8 ± 5.7 (12)	59.0 ± 9.4 (12)	54.9 ± 7.0 (24)	56.5 ± 7.7 (24)
30-39	53.5 ± 8.6 (8)	50.6 ± 10 (8)	53.8 ± 7.1 (31)	53.8 ± 9.7 (31)
40-49	53.2 ± 8.4 (14)	54.9 ± 8.4 (14)	54.5 ± 6.3 (18)	56.2 ± 10.5 (8)
> 50	52.0 ± 6.9 (16)	53.3 ± 8.8 (16)	53.9 ± 5.7 (17)	56.2 ± 7.7 (17)
Total	54.4 ± 7.9 (50)	53.4 ± 8.8 (50)	54.3 ± 6.9 (90)	55.4 ± 9 (90)

Note. Mean and *SD*, cm.

Discussion and Conclusion

Technological development in industry has played an important role in creating certain negative influences. Following mechanization, the physical requirement at work has decreased. Work that previously required movement and physical activity is performed now by automatic and computerized machines. This study tried to affect the physical condition of the employees in such an industry by raising the level of certain physical fitness components through systematic and controlled daily physical activity during working hours and thus lower stress, reduce the level of emotional burnout, anxiety, and depression, decrease health problems (including risk factors for cardiovascular diseases), improve job satisfaction and motivation at work, reduce absenteeism due to illness, and modify smoking habits (Keir, 1972; Pauly, 1982; Shepard, 1986). All of these will be reported separately. This report is limited to the issue of the appropriate kind of intervention through controlled and systematic physical activity.

In order to motivate workers to participate in physical activity programs, an increased level of awareness was necessary to stress the importance of and the need for these activities during working hours. The high adherence rate (90%) reached in the study proved that this process was conducted successfully. Another important consideration was the implementation of a system that would be available without direct cost for industry by the use of employees as trained physical instructors in a very basic and simple program of activities. These trained employees instructed their fellow workers in small units in accordance with this simple, structured, and systematic program during the employer's time.

Compared to the active Israeli population, the physical fitness level of the subjects in this study was found to be moderate to low. As a result of the intervention, changes were recorded only in flexibility and muscular strength, and no changes were found in aerobic capacity. Although the activity program was quite simple, a medical and physiological screening test was conducted by the researchers in order to detect employees with chronic diseases and measure the effects of health problems.

It should be noted that the program lasted for 7 months only and served mainly for the development of a model for future implementation. The researchers did not expect this to constitute sufficient time to affect significant physiological changes. Also, a period of 15 min in which only 3-4 min were devoted to aerobic exercise was not expected to create a cardiovascular endurance training effect, as the results of the study indeed proved (Åstrand, 1972; Shephard, 1968, 1982). Therefore, the main significant effects were in muscular strength and flexibility. It is also important to note that whenever an aerobic effort is being introduced to such a program, there must be medical-physiological screening available, and this may increase the cost of such a project or prevent a larger number of employees from participating in such a program for different reasons. However, if an activity program excludes an aerobic component, which requires at least a daily duration of at least 15 min, it may enable the implementation of such a program under less restricting conditions, helping both management and employees to enter more willingly into such a program.

The researchers thus recommend that the issue of an aerobic component in employee physical fitness programs be further explored, and until more evidence is available regarding its feasibility, a short program of 15 min of the employer's time should include mainly selected muscular strength, flexibility, and relaxing exercises. The program should avoid the exposure of employees of different sexes, age groups, and health levels to strenuous aerobic and cardiovascular endurance exercises, which demand more screening and control and may not be available in an extensive and mass employee fitness program.

Daily Physical Activity Program
for Industrial Employees

S.T. Halfon, O. Rosenfeld, H. Ruskin, and G. Tenenbaum
Department of Medical Ecology and Occupational Health, Hebrew
University—Hadassah School of Public Health and Community Medicine,
Jerusalem and Cosell Physical Education Center, Hebrew University,
Jerusalem, Israel, Wingeit Institute for Physical Education and Sport,
Netania, Israel

In many countries physical activity during work was found to be a contributing factor in the improvement of the functioning and health of employees. The aim of the present study was (a) to introduce a program for physical activity during work and to evaluate the contributions to health and (b) to establish an organizational model of physical activity that could be adapted to the socioeconomic system in Israel and adopted by Israel industries. The project was carried out during 1985-1986 in two TEVA pharmaceutical factories. In technologically developed countries, extensive physical effort has been replaced by machines. Furthermore, modern lifestyle has been characterized by a low level of physical activity, increased mental tension, and anxiety and pressure on muscles due to more static work (7). Physical activity has a beneficial influence on the psychological state and induces a temporary feeling of well-being (8, 9). Epidemiological studies have indicated a low level of risk factors for cardiovascular disease in subjects involved in physical activity (5). It was shown that physical activity programs during work increased productivity (11), and the feeling of job satisfaction and efficiency at work (6).

The study group comprised workers of two pharmaceutical factories (TEVA), 264 from Factory 1 and 276 from Factory 2. The male:female ratio was 1:15 and 0:79, respectively. Approximately half of the employees in both factories were under the age of 40 while the other half were older than 40. Classification by occupation showed a similar distribution of employees among various occupations in both factories.

Methods

The study was carried out over 7 months during 1985-1986. The influence of physical activity programs on sports motivation, work load, and feelings of fatigue during work was evaluated by questionnaires. The perception of work load (WL) and fatigue during work (WF) were self-reported in the questionnaires. The information was obtained three times: before the study, 3 months after the study was initiated, and at the end of the study. Each answer was an employee estimation of the mean WL and WF during the 3-month period preceding the collection of the data. The answers on WL and WF were ranked on a scale of 1 (high) to 6 (low). The mean WL and mean WF for the group were calculated from the individual reporting. Work efficiency (WE) was calculated from the equation WL/WF. If WL increased and WF decreased, the WE also increased and vice versa.

Mental Fatigue

The index of mental fatigue was based on 27 questions in which personal feelings during work were reported. The questionnaire was given twice (before and after the test) to each participant in the study. The answers were based on personal feelings during the past 4 months. The questions related to lack of concentration during work, feelings of monotony at work, lack of job satisfaction, bad temper, insomnia, anxiety, low self-esteem, physical complaints, and low work capacity. Each variable was examined on a scale of 6; the individual maximum score was 162. For the analysis, the mean score for the group was calculated. The homogenicity coefficient for all the questions was alpha = 0.87.

Physical Fatigue

This was reported in 14 questions consisting of information on chest and back pains, fatigue during work, finger tremors, health problems including cardiovascular disease, cancer, and other chronic conditions. Each variable was ranked on a scale of 6. The sum of all the answers for each subject gave a score of 84. The homogenicity coefficient was alpha = 0.79. Job satisfaction was examined in 28 questions related to job satisfaction, safety of work, lack of interest, low productivity, importance of work, working conditions, fatigue, monotony of work, and plans for change of work place. The maximum individual score was 168 and the homogenicity coefficient was alpha = 0.78.

The physical activity program was held 15 min before lunch time 5 days a week over 7 months. The program included a warm-up, stretching and relaxation exercises for trunk muscles, muscular strengthening exercises, and cardiopulmonary activities consisting of runs for 3-7 min.

The control group program consisted of social games and activities requiring a seated position, which were given during the same period of time (i.e., 15 min before lunch) and which included cards, chess, checkers, and reading newspapers or journals. The employees in the control group were forbidden to do any physical work during the 15 min of the program.

Results

The differences between the study and control groups in pre- and posttesting were examined by an analysis of variance for repeated measurements.

Work load (WL)—The feeling of WL increased progressively during work hours and throughout the study period. The study group reported higher WL than the control group ($F = 25.9$, $df = 400$, $p < .001$). The WL at the end of study periods during the work day can be seen in Figure 1. In both groups, females reported more WL than males during the study period. ($F = 3.9$, $df = 400$, $p < .005$).

Work fatigue (WF)—work fatigue before the initiation of the program was reported to be similar by both the study group and the control group during the work day. At the end of the study, the feeling of WF increased in both groups, but in the controls the WF increased more during the work days, especially after lunch. In the study group the increase in WF only slowly increased after lunch. The differences between the study and control groups were examined by an analysis of variance for repeated measurements, and it was found that both were statistically significant ($F = 53.9$, $df = 400$, $p < .001$; $F = 62.9$, $df = 400$, $p < .001$).

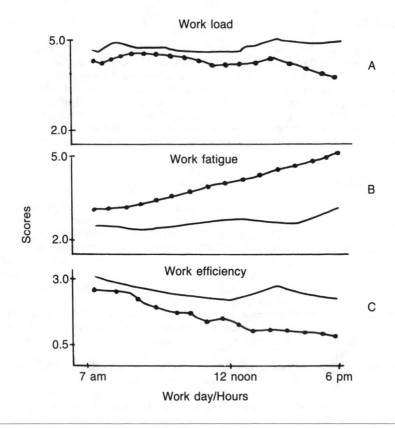

Figure 1.   Changes in work load, work fatigue, and work efficiency (posttest): ———— study group, •—•—•—• control group.

Work efficiency (WE)—The participants in the physical activity program reported higher WE than the control group ($F = 91.4, p < .001$). The differences between the two groups were higher, especially during the afternoon work hours compared with the morning work hours ($F = 19.0, p < .001$). The differences between male and female employees in WE were not statistically significant ($F = .36$ ns). A significant interaction was observed between the variables of group, period, and work hours ($F = 16.7, p < .001$).

Mental and physical fatigue (see Figure 2)—Before the physical activity program was introduced, both the study and control groups showed a similar mean score for mental fatigue ($F = 2.6$ ns). During the study period, mental fatigue increased and subjects reported lower scores than in the pretest. However, the mean score for the control group was significantly lower then the mean score for the study group ($F = 4.5, p < .03$). Physical fatigue showed similar patterns: a decrease in the mean score of both groups during the study. Among the controls, the score decreased significantly more in the posttest than among the study group ($F = 16.4, p < .001$).

Job satisfaction and motivation for work (see Figure 3)—In the pretest, both groups showed similar scores. At the end of the study, clear mean differences were observed between the study and control groups. Among controls, the mean score was significantly lower than in the study group ($F = 7.5, p < .01$).

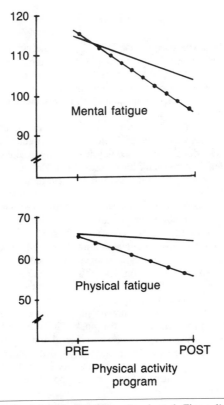

Figure 2. Changes in mental and physical fatigue (see legend, Figure 1).

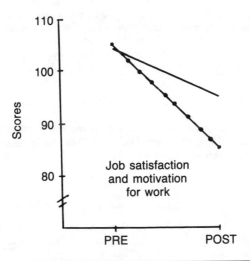

Figure 3. Changes in job satisfaction (see legend, Figure 1).

Discussion

The results of the present study show that daily physical activity programs incorporated within working hours are acceptable by both employer and employees. In modern industry, one of the problems concerning health is the sedentary nature of the work. The selection of pharmaceutical industries for physical activity programs was based on this problem. The high level of professional education and discipline was another factor in the selection of pharmaceutical factories for the study.

The initial and probably the most important motivation in introducing physical activity programs for the employees was the inverse relationship between physical fitness and risk profiles for coronary heart disease. Increased physical activity in adults has beneficial effects on lowering the incidence of coronary heart disease (3). Previous studies in Israel have reported that the fatal coronary heart disease rate was 2-4 times higher among sedentary workers than among non-sedentary workers in rural collective settlements (kibbutzim) (1). The concept of industry-supported physical fitness programs is receiving increasing attention and several programs have reported beneficial effects on employees.

The results of the present study clearly indicate that physical activity programs introduced during work decrease the feelings of fatigue and increase work efficiency. Other studies have also associated this reduction of fatigue with an increased work capacity (10), reduction in body fat, increased job satisfaction, less absenteeism due to illness (6), and fewer work accidents (11).

The results of the study showed a progressive increase in work load reported by the employees. These were reflected by an increase in physical and mental complaints and decrease in job satisfaction and motivation for work. The effects of the regular physical activity program were measured by a decrease in mental and physical fatigue compared to the control group. Current research has demonstrated that regular aerobic and physical exercises have a positive influence on mental health, anxiety, depression, self-confidence, and body image (2). This beneficial effect in mental health was followed by improved work performance (13).

In other studies, physical activity was a compensation for monotonous work and lack of satisfaction (4). Physical activity has a protective effect on physical complaints. During the period when work load and work fatigue increased, the employees participating in the physical activity program reported fewer physical complaints such as back pains, headaches, or insomnia. These confirmed previous findings that physical activity during work improves employees' mental and physical health. One of the problems of physical activity during work in industries is how to increase employees' sports motivation. The interest in sports activities is limited, generally due to fatigue after work or family problems.

Acknowledgments

The National Committee for the Preventive Action and Research of Health in Labor; Ministry of Labor and Welfare, The State of Israel; and factories of TEVA pharmaceutical complex in the cities of Jerusalem and Kfar Saba.

References

1. Brunner, D., Manelis, G., Modan, M., Levi, S. Physical activity at work and the incidence of myocardial infarction, angina pectoris and death due to ischemic heart disease. J. Chron. Dis. 27:217-233, 1974.

2. Buffone, G.W. Exercise as a therapeutic adjunct. In: Silva, J.M., Weinberg, R.S., eds. Psychological foundations of sport. Human Kinetics, Champaign, IL, 1984: 445-451.

3. Cooper, K.H., Pollock, M.L., Martin, R.P., White, S.R., Linnerud, A.L., Jackson, A. Physical fitness levels vs. selected coronary risk factors: a cross sectional study. J. Am. Med. Assoc. 236:166-169, 1977.

4. Folkins, C.H., Sime, W.E. Physical fitness training and mental health. Am. Psychol. 36:373-389, 1981.

5. Goode, R.C., Firstbrook, J., Shephard, R.J. Effects of exercise and a cholesterol-free diet on human serum lipids. Can. J. Physiol. Pharmacol. 44:575-580, 1966.

6. Heinzleimann, F. Response to physical activity programs and their effects on health behavior. Pub. Health Rep. 85:905-911, 1970.

7. Howard, J., Mikalacki, A. Fitness and employee productivity. Can. J. Appl. Sport Sci. 43:190-197, 1979.

8. Layman, R.M. Psychological effects of physical activity. Ex. Sports Sci. Rev. 2:33-70, 1974.

9. Michael, E.D. Stress adaptation through exercise. Res. Q. 28:50, 1957.

10. Shephard, R., Cox, M., Corey, P. Fitness program participation: its effect on worker performance. J. Occup. Med. 23:359-367, 1981.

11. Vermeersch, J.A., Feeney, M.J., Wesner, K.M., Dahl, T. Productivity improvement and job satisfaction among Public Health Nutritionists. J. Am. Diet. Assoc. 57:637-640, 1979.

The Effect of Physical Intervention on Industry Workers: Their Needs, Habits, and Desire for Recreational Physical Activity

O. Rosenfeld, H. Ruskin, S.T. Halfon, and G. Tenenbaum

Hebrew University, Jerusalem, and Wingate Institute, Netanya, Israel

Intervention programs in industry have shown that physical activity positively affects the willingness of the worker to take part in motor activity during work and leisure times (2, 8, 15, 17). Perceived willingness, necessity, habits, and intensity of physical activity are divided into two dimensions: realistic and ideal (7). Haller and Miller (7) maintained that the ideal aspiration for physical activity should not be affected by environmental and social constraints. However, realistic aspirations are more self- and environment dependent.

An additional dimension that affects motor outcome is the intensity in which one is engaged in motor activity. Sharkey (14) has suggested that intensity is a function of duration, load, and frequency. The higher each of these components is, the higher the overall intensity of the activity. The index of physical intensity has rarely been taken into account in studies of the industrial worker, and therefore the effect of intervention programs on this is unknown.

The main purpose of this study was to examine the effect of a 7-month structured physical activity (PA) program upon perceived willingness and the necessity for physical activity at work and leisure and to examine real-ideal dimensions of PA aspirations compared to the affect of social activity (SA) upon the same variables.

Methods

Sample

Five hundred twenty-two workers from two pharmaceutical industries began the program, of whom 267 were females and 255 males. The age mean was about 40 years. During the 7 months, 11.7% dropped out as a result of chronic disease, resignation from work, and refusal to take part in the program.

Variables and Instrumentation

Perceived willingness and necessity for physical activity (PA) was the second factor derived from the Worker's Functioning Questionnaire (WFQ) using an oblique rotation through a factor-analysis procedure. Each item contained ratings ranging from 1 (never) to 6 (always). The total scores were between 9 and 54. The higher the score, the higher the perceived willingness and necessity for PA.

Two additional items were related to the actual and ideal dimensions of PA during leisure time. The workers were asked to rate each from 1 (not active at all) to 9 (very active). The gap between the actual and ideal dimensions was added into the analysis.

The intensity of the PA was calculated by multiplying the difficulty level by time (duration) and frequency. This index was applied to ball games, jogging, gymnastics, swimming, and tennis.

Treatment, Procedure, and Analysis

The subjects were randomly assigned to two groups within each factory. The experimental group was exposed to a physical program consisting of mobilization and relaxation of strained body muscles. The exercises were carried out for 15 min five times a week during work hours. The control group was exposed to static social activity at the same time as the physical activities of the experimental group.

The physical program was carried out by workers within the factories who were trained to serve as physical instructors. The instructors were chosen on the basis of popularity, leadership, and acceptance by fellow workers.

The physical program was designed to fit the characteristics of the workers' conditions at work. The program consisted of three components: aerobics, strength, and flexibility. The exercises were performed 15 min prior to lunch time. Approximately one third of the time was allocated to each of the PA components.

The behavioral components were examined at the beginning, middle, and end of the experiment. Thus, a repeated measures MANOVA by group (physical vs. social), period (beginning, middle, and end), and gender (male vs. female) was applied to the data.

Results

The repeated measures MANOVA applied to the perceived willingness and necessity for PA showed a significant effect for period (pre- and posttest) [$F(1,386) = 36.9; p = .000$] and a significant Group $\times$ Period interaction [$F(1.36) = 27.3; p = .000$]. These two effects are demonstrated in Figure 1.

After 7 months, perceived willingness increased by 5% (from 62.1% to 67.0% of the maximal rate). However, the significant interaction indicates that the main increase was obtained by the physical workers ($\Delta = 9.7\%$) as opposed to the social workers ($\Delta = 0.21\%$).

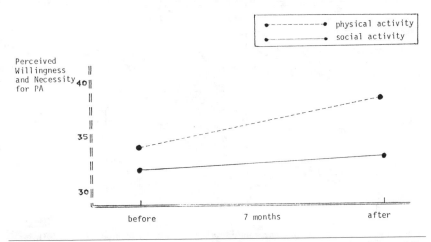

Figure 1. Perceived willingness and necessity for PA by period and intervention (PA vs. SA).

The two groups (PA and SA) and the two periods (pre- and posttest) were not related to gender and age.

Considering the ideal and real dimensions of physical activity, the MANOVA has indicated only a period effect for the ideal dimension. Both groups expressed higher ideal aspirations at the end (61.1%) of the intervention as compared to the beginning stage (57.8%). However, the same analysis on the realistic aspirations for PA indicated a period effect [$F(1,393) = 59.2; p = .000$], Group $\times$ Period effect [$F(1,393) = 20.1; p = .000$] and Group $\times$ Gender $\times$ Age $\times$ Period effect [$F(3,393) = 2.6; p = .05$]. For reasons of simplicity, the four-way interaction is presented in Figure 2.

Both groups expressed an increase in real PA of 7.7% from the start to the end of the study. The physical group increased by 13.3% while the social group by only 2.2%. The four-way interaction shows that out of all the participants in both groups, females aged 20-29 (the youngest) who exercised reported the most substantial positive change in PA from the start to the end of the study ($\Delta = 26.6\%$) followed by females aged 30-39 ($\Delta = 16.6\%$) who exercised, males aged 30-39 ($\Delta = 15.6\%$) who exercised, and males aged 50-65 ($\Delta = 12.2\%$) who exercised. In contrast, males aged 50-65 in the social group decreased in PA ($\Delta = -8.8\%$) followed by the social group females aged 30-39 ($\Delta = -3.4\%$), social group females aged 40-49 ($\Delta = -2.3\%$), and social group males aged

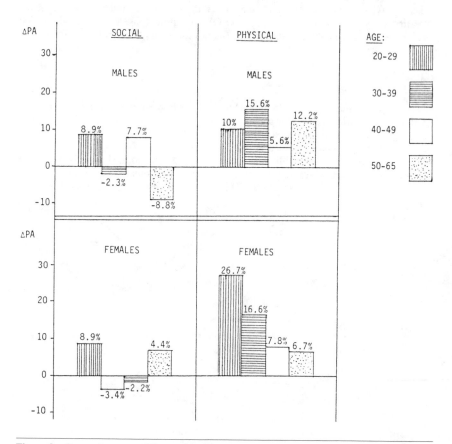

Figure 2.   Pre- and posttest differences in leisure physical activity by group (PA vs. SA), gender, and age.

30-39. As a result, the gap between the ideal and the real PA dimensions decreased substantially more in the physical group compared to the social group at the end of the study in relation to the beginning of the study [$F(1,392) = 6.5$; $p = .01$] (see Figure 3).

MANOVA applied to the intensity of PA in males and females separately has indicated that in females, Period × Group effects were statistically significant [$F(1,233) = 3.26$; $p = .05$]. This interaction is presented in Figure 4.

The results indicate that females engaged in PA increased leisure PA intensity during the study by 6% compared to SA females, who decreased −0.91%. A similar analysis

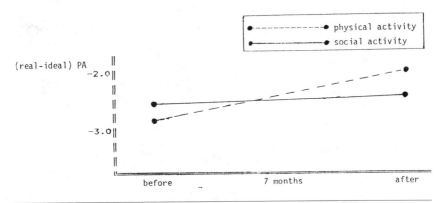

Figure 3.   PA (real-ideal) before and after interventions by group (PA vs. SA).

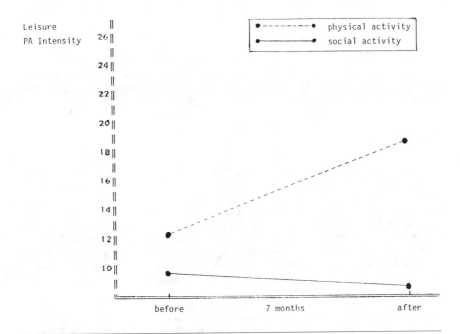

Figure 4.   Leisure intensity in females by intervention (PA vs. SA) and period (pre- and posttest).

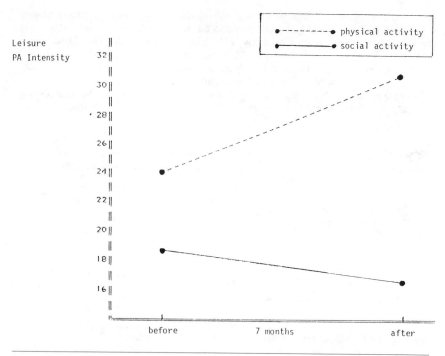

Figure 5. Leisure PA intensity in males by intervention (PA vs. SA) and period (pre- and posttest).

for males revealed significant Group × Period effects [$F(1,222) = 4.99; p = .03$]. This is presented in Figure 5. The results indicate that males engaged in PA increased their leisure PA intensity during the study by 7.3% while those engaged in SA decreased by −2.2%.

Discussion

The results of the study clearly indicate that physical intervention in the pharmaceutical industries increases the willingness and necessity for PA more than SA. Physical intervention was also found to modify burnout, anxiety, stress, and the depression of workers (13). This has probably affected the willingness to perform motor tasks more than social intervention. Physical intervention was also found to decrease health disorders, fatigue, and work-perceived efficiency (14). The results obtained in this study were also evident in other studies conducted in the industry (1, 5, 11, 17, 19). It is also believed that PA was associated with positive feedback from these workers. Together with physiological, psychological, and social need fulfillment, there was a stronger willingness and necessity to participate and continue in leisure PA.

The exposure to physical and social interventions causes a positive change in ideal PA. However, the most substantial change has occurred in the real dimension, particularly in workers who were exposed to physical intervention. These findings are supported by Parker's (12) theory, which clarifies such a behavioral pattern by two mechanisms: (a) spillover—exposure to PA has been extended to similar leisure activity and (b) compensation—increased

PA resulted from absence of activity during working time. These findings are supported by other studies as well (6, 9, 19). Since SA workers were not exposed to any physical activity during work hours and still reported on a minor real PA increase, their behavior may be explained better by the spillover mechanism rather than compensation mechanisms. It is also the physical and not the social intervention that modified psychological stress and burnout thus causing a positive attitude change toward physical activity, particularly in the real dimension. However, it seems that social and educational intervention support an alteration of PA habits (3, 6, 9) but not as dramatically as physical intervention. This explains the reduction of the real-ideal PA gap in the physical group compared to the social group. This is theoretically supported by Shephard (16).

Both males and females of the physical group improved their leisure PA activity (LPAA) compared to the social workers. Males who usually enjoy more leisure time after working hours increased their absolute PA intensity similarly to females. However, in absolute terms their PA was much more intensive. It should be noted that social workers have shown a small decrease in LPAA, which supports the notion that LPAA requires more time and experience to be positively altered (4, 10).

References

1. Allen, R.J. Human stress: its nature and control. University of Maryland: Burgess, 1969.
2. Collis, L. Employee fitness. Ottawa: Department of Health and Welfare, 1977.
3. Deci, E.L. Intrinsic motivation. New York: Plenum Press, 1975.
4. Eitzenen, D., Sage, H. Sociology of American sport. Dubuque, IA: Brown, 1978.
5. Fielding, J. Effectiveness of employee health improvement programs. J. Occup. Med. 24:910-912, 1982.
6. Groves, D.L. A system analysis of benefits from the industrial recreation environment. J. Environ. Sys. 10:1-15, 1980.
7. Haller, A.O., Miller, I.W. The occupational aspiration scale: theory, structure and correlates. Cambridge, MA: Schenkman, 1971.
8. Heinzelman, F., Bagley, R. Response to physical activity programs and their effects on health behavior. Pub. Health Rep. 25:905-922, 1970.
9. Hunt, S., Brooks, K. Perceptions of work and leisure—a study of industrial workers. Rec. Manag. 213:31-35, 1980.
10. Luschen, G., Sage, G. Handbook of science of sport. Stipes, 1981.
11. McPherson, P. Psychological effects of an exercise program for post-infarct and normal adult men. J. Sports Med. Phys. Fit. 7:61-66, 1976.
12. Parker, S.R. The future of work and leisure. MacGibbon & Kee, 1971.
13. Rosenfeld, O. The effect of physical activity on the functioning of industrial workers. Jerusalem, Israel: Hebrew University: 1988. Dissertation.
14. Sharkey, J.B. Fitness and work capacity. Washington, DC: Forest Service, Department of Agriculture, 1977.
15. Shephard, R.J. Fitness and health in industry. Toronto, Ontario, Canada: School of Physical & Health Education, University of Toronto, 1986.
16. Shephard, R.J., Corey, P., Cox, M. Health hazard appraisal: the influence of an employee fitness programme. Can. J. Pub. Health 73:183-187, 1972.

17. Shephard, R.J., Morgan, P., Finncance, R., Schimmelfing, L. Factors influencing recruitment to an occupational fitness program. J. Occup. Med. 22:389-398, 1980.

18. Staines, G.L. Spillover vs. compensation: a review of the literature on the relationships between work and non-work. Hum. Relat. 33:111-130, 1980.

19. Wright, C.C. Cost containment through health promotion programs. J. Occup. Med. 24:965-968, 1982.

Physical Fitness of Nursery Governesses

M. Shimaoka, S. Hiruta, Y. Ono, K. Shimaoka, and K. Yabe

Nagoya University, Furocho, Chikusa-ku, Nagoya, Japan

The literature of cross-sectional studies of normal persons after 30 years of age clearly indicates a decline in physical fitness with increasing age (1, 2, 7, 10, 12), but change with age in physical fitness of working women doing the same job has not been clearly studied. We have previously reported that nursery governesses describe their occupational activities as a moderate to heavy level of daily physical activity in energy expenditure (14, 15). Accordingly, this study was designed to examine physical fitness of nursery governesses and to compare the findings with those for other groups of the population.

Methods

Two hundred sixty-seven nursery governesses aged 20-47 in Nagoya city participated as subjects in this study. The subjects underwent a medical exam and anthropometric and physical fitness measurements during July 4-7, 1987. Height and weight were measured and skinfold thicknesses were obtained from the sum of thicknesses at the triceps and subscapular. Each subject performed 9-minute submaximal rides on a bicycle ergometer (Combi Aerobike 700) to calculate maximal oxygen uptake ($\dot{V}O_2max$). The subjects began pedaling at 25 watt load (50 rpm) and the work load, controlled by computer program not to exceed 70% HRmax, was increased every 3 min. Right and left grip strength and back strength were measured. Explosive strength was measured by measuring height of vertical jump by using a jump meter (Takei Co. Ltd.). Flexibility was measured by measuring the length of trunk extension and standing trunk flexion. The number of subjects for every measurement in each age group was presented in Table 1.

Differences between the mean of nursery governesses (MNG) and the norm of Japanese women (NJW) reported by Physical Fitness Laboratory, Tokyo Metropolitan University (12). was evaluated by a test of hypothesis concerning mean for each measurement. Difference between the MNG of two different age groups was evaluated by a t-test for each measurement.

Results

Age, years of employment, and the physical feature of subjects in each age group are presented in Table 2, along with the NJW for height, weight, and skinfold thickness. The MNG for height and weight were similar to the NJW in the same age group except height in the 25-29 age group and weight in the 30-34 age group. The MNG for skinfold thickness was lower than the NJW in each age group except for the 20-24 age group and significantly lower in the 30-34 age group. The means and standard deviations (SD) of physical fitness variables achieved by the subjects are presented in Table 3 along with the NJW. The MNG for trunk extension, standing trunk flexion, and vertical jump tended to decrease

Table 1   The Number of Subjects in Each Age Group

Measurements	Age group (yr)						
	20-24	25-29	30-34	35-39	40-44	45-49	Total
Height	68	70	54	49	18	6	267
Weight	68	70	54	49	18	6	267
Skinfold thickness	65	67	54	47	18	6	259
Back strength	68	69	49	48	18	6	259
Grip strength	68	70	54	49	17	6	266
$\dot{V}O_2$max	61	59	45	44	15	4	230
$\dot{V}O_2$max/W	61	59	45	44	15	4	230
Vertical jump	65	66	52	45	18	6	254
Standing trunk flexion	68	69	51	49	18	6	263
Trunk extension	68	69	50	48	18	6	261

Table 2   Age, Years of Employment, and Physical Features of Subjects

	Age group (yr)					
	20-24	25-29	30-34	35-39	40-44	45-49
Nursery Governesses						
Age (yr)	22.4	26.7	32.2	36.8	42.0	45.7
	1.3	1.4	1.4	1.4	1.3	0.7
Years of employment	1.8	5.8	10.8	12.8	14.8	19.8
	1.5	1.8	2.1	4.6	5.0	4.5
Height (cm)	156.8	154.6*	155.0	154.5	153.9	153.5
	5.6	4.9	5.1	5.4	5.0	3.8
Weight (kg)	50.6	49.7	49.8*	51.7	52.7	53.5
	6.1	6.6	6.3	6.5	6.8	7.4
Skinfold thickness (mm)	33.3	31.5	30.7**	35.7	35.4	39.2
	9.2	11.3	8.1	11.2	11.8	8.4
Norm						
Height (cm)	156.4	155.9	155.0	154.2	153.5	152.5
	4.7	4.7	4.7	4.7	4.6	4.6
Weight (kg)	50.6	50.9	51.6	52.2	52.4	52.5
	5.4	5.7	6.1	6.3	6.4	6.4
Skinfold thickness (mm)	31.5	34.0	36.8	36.8	40.4	40.4
	9.8	12.5	13.1	13.1	13.6	13.6

Note. Values are means (upper) and *SD*s (lower). Skinfold thickness is the sum of thick-nesses at triceps and subscuplar.

*$p < .05$, **$p < .01$, significant compared to the norm.

with age. On the other hand, the MNG for grip strength and back strength did not decrease until subjects reached the 35-39 age group. The MNG for $\dot{V}O_2$max/w did not decrease until subjects reached the 40-44 age group. The MNG for back strength in the 40-44 age group was significantly lower than in each group in the 20-39 age range, respectively. The MNG in the 45-49 age groups were lower than those in the other age groups for all fitness measurements except standing trunk flexion.

In comparison with the NJW, the MNG for back strength was higher in every age group and significantly higher in the 20-39 age range. On the other hand, the MNG for standing

Table 3 Physical Fitness Measurements of Subjects

	Age group (yr)					
	20-24	25-29	30-34	35-39	40-44	45-49
Nursery governesses						
Back strength (kg)	88.7*	91.2**	89.4**	89.7**	77.4	78.7
	19.5	21.0	20.2	23.2	19.5	10.0
Grip strength (kg)	28.8*	29.4	29.7	29.0	28.3	26.9
	4.2	4.1	4.1	4.4	4.0	4.0
$\dot{V}O_2$max (L/min)	1.70	1.67	1.73**	1.82**	1.84**	1.61*
	0.36	0.31	0.43	0.42	0.37	0.24
$\dot{V}O_2$max/W (ml/kg/min)	33.6*	33.5	34.6**	35.1**	34.0**	31.1*
	6.3	5.8	6.6	6.9	5.4	5.2
Vertical jump (cm)	40.3**	40.5	38.2	37.2**	34.6	30.3
	4.9	5.0	4.3	5.2	4.7	4.6
Standing trunk flexion (cm)	12.9**	13.6	12.2	10.8**	9.1**	9.9
	6.5	6.8	6.3	6.8	7.8	4.5
Trunk extension (cm)	48.3**	46.8**	42.6**	40.7**	36.7**	30.0
	6.7	8.0	6.6	10.2	8.3	6.1
Norm						
Back strength (kg)	83.0	80.0	79.0	77.0	72.0	68.0
	18.9	19.0	18.9	19.0	18.0	16.5
Grip strength (kg)	30.3	30.2	30.1	29.7	28.7	27.6
	5.0	5.1	5.1	5.0	4.8	4.7
$\dot{V}O_2$max (L/min)	1.80	1.65	1.51	1.38	1.30	1.20
	0.34	0.34	0.34	0.34	0.34	0.34
$\dot{V}O_2$max/W (ml/kg/min)	35.7	33.5	30.8	28.5	26.4	24.8
	5.4	6.0	6.0	6.0	6.0	6.0
Vertical jump (cm)	44.0	40.5	37.0	34.5	33.0	31.0
	6.5	6.2	6.3	6.1	6.3	5.6
Standing trunk flexion (cm)	16.4	14.7	13.5	12.6	12.1	11.9
	6.3	6.2	6.2	6.1	6.0	5.8
Trunk extension (cm)	55.6	51.9	45.2	37.0	31.2	27.5
	8.2	8.1	6.8	5.4	4.8	4.3

Note. Values are means (upper) and *SD*s (lower).

*$p < .05$, **$p < .01$, compared to the norm.

trunk flexion was lower in every age group and significantly lower in the 20-24, 35-39, and 40-44 age groups. For grip strength, the MNG was significantly lower in the 20-24 age group. For vertical jump, the MNG was significantly lower in 20-24 age group and significantly higher in the 35-39 age group. For trunk extension, the MNG was significantly lower in the 20-34 age range and significantly higher in the 35-44 age range. For $\dot{V}O_2max/W$, the MNG was significantly lower in the 20-24 age group and significantly higher in the 30-49 age range.

Discussion

The MNGs for trunk extension, standing trunk flexion, and vertical jump tended to decrease with age, as found in the other cross-sectional studies (12, 17). The MNG for $\dot{V}O_2max/W$ tended to be stable from 20 to 44 years of age and that in the 45-49 age group was the lowest of all age groups. Several reports showed that the levels of physical fitness in the habitually active were superior to the sedentary in the same age group (2, 5, 9). Profant et al. (13) reported that mean $\dot{V}O_2max/W$ of active women in the 40-59 age range was higher than or similar to that of sedentary women 10 years younger. Drinkwater et al. (6) reported that habitual levels of activity rather than age per se determines levels of $\dot{V}O_2max$ for women in the 20-49 age range. In addition, the percentage of the subjects having habitual training and sports in each age group was only between 9% and 24% (mean 14%). Therefore, from the findings in this study that nursery governesses had a stable mean $\dot{V}O_2max/W$ in 20-44 age range, it is suggested that they have about the same level of physical activities in their daily work regardless of age.

The mean of some physical fitness variables of nursery governesses in this study differed from the norms. The MNG for $\dot{V}O_2max/W$ in the 20-24 age group were significantly lower than the NJW and were similar to the means of students (19-20 years) (3, 8), sedentary group (20-29 years) (2) and average group (20-24 years) (10) as previously reported. On the other hand, the MNG for $\dot{V}O_2max/W$ in the 30-49 age range was significantly higher than the NJW and the MNG in the 30-39 age range is higher than the level for the physically active (29-39 years) (2, 13) or equal to those with scores evaluated as "very good" (35-39 years) (10). In our previous study, energy expenditures of nursery governesses (17 women, 20-39 years old) were 2,034 kcal (0.0291 kcal/kg/min) in a day and 906 kcal (0.0390 kcal/kg/min) during work (15). Their intensity of daily energy expenditure is found classifiable as moderate to heavy according to a report of The Ministry of Health and Welfare (18). Several reports described that members of primitive societies and physical laborers having a physically active life had higher scores for $\dot{V}O_2max/W$ or fitness measurements concerning aerobic power than sedentary groups (4, 11, 16). In addition, our previous study showed that four 20-year-old beginning nursery governesses having lower $\dot{V}O_2max/W$ than the average got about 10% higher $\dot{V}O_2max/W$ than those initial scores when tested one year later (14). Therefore, it was suggested that higher mean $\dot{V}O_2max/W$ of subjects in 30-49 age range might be caused by their relatively intense physical activities in their daily work for over 10 years.

The MNG for back strength for each group in the 20-39 age range remained stable at 89-91 kg and was significantly higher than the norm. The scores were similar to the mean back strength of women working in the primary industry in 21-24 age range (17). According to our previous studies, such nursery governesses spent 31% of their working time in a bending posture and another 11% holding children (15). Therefore, such work may account for the higher back strength of the subjects regardless of age.

In this study, the reason some fitness scores of nursery governesses in the 20-40 age range remained stable and why they scored higher than the norm for some fitness measurements in the 30-44 age range appears to be related to their work. It would then appear that levels of physical fitness for nursery governesses are determined by habitual levels of occupational activity rather than by age.

References

1. Åstrand, P.-O., Åstrand, I.H., Kilbom, A. Reduction in maximal oxygen uptake with age. J. Appl. Physiol. 35:649-654, 1973.

2. Atomi, Y., Miyashita, M. Maximal aerobic power of Japanese active and sedentary adult females of different ages (20 to 62 years). Med. Sci. Sports 6:223-225, 1974.

3. Bale, P., Colley, E., Mayhew, J.L. Relationships among physique, strength, and performance in women students. J. Sports Med. 25:98-193, 1985.

4. Beall, C.M., Goldstein, M.C., Feldman, E.S. Social structure and intracohort variation in physical fitness among elderly males in a traditional third world society. J. Am. Geriatrics Soc. 33:406-412, 1985.

5. Dehn, M.M., Bruce, R.A. Longitudinal variations in maximal oxygen intake with age and activity. J. Appl. Physiol. 33:805-807, 1972.

6. Drinkwater, B.L., Horvath, S.M., Wells, C.L. Aerobic power of females, ages 10 to 68. J. Gerontol. 30:385-394, 1975.

7. Hodgson, J.L., Buskirk, E.R. Physical fitness and age, with emphasis on cardiovascular function in elderly. J. Am. Geriatrics Soc. 15:385-392, 1977.

8. Ikegami, H., Shimaoka, K., Ikegami, Y. Relationship between daily physical activity and physical fitness of female university students. Bull. Nagoya Holy Spirit Junior College. 8:56-64, 1986.

9. Kasch, F.W., Wallace, J.P., Van Camp, S.P., Verity, L. A longitudinal study of cardiovascular stability in active men aged 45 to 65 years. The Physician and Sportsmed. 16:117-126, 1988.

10. Kobayashi, K. Aerobic power of the Japanese. Tokyo: Kyorin Shoin, 1982: 311-316 (Part III).

11. Konno, M., Chiwata, T., Yasunaga, M. Maximal aerobic power and heart rate during usual activities of sedentary workers in urban districts. J. Phys. Fit. Japan 27:135-139, 1978.

12. Physical Fitness Laboratory, Tokyo Metropolitan University. Physical fitness standards of Japanese people. 3rd ed. Tokyo: Fumaido, 1980.

13. Profant, G.R., Early, R.G., Bruce, R.A. Responses to maximal exercise in healthy middle-aged women. J. Appl. Physiol. 33:595-599, 1972.

14. Shimaoka, M., Hiruta, S., Shimaoka, K. Effect of levels of daily physical activity on physical fitness in new nursery governesses. Nagoya J. Health, Phys. Fit. & Sports 10:103-113, 1987.

15. Shimaoka, M., Hiruta, S., Shimaoka, K., Kobayashi, K. Energy expenditure in a day and during working time for nursery governesses. Nagoya J. Health, Phys. Fit. & Sports 8:115-128, 1985.

16. Slattery, M.I., Jacobs, Jr., D.R. The interrelationships of physical fitness and body measurements. Med. Sci. Sports and Exer. 19:564-569, 1987.

17. The Ministry of Education, Culture and Science. Annual report of physical fitness and motor performance. Tokyo: The Ministry of Education, Culture and Science, 1987.

18. The Ministry of Health and Welfare. The required nutrition of Japanese. Tokyo: Daiichi Shuppan, 1984.

Workload and Physical Fitness

N. Onishi

Division of Work Physiology and Psychology, Institute for Science of
Labour, Sugao, Miyamae-ku, Kawasaki, Japan

Recently, the incidence of such adult diseases as cancer, cerebrovascular disease, and heart
disease has increased. This is mainly because of an increase in the percentage of the aged
population. But there are not a few cases of adult diseases among workers in their prime.
It seems that workers pay more attention to their health when they are aware of a decline
in physical fitness or have some actual health problems. As part of worker safety and health
education, we should place stress on the necessity of proper exercise for preventing a
degenerative decline in physical functions. But workers never support such exercise programs that aim at keeping physical fitness strong enough to stand constrained work for
long hours under bad working conditions.

In this study, workload and physical capacity were examined to improve working conditions particularly for female workers, among whom muscloskeletal disorders are
predominant.

Working Operations

Two groups of female workers were examined: (a) workers engaged in school lunch service
at primary or middle schools and (b) workers in a food processing factory. The Group
A workers worked 39 hr a week, daily from 8:00 a.m. until 4:00 p.m. with a 1-hr lunch
recess. Their tasks consisted of several processes, including cleaning and preparing
materials, cooking, distributing meals for each class, and cleaning cooking and eating
utensils. The Group B workers were part-timers, working for 4 hr per day with a 19-min
break. Their duties were cutting fish and meat and prepacking prepared food.

Methods

1. A questionnaire study concerning subjective symptoms and experience of low back
pain: Questionnaire sheets were distributed to 167 workers of Group A and 385 workers
of Group B. Of the handout, the numbers of questionnaires returned were 160 (or 95.8%)
and 344 (or 89.4%), respectively. The ages of the respondents were 27-59 years for Group
A and 25-57 years for Group B, the average age being 46.2 years and 42.6 years, respectively.

2. Measurement of physiological changes at work and working posture analysis: Of
the workers of Group A, six workers of an average age of 45.1 years were selected for
measurement of surface electromyograms during their operations, measurement of leg
circumference before and after the work, working posture analysis by 30-s snap time study,
and subjective fatigue feeling survey. Of the workers of Group B, 12 workers of the average age 44.3 years were also selected for the same examinations.

3. Physical fitness tests: Physical build, muscle strength, and other physical functions were measured in 109 workers of Group A and 124 workers of Group B. Parameters measured were as follows: body weight, body height, and skinfold thickness; grip strength, elbow flexion strength, knee extension strength, and back muscle strength; and one-leg standing with closed eyes, vertical jumping height, repeated side-step jumping, and vital capacity.

Results

In the school kitchens, cleaning and preparing materials and cooking were done under time pressure in order to get meals ready by 12:20 p.m. After a 1-hr lunch recess, cooking and eating utensils were cleaned. During 4-hr operations in the food processing factory, high density work of repetitious motions in constrained postures was done with a 19-min break and three short pauses.

Figure 1 shows the relative frequency of working postures in the two groups. Standing posture amounted to 70-80% of the working time, and 20-27% of it was spent in carrying and walking. Moreover, deep forward bending of more than 45° during standing was also observed. The workers complained most frequently about the load in the low back and shoulder/upper limb region.

The rates of those who had experienced low back pain severe enough to hinder their movements at work or in daily life were as much as 52.8% of Group A and 22.5% of Group B. Both groups told that they had experienced low back pain since the present employment.

Further, the results show the rates of those who had experienced sick leave due to severe stiffness or pain in the shoulder/upper limb region. More than 60% of all the workers surveyed reported that they had experienced stiffness or pain in the shoulder/upper limb region. Cumulative days of sick leave per person in a year were about 3 weeks for Group A and 1.1 days for Group B on average. The frequency of these musculoskeletal disorders is higher in the workers of Group A. But it can be said that in the case of the workers of Group B, the frequency was rather high considering their shorter working hours.

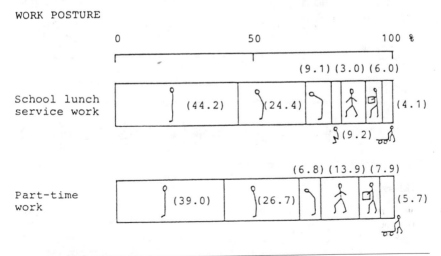

Figure 1. Frequency of working postures during operations, Groups A and B.

Figure 2 illustrates examples of electromyographic activities of m. forearm extensor, m. trapezius, and m. erector trunci during the working operations in Group A and Group B. In the case of Group A, electromyograms were recorded in the operations of transferring utensils from a dishwashing machine into baskets, shaking water from the baskets, and putting them into a case with heat disinfection equipment. Since the workers had to raise the basket, weighing 4-5 kg, to the shoulder height level, the electromyographic activities of the bilateral trapezius muscles amounted to as much as 0.7-0.8 mv. Those of the erector trunci were somewhat lower, 0.2-0.3 mv, but continuous. In the case of Group B, electromyograms were recorded during the operations of continuously cutting salmon into 2 cm pieces. The electromyographic activities of the right forearm extensor muscles and the right trapezius muscles were large.

This was because the subject was holding a knife with the right hand during the operation. When fish was being cut, the highest electromyographic activities of the right forearm extensor muscles were recorded, and when the knife was being raised for the next cutting procedure, the electromyographic amplitude became higher.

The data have disclosed that the workload of the school kitchen work, including the manual carrying and lifting of heavy objects, was generally higher than that of the food processing work. But large loading of the right forearm extensor muscles was observed in group B due to the operations requiring rapid and repetitive movements of the right hand.

Figure 3 shows the results of measurements of physical structure and physical capacity by age in each group. Mean body height and %FAT of Group B were slightly greater than those of Group A. Mean grip strength was found to be slightly higher for Group A workers than for Group B workers. But physical functions in terms of vertical jumping height, side step jumping, and one-leg standing with closed eyes and vital capacity were better for Group B workers. Blood pressure and %FAT by age were significantly higher in the group in their 50s than in the group in their early 30s or younger. A decline in muscle strength and physical functions was much more remarkable in the group in their 50s than in the group in their early 30s or younger.

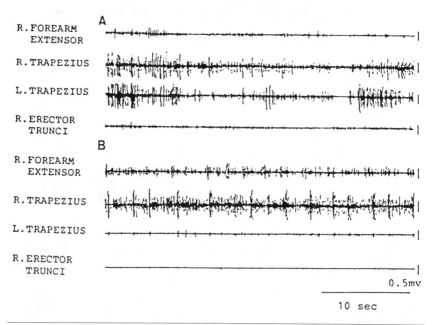

Figure 2.   An example of electromyographic activities of arm, shoulder, and low back muscles during the working operations in Groups A and B.

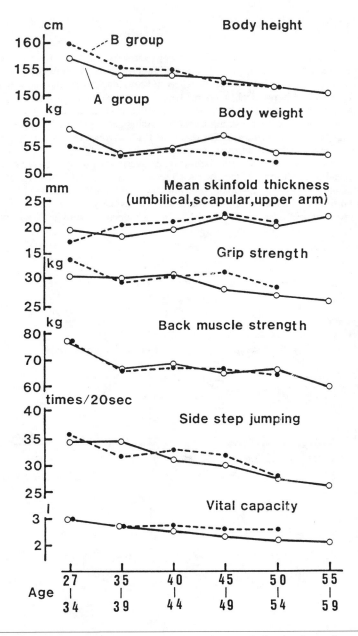

Figure 3. Mean values of physical structure and muscle strength, by age, for workers of the Groups A and B.

A decreasing tendency by age of muscular strength and physical function was prominent, particularly in vertical jumping height and side step jumping scores. Compared with strength and elbow flexion strength, knee extension strength and back muscle strength decreased to a larger extent.

Discussion

Workers' physical capacity is influenced mainly by their tasks at their work places. Ishii (1) found that workers whose tasks were in the medium level of RMR were most prominent in physical capacity and that workers doing very heavy muscular tasks had a hastened degenerative decline in physical functions. Onishi (2, 3) reported that forestry workers were stronger in back muscle strength than sedentary office workers and that in the latter group, a decline in back muscle strength was more remarkable and bodily fat deposit was more prominent with increasing age. The reason why office workers are said to be suffering from insufficient exercise syndrome would be these physical factors.

In the present study, there were no significant differences in physical capacity between Groups A and B. But loading of the low back muscles in Group A and that of the shoulder and upper limb muscles in Group B were remarkable during working operations.

Figure 4 shows the scatter diagrams of grip strength and back muscle strength by those with and without pains or stiffness of the shoulder and upper limb muscles. The right side

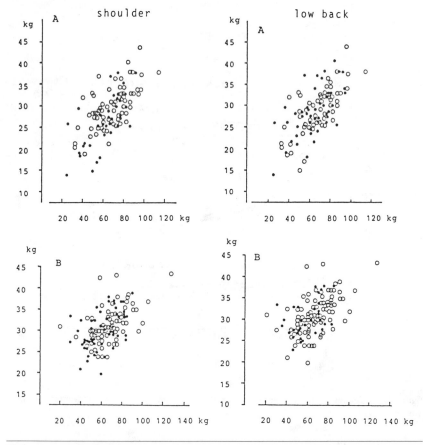

Figure 4.   Relationship between grip strength and back muscle strength. Black dots indicate those workers who had pain or stiffness in the shoulder/upper limb region (left) and those workers who had experience of low back pain (right).

displays the scatter diagrams of grip strength and back muscle strength by those with and without low back pain experience. Small black dots represent those workers who experienced low back pain and workers having shoulder pain. The fact that those having stronger muscle strength had less prevalence of pain or stiffness of the shoulder and upper limb muscles was not observed. But it can be said that such complaints were higher for those having grip strength of less than 25 kg and back muscle strength of less than 60 kg. This data suggested that preservation of muscle strength in some degree was needed for these operations.

Values of muscle strength for those with low back pain experience were also widely distributed on the rating scale of muscle strength levels. Those having stronger muscle strength experienced low back pain almost to the same degree. Moreover, in workers handling heavy objects and having stronger muscle strength, complaint rates of tiredness in low back muscles were observed to be higher.

The back muscle strength was found to be significantly lower for those with low back pain experience in Groups A and B, and the knee extension strength was also found to be significantly lower for those with pain or stiffness of the shoulder and upper limb muscles. Fatigue caused by tasks is dependent on two basic factors: degree of workload and a worker's physical work capacity. Workers who have a higher physical work capacity are generally strong enough for hard work. But under widespread mechanization and automation in factories and offices, the nature of things is not so simple. With an increase of tasks requiring high density, repetitive work in constrained postures, localized, cumulative muscle fatigue in the shoulder/upper limb region and in the low back has come to be prevalent. For example, as the author has already mentioned, forward bending postures during the operations in each group surveyed were frequently observed.

These postures were related to the working surface height and workers' body height. In fact, workers who were taller had higher rates of fatigue in the shoulder muscles and low back region. One of the causes was obviously a working surface height unsuitable for such workers. Actually, by addressing working postures, tool design, equipment, and general work practices, many of the risk factors can be eliminated. General health promotion considerations should dictate these kinds of changes.

References

1. Ishii, Y. Study on the physique and physical strength of workers (1). J. Sci. Labour 30:18-24, 1954.

2. Onishi, N., Monura, H. Low back pain in relation to physical work capacity and local tenderness. J. Hum. Ergol. 2:119-132, 1973.

3. Onishi, N., Momura, H. A comparative study on the physical fitness of workers in various industries. J. Sci. Labour 50:319-331, 1974.

Physiological Responses To Heat Stress

S.E. Terblanche, A. van der Linde, A.J. Kielblock, and D. Van Gerven

Department of Biochemistry, University of Zululand, Kwa Dlangezwa and the Research Organization of the Chamber of Mines of South Africa, Johannesburg, South Africa; Institute of Physical Education, Catholic University Leuven, Leuven, Belgium

Most people have been exposed to heat stress at one time or another. Its effects may vary from slight discomfort to serious disorders and even death. Total prevention of heat stroke is in reality impossible (6). Heat stroke has been defined as a heat disorder characterized by a high body temperature (8, 10). Body temperature is determined by the balance of heat absorbed into and generated within the body and the heat lost to the environment (11).

Changes in serum enzyme levels as indicators of tissue damage in heat were first reported by Bedrak (1). During heat stroke, plasma enzyme levels (especially lactate dehydrogenase and creatine kinase) increase until peak levels are reached in approximately 48 hr. Plasma enzyme levels may remain above normal for lengthy periods (14 days) (5).

The aim of this study was to ascertain the effects of exercise and hyperthermic stress separately and collectively on body temperatures and plasma enzyme levels of lactate dehydrogenase (LD) and creatine kinase (CK) in rats. The choice of the rat as the experimental animal was based on several factors but especially the attendant risk of mortality associated with acute heat stress, which could manifest itself in heat stroke. Until relatively recently, the major objection to using an animal as a heat stroke model stemmed from the definition of heat stroke, in particular from the fact that the pathogenesis of heat stroke depended on sweat cessation. This has since been questioned (14) and in subsequent definitions of heat stroke the term *sweat cessation* has been omitted. Cardiovascular responses (7) and organ systems (2) have been qualitatively extrapolated from animal to man.

Methods

Male Long Evans rats were housed at 22 °C $\pm$ 1 °C on a 12-hr day/night regimen. They were subdivided into three groups consisting of 6, 15, and 20 rats respectively. Group 1 (6 rats) acted as a control group. The animals fasted for 24 hr before experimentation to minimize any subtle effects of nutritional status on performance or resistance to stress. Group 2 (15 rats) and Group 3 (20 rats) were subjected to a program of treadmill running until exhaustion or when a body temperature of 43 °C was reached. Groups 2 and 3 were exercised at 26°C and 38 °C respectively (relative humidity was 60% in both cases).

The rats were exercised at 27 • min^{-1} up a 15% gradient. Eight of the rats in both groups 2 and 3 were anaesthesized and sacrificed within 5 min following exercise. A blood sample was collected from the abdominal aorta. The remaining rats in Groups 2 and 3 were first allowed to recover at 26 °C and 38 °C respectively for 1 hr and then were caged at an ambient temperature of 22 °C with access to water ad libitum but not too food. Venous blood (1 ml, tail vein) was sampled at 6 hr post stress followed by sacrifice and blood sampling (abdominal aorta) at 24 hr. All exposures (exercise at 26 °C and 38 °C) were conducted in an environmental chamber specifically designed for this purpose.

Physiological Measurements

Core temperature (Tc) (rectal probe inserted 6.5 cm into the rectum) and skin temperature (Ts) (measured at base of the tail on its anterior surface) were measured to within 0.1 °C using 0.1 mm copper-constantan thermocouples in conjunction with a thermocouple reference oven (Julabo, Model VL), a microvolt meter (Dorig, Model DS 100), and a 1 millivolt chart recorder (Varian Techtron, Model 1800). The skin probe was insulated from the environment by wrapping with cotton wool placed on the skin and kept in position with adhesive tape.

Blood Measurements

Packed cell volume (PCV) was measured with the aid of a microcentrifuge and haemoglobin (Hb) by the cyanomethaemoglobin method (Boehringer Mannheim). Lactate dehydrogenase (LD) and creatine kinase (CK) in plasma were assayed by means of a semimicromethod using Boehringer Optimized Monotest combinations. CK was stabilized by the addition of N-acetyl cystein. The Boehringer LD optimized test combination kit utilized the rate of oxidation of $NADH + H^+$ in the conversion of pyruvate to lactate with LD as a catalyst $(LDp \rightarrow \ell)$. All total enzyme activities were determined in a PYE-UNICAM SP 8-200 split beam ultraviolet spectrophotometer equipped with a temperature-controlled cell housing. Assays were performed at 30 °C in keeping with the recommendations of the Commission on Enzymes of the International Union of Biochemistry.

Heat Stress

In their review on heat stroke Shibolet et al. (15) emphasized that the effect of heat, like other physical agents, is determined by both its intensity and duration. Thermal load was calculated as the hyperthermic area in °C • min of core temperature (Tc) and mean body temperature (Tm) for all increments above 40.4 °C during both the heating (exposure) and cooling (recovery) phases of the temperature (Tc or Tm) curve. The choice of the baseline was based on the documented experience of Hubbard (4), who found that 50% of rats exposed to 41.5 °C core temperature during running died within 24 hr (LD_{50} = 41.5 °C Tc). The minimum lethal dose (LD_0) where all rats survived longer than 24 hr following running (11m • min^{-1}, 6° incline) was a Tc of 40.4 °C, which corresponds closely to a LD_0 of 40.6 °C core temperature in humans. The integrated hyperthermic exposure (ΣTc or ΣTm) was calculated according to the following formula:

$$\Sigma Tc \text{ or } \Sigma Tm = \frac{(T1 + T2)\, t1}{2} + \frac{(T2 + T3)\, t2}{2} + \ldots$$

$$\frac{(Tn - 1 + Tn)\, t\, (n - 1)}{2} \qquad °C • min$$

T = Core or mean body temperature in °C
t = Time interval in minutes

The mean body temperature was derived by the use of the following equation:

Tm = 0.8 Tc − 0.2 Ts
Tm = Mean body temperature
Tc = Core temperature
Ts = Tail skin temperature

Results

Body Temperatures

Exercise until exhaustion at 26 °C (60% humidity) resulted in significant elevations in body temperature above the resting level (see Figure 1). However, the prevailing environmental temperature (26 °C) seemed to have provided sufficient cooling to prevent core temperature from increasing to the "danger zone" of 40.4 °C and higher where the risk of hyperthermic injury in rats becomes progressively greater.

Exercise at 38 °C caused much higher hyperthermic stress levels than exercise at 26 °C as judged by Tc or Tm (see Figure 2). Because ΣTc increased quantitatively more than ΣTm during exercise at 38 °C, it was the more sensitive indicator of the stress level. Also, because core temperature is in practice more readily measured, ΣTc instead of Tc, Tm, or ΣTm was used as the measure of hyperthermic load in dose-response relationships.

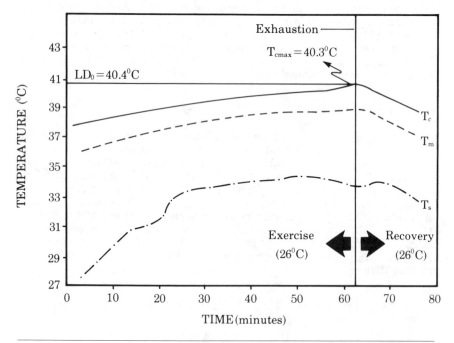

Figure 1. Body temperature responses to exercise at 26 °C. Tc_{max} = maximum core temperature, Tm = mean body temperature, Ts = tail skin temperature, Tc = core temperature.

Temperature Responses

For the purpose of this investigation complicated hyperthermia (CH) was defined as a condition that resulted in enzyme elevations at 24 hr above those measured at 6 hr following stress and vice versa. Uncomplicated hyperthermia (UCH) was a condition during which recovery of the plasma enzyme activities was observed over the same period.

The hyperthermic exposure as measured by ΣTc in rats that suffered CH following exercise at 38 °C was greater than the hyperthermic exposure of rats that suffered UCH only.

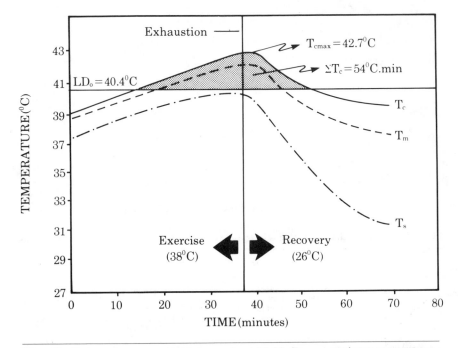

Figure 2.   Body temperature responses to exercise at 38 °C. Tc_{max} = maximum core temperature, ΣTc = integrated area of Tc > 40.4 °C, Tm = mean body temperature, Ts = tail skin temperature, Tc = core temperature.

It was observed that while the rate of increase in core temperature in CH and UCH was equal at a constant level of stress, rats that suffered CH also endured each stress condition for a longer period (see Figure 2). In addition, the cooling rate following the termination of exposure at exhaustion at 38 °C was slower in the CH group compared to the UCH group, which led to longer hyperthermic exposure (Tc > 40.4 °C) of the CH group.

Dehydration

The level of dehydration at the termination of stress as indicated by decreases in mass and relative changes in plasma volume was significantly higher in the exercise at 38 °C group ($\Delta PV = -20.8\%$) compared to the exercise at 26 °C group ($\Delta PV = -6.3\%$). The CH group of rats also dehydrated more than rats in the UCH group after exercise at 38 °C.

Temporal Changes in Plasma LD and CK

LD and CK plasma levels were measured at the termination of stress and at 6 and 24 hr following the termination of stress in the animals exercised at 26 °C and 38 °C and after 6 and 18 hr of fasting in the control animals (see Figures 3 and 4). Plasma LD and CK in some of the rats exposed to exercise at 38 °C displayed a progressive increase between the termination of stress and sacrifice at 24 hr following stress. These rats were regarded to have suffered complicated hyperthermia (CH). In the remainder, an increase in plasma enzymes was noted until 6 hr poststress followed by a decrease until sacrifice at 24 hr. These rats were regarded to have suffered uncomplicated hyperthermia (UCH).

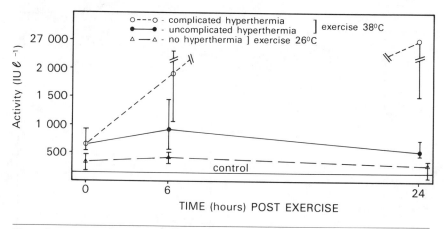

Figure 3.   Temporal changes in plasma lactate dehydrogenase (LD) activity levels after exposure to exercise at 26 °C and 38 °C.

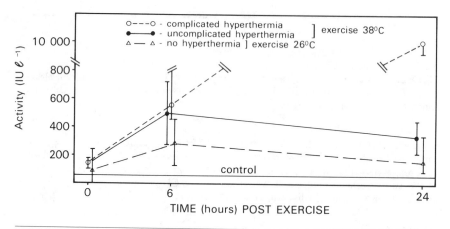

Figure 4.   Temporal changes in plasma creatine kinase (CK) activity levels after exposure to exercise at 26 °C and 38 °C.

In control rats, a decreased tendency in the levels of activity of both LD (196 to 153 IU · ℓ^{-1}) and CK (75 to 69 IU · ℓ^{-1}) was observed 6-18 hr after fasting. At the termination of stress, plasma LD was the most sensitive indicator of the level of stress, being significantly elevated above control levels following exercise at 26 °C ($p = .021$) and 38 °C ($p < .001$). Exercise at 38 °C also resulted in a significantly elevated response when compared to exercise at 26 °C ($p < .001$). Exercise at 38 °C also resulted in significantly higher CK activity levels when compared to control levels ($p < .001$) and the levels after exercise at 26 °C ($p < .014$).

Both the LD and CK activities measured at 6 hr following exercise at both 26 °C and 38 °C were significantly elevated above the respective levels measured at the termination of stress. In the case of CH, the increase in the activity levels of CK and especially LD was more pronounced compared to UCH.

At 24 hr following exercise at 38 °C, the activity levels of both LD and CK in the CH group were significantly elevated in comparison with the UCH group. Contrary to the UCH group, the activity levels of both LD and CK in the CH group were significantly higher 24 hr following stress compared to after 6 hr.

Discussion

An uneven distribution of heat within the body during heat exposure has been demonstrated (12), which is probably due to combinations of metabolic activity in and blood flow to various organs. Vasoconstriction in the splanchnic and renal area and repartitioning of cardiac output (13) occur, and obviously this may have a bearing on the outcome of any exposure to work in heat.

In the above context, ΣTc, which incorporates both the intensity (Tc) and duration of hyperthermia, was the better indicator of hyperthermic exposure compared to Tc, Tm, and ΣTm. ΣTc also correlated best with indicators of cellular damage, a finding supported by the results obtained by Hubbard (4) under comparable experimental conditions.

Rats suffering complicated hyperthermia were exposed to significantly higher levels of hyperthermic stress (ΣTc) than the rats that suffered uncomplicated hyperthermia. The correlation between ΣTc and period of exercise at 38 °C ($r = .67$) suggests that endurance to hyperthermic stress may, ironically have been the most important causal factor of heat stroke in this study.

During the present study it was observed that peak plasma enzyme levels did not coincide on a temporal scale. As the enzyme release patterns are of cardinal importance in the interpretation of data, consideration of the mechanism of enzyme release into the plasma is of particular relevance. Enzymes measured in this study are transported into plasma largely via the lymph. The delay in peak activity (6 hr) following exercise stress and uncomplicated hyperthermia could therefore result from the slow time course of lymphatic transportation (9).

The nature of enzyme release into the plasma from cells that have undergone a pathological change (ranging from simple modification of cellular permeability to necrosis) is not related to the etiological agent but to the type of lesion (3). This view finds support in the present study when it was observed that total plasma LD and CK activity levels were insensitive to the type of stress (exertional or hyperthermic stress) until 6 hr following stress.

Complicated hyperthermia (CH) might be described as a condition (hyperthermia) that provokes a collapse of cellular metabolism during heat exposure to the extent that secondary complications develop subsequent to the termination of stress. Cellular injury, as in the prodromal period and in uncomplicated hyperthermia, is mild (permeability changes) and rapidly reversible compared to the cellular injury in complicated hyperthermia (16).

In this study, rats regarded to have suffered complicated hyperthermia by way of their plasma enzyme responses most likely suffered heat stroke. A continuous deterioration of cellular integrity and secondary complications (indicated by an increased plasma enzyme activity) occurred in these animals. As in heat stroke, marked increases in plasma enzyme levels occurred at 24 hr following stress in the CH group.

From the present study it can be concluded that ΣTc, which incorporates both the intensity and duration of hyperthermia, was the better indicator of hyperthermic exposure when compared to Tc, Tm, and ΣTm. Furthermore, LD and CK activity levels 24 hr after the cessation of stress could be useful indicators in distinguishing between complicated and uncomplicated hyperthermia. However, it is strongly recommended that LD and CK plasma isoenzyme release patterns be investigated in an attempt to derive more sensitive indicators regarding the level of stress as well as possible cellular damage associated with hyperthermia.

Acknowledgment

Financial support from the Chamber of Mines of South Africa is gratefully acknowledged.

References

1. Bedrak, E. Effect of muscular exercise in a hot environment on canine fibrinolytic activity. J. Appl. Physiol. 20:1307-1311, 1965.

2. Bynum, G., Patton, J., Bowers, W., Leav, I., Wolfe, D., Hamlet, M., Marsili, M. An anaesthetized dog heat stroke model. J. Appl. Physiol. 43:292-296, 1977.

3. De Ritis, F.D., Giusti, G., Piccinino, F., Cacciatore, L. Biochemical laboratory tests in viral hepatitis and other hepatic diseases. World Health Bulletin 32:59-72, 1965.

4. Hubbard, R.W. Effects of exercise in the heat on predisposition to heat stroke. Med. Sci. Sports 11:66-71, 1979.

5. Kew, M.C., Bersohn, I., Seftel, H. The diagnostic and prognostic significance of the serum enzyme changes in heat stroke. Trans. Roy. Soc. Trop. Med. Hyg. 65:325-330, 1971.

6. Khogali, M., Al-Marzoogi, A. Prevention of heat stroke: is it possible? In: Khogali, M., Hales, J.R.S., eds. Heat stroke and temperature regulation. New York: Academic Press, 1983, 293-302.

7. Kielblock, A.J. Cardiovascular function during experimental hyperthermia with specific reference to circulatory failure. Potchefstroom: Potchefstroom University for C.H.E., 1979. Doctoral thesis.

8. Knochel, J.P. Environmental heat illness: an electric review. Arch. Intern Med. 33:841-864, 1974.

9. Lindena, J., Küpper, W., Trautschold, I. Enzymatic composition of canine leg lymph. Enzyme 28:18-27, 1982.

10. Malamud, N., Haymaker, W., Custer, R.P. Heat stroke: a clinicopathologic study of 125 fatal cases. Milit. Surg. 99:397-449, 1946.

11. Mount, L.E. Adaptation to thermal environment. London: Edward Arnold, 1979.

12. Rowell, L.B., Blackman, J.R., Martin, R., Mazzarella, J.A., Bruce, R.A. Hepatic clearance of indocyanine green in man under thermal heat stress. J. Appl. Physiol. 20:384-394, 1965.

13. Rowell, L.B., Marx, H.J., Bruce, R.A., Conn, R.D., Kusumi, F. Reductions in cardiac output, central blood volume and stroke volume with thermal stress in normal men during exercise. J. Clin. Invest. 45:1801-1816, 1966.

14. Shibolet, S.R., Coll, R., Gilat, T., Sohar, E. Heat stroke: its clinical picture and mechanism in 36 cases. Q. J. Med. 36:525-548, 1967.

15. Shibolet, S., Lancaster, M.C., Danon, Y. Heat stroke: a review. Aviat. Space Environ. Med. 47:280-301, 1976.

16. Wyndham, C.H., Kew, M.C., Kok, R., Bersohn, I., Strydom, N.B. Serum enzyme changes in unacclimatized and acclimatized men under severe heat stress. J. Appl. Physiol. 37(5):695-698, 1974.